WORKBOOK TO ACCOMPANY

ADMINISTRATIVE MEDICAL ASSISTING

Eighth Edition

Linda L. French, CMA-C (AAMA), NCICS, CPC

**Formerly, Instructor and Business Consultant,
Administrative Medical Assisting, Medical Terminology,
and Medical Insurance Billing and Coding**

Simi Valley Adult School and Career Institute, Simi Valley, California
Ventura College, Ventura, California
Oxnard College, Oxnard, California
Santa Barbara Business College, Ventura, California
Harbor College of Court Reporting, Ventura, California
University of California Santa Barbara Extension, Ventura, California

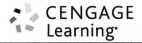

CENGAGE
Learning·

Australia • Brazil • Mexico • Singapore • United Kingdom • United States

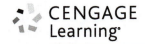

Administrative Medical Assisting Workbook, Eighth Edition
Linda L. French

SVP, GM Skills & Global Product Management: Dawn Gerrain

Product Director: Matthew Seeley

Product Team Manager: Stephen Smith

Senior Director, Development: Marah Bellegarde

Senior Product Development Manager: Juliet Steiner

Product Assistant: Mark Turner

Vice President, Marketing Services: Jennifer Ann Baker

Marketing Manager: Jessica Cipperly

Senior Production Director: Wendy Troeger

Production Director: Andrew Crouth

Senior Content Project Manager: Thomas Heffernan

Managing Art Director: Jack Pendleton

Cover image(s): antishock/Shutterstock.com

For product information and technology assistance, contact us at
Cengage Learning Customer & Sales Support, 1-800-354-9706
For permission to use material from this text or product,
submit all requests online at **www.cengage.com/permissions**.
Further permissions questions can be e-mailed to
permissionrequest@cengage.com

Library of Congress Control Number: 2016950837

ISBN: 978-1-305-85918-0

Cengage Learning
20 Channel Center Street
Boston, MA 02210
USA

Cengage Learning is a leading provider of customized learning solutions with employees residing in nearly 40 different countries and sales in more than 125 countries around the world. Find your local representative at **www.cengage.com.**

Cengage Learning products are represented in Canada by Nelson Education, Ltd. To learn more about Cengage Learning, visit **www.cengage.com** Purchase any of our products at your local college store or at our preferred online store **www.cengagebrain.com**

Printed at CLDPC, USA, 01-21

CONTENTS

APPENDICES

A C K N O W L E D G M E N T S

This *Workbook* has grown to include hundreds of chapter review questions, expanded critical thinking exercises, and more than 150 Job Skills, updated and revised to follow the chapter content. With this edition, the revenue cycle is introduced in Chapter 13 (*The Revenue Cycle: Fees, Credit, and Collection*) and all ledger-posting exercises have been moved to Chapter 15 (*Bookkeeping*). The coding chapter has been split into *Procedure Coding* (Chapter 16) and *Diagnostic Coding* (Chapter 17), with the insurance chapter following—*Health Insurance Systems and Claim Submission* (Chapter 18).

I wish to express my gratitude for the help and encouragement provided by friends, colleagues, and family, and the staff of Delmar Cengage Learning. And to the people and organizations that so willingly and enthusiastically contributed to the contents of this book, I am ever grateful. Without their expertise, comments, and suggestions, the work would not be as complete as it is.

I extend my sincere thanks to all of the companies that granted permission to use the various forms that are now offered online at www.cengagebrain.com and are an integral part of this *Workbook*, including Bibbero Systems, Inc. and Carolyn Talesfore, Advertising and Promotion Manager, whose has helped develop forms used in the *Workbook* for many years. The realistic forms allow students to complete and master Job Skills so they are ready to enter the workforce. This is our ultimate goal!

INSTRUCTIONS TO THE STUDENT

This *Workbook* has been prepared for those who use *Administrative Medical Assisting* as a text. The *Workbook* job skills combined with the theory learned in the *textbook* meet the educational entry-level competencies outlined in 2016 by the Commission on Accreditation of Allied Health Education Programs (CAAHEP) and in 2017 by the Accrediting Bureau of Health Education Schools (ABHES) as well as the Certification and Examination Content from the American Association of Medical Assistants for the CMA (AAMA) from 2014, the American Medical Technologists (AMT) Medical Assisting Task List of 2015, the Certification Examination Competencies for the Registered Medical Assistant (RMA) of 2009, and the AMT Examination Specifications for the Certified Medical Administrative Specialist (CMAS) of 2008.

The following components have been developed to make the *Workbook* a complete learning tool, which allows practical application of job skills that will be performed in a physician's office. An asterisk (*) indicates features new to or enhanced for this edition.

Chapter Exercises*

- **Abbreviation and Spelling Review** incorporates medical terminology into a short chart note for each chapter, giving students an opportunity to write definitions for abbreviations and spell medical terms. Answers are found in the *Instructor's Manual*.
- **Review Questions*** cover key points in chapters and address areas not covered by the exam-style review questions in the *textbook*. Review questions help students prepare for a multiple-choice theory test on each chapter studied. Answers are found in the *Instructor's Manual*.
- **Critical Thinking Exercises*** offer students an opportunity to address situations and solve problems realistic to an office setting.
- **Job Skills*** have been enhanced to include up-to-date forms and technical information to cover and cross-reference the 2016 CAAHEP* and the 2017 ABHES* competencies. They are designed to include a Performance Evaluation Checklist with the directions, thus eliminating the need for a separate form to grade each job skill. *The format has been changed to include a simplified list of what is needed and referred to in each job skill.

The *textbook* lists objectives for all job skills—both in a comprehensive list and chapter by chapter. These job skills are also listed at the beginning of the *Workbook*. Read through each job skill entirely before attempting to begin the assignment. Follow the directions in the *Workbook* where noted, locate the needed materials and forms online at www.cengagebrain.com with student resources, and refer to *textbook* figures for visual examples and the Procedure in the *textbook* for step-by-step directions. These directions are comprehensive and written to assist students with the office task, not just the job skill in the *Workbook*.

Performance objectives are stated for each exercise. Your instructor will indicate which standards are expected, the time frame for the completion of each exercise, and the accuracy required for individual exercises. Points are assigned for each job skill for the first, second, and third attempt according to the steps required and difficulty of the task. These may be adjusted by your instructor.

Appendices

Two important appendices are provided to help you successfully complete the activities in this workbook.

Appendix A: Practon Medical Group, Inc.

Important information is listed in the Practon Medical Group, Inc., reference file, which includes detailed office protocols. Before beginning the job skills, tear out the appendix, place it in a three-ring binder, and add section indexes so you can access information quickly to help you complete the *Workbook* Job Skills. The appendix includes (1) medical practice reference material with physician/office contact information and important federal identification numbers; (2) office policies, including information about the daily routine in the office, office hours, appointment protocols, information regarding telephone calls, and filing routines; (3) payment policies and health insurance protocols to be used as guidelines when filing insurance claims; and (4) directions for using the office fee schedule. Figure A-1 provides a mock fee schedule that lists procedure codes (by sections) in the same order in which they are listed in the *CPT* codebook, descriptions of services, and fees you will need when answering questions that patients might ask and for posting to patient accounts and completing insurance forms. Also included are (5) a listing of *CPT* code modifiers with brief descriptions and (6) a sample listing of Medicare *HCPCS Level II* codes with fees.

Appendix B: Abbreviation Tables

Abbreviation tables that appear in the *textbook* are conveniently listed to easily locate medical definitions and help decode abbreviations when completing the *Workbook* Abbreviation and Spelling Review lessons, answering questions, and performing Job Skills.

Forms

To complete many of the activities and job skills in this workbook, you will need to refer to the editable forms provided on the free online companion site located at www.cengagebrain.com with student resources. These blank forms are similar to those found in medical offices. They are available to complete electronically and email to your instructor or as downloadable PDFs that you can fill out manually and print. Your student companion site resources can be quickly and easily accessed:

1. Go to www.cengagebrain.com.

2. Create a student account.

3. Search for Administrative Medical Assisting Eighth Edition.

4. Click on Free Study Tools and explore the forms and other resources available to you.

Additional Items Needed

If you do not have a background in medical terminology, you need to obtain and use a good medical dictionary. It is also suggested that you obtain the following items. Check them off as you acquire them for your coursework.

_____ 1 three-ring binder with index tabs

_____ 1 folder with pockets to hand in assignments

_____ 3 manila file folders

_____ 3 name labels for manila folders

_____ 50 sheets of 8½" by 11" white multiuse copy paper

_____ 60 3" by 5" white file cards

_____ 2 white number 10 envelopes (9½" by 4")

_____ rubber bands, paper clips, pens, highlighter pen set (5 colors), pencils, transparent tape

Optional items:

_____ 7 white number 10 envelopes (large)

_____ 7 white number 6 envelopes (small)

Notebook Content Suggestions

It is a good idea to remove the Appendix A (Practon Medical Group, Inc. reference file) and the Abbreviation Tables (Appendix B) from the *Workbook* and place them in a notebook. You may want to print the blank forms from the student companion site at www.cengagebrain.com, which may be photocopied prior to use. Following are several items from the *textbook* that you may also want to include:

List of Evaluation and Management *CPT* Codes	Tables 16-3 and 16-4
Comprehensive List of *CPT* Modifiers	Table 16-5
Insurance Form Template for Medicare	Figure 18-15
Insurance Form Template for Medicare/Medigap	Figure 18-17
Insurance Form Template for TRICARE	Figure 18-18
CMS-1500 Claim Form Field-by-Field Instructions	Appendix A
Commercial Insurance Template	Figure A-1
Glossary Pages	748

Portfolio

Saving your completed work in a portfolio is strongly suggested. You may wish to take it to a job interview in order to present the type of job skills you have acquired and the level of work you have performed during your course of study. You will need a three-ring binder with indexes to organize the material and develop a table of contents. You should add items to this folder as you progress through the course. There are several ways to accomplish this, but a simple way would be according to job duties (e.g., appointment scheduling, telephone techniques, insurance coding and claim forms, letter composition, bookkeeping, and payroll). Your instructor may suggest additional items to include or a specific arrangement of all items.

The content of this portfolio is evidence of your administrative skills and is a good indication of your organizational abilities as well as the neatness and completeness of your work.

WORKBOOK JOB SKILL EXERCISES

C H A P T E R **1**

A Career as an Administrative Medical Assistant

STOP AND THINK CASE SCENARIOS

Refer to the end of Chapter 1 in the *textbook* for the following scenarios:

- Listen and Observe
- Positive Attitude
- Patient Education
- Aggressive versus Assertive Response

EXAM-STYLE REVIEW QUESTIONS

Refer to the end of Chapter 1 in the *textbook*.

Review Questions

Review the objectives, glossary, and chapter information before completing the following review questions.

1. In a customer-service-oriented practice, the elements of customer service are demonstrated by the
   _____, _____, and _____.

2. True or False. Each employee and patient has the same idea about what "good" service means.
   _____

3. Define "patient navigator." _____
   _____
   _____
   _____

4. Define "flextime." _____

5. Name some specialty areas in which administrative skills may be used in a health care career.

   a. _____

   b. _____

   c. _____

   d. _____

   e. _____

6. A medical transcriptionist is now also known as a _____ or

   _____.

7. Of the duties an administrative medical assistant might perform:

   a. List two that require interpersonal skills.

   _____

   _____

   b. List five that require keyboard input skills (assume you work in a computerized office).

   _____

   _____

   _____

   _____

   _____

   c. List five that require basic math skills.

   _____

   _____

   _____

   _____

   _____

   d. List five that require other clerical skills.

   _____

   _____

   _____

   _____

8. In addition to the many duties that an administrative medical assistant performs, there are various interpersonal skills required. Name five that you would like to be known for.

   a. _____

   b. _____

   c. _____

   d. _____

   e. _____

9. When trying to understand a viewpoint or evaluating a patient's behavior, it is important to

   _____ and _____.

10. An emergency has occurred in Dr. Practon's office. Name the behavior the medical assistant must exhibit to patients.

    a. _____

    b. _____

    c. _____

    d. _____

    e. _____

11. List some attributes an employee needs for good team interaction.

    a. _____

    b. _____

    c. _____

    d. _____

    e. _____

    f. _____

12. What must a health care worker be aware of and understand in order to avoid work-related emotional

    and psychological problems? _____

13. When patients receive unfortunate news about themselves or loved ones, how should medical assistants

    act, and what are some things that can be done to help? _____

    _____

14. List the stages of dying.

    a. _____

    b. _____

    c. _____

    d. _____

    e. _____

15. What is the name of the national foundation that offers medical care and support to patients and family members dealing with a terminal illness or the loss of a loved one?

    _____

16. Define "stress," and name one thing that has caused stress in your life.

    _____

    _____

17. How does a medical assistant's excellent grooming reflect the image and management of the medical office?

    _____

    _____

18. Give the names of two national organizations that certify or register medical assistants trained in both clinical and administrative areas.

    a. _____

    b. _____

19. Name five ways a medical assistant can keep knowledge of research and new techniques current.

    a. _____

    b. _____

    c. _____

    d. _____

    e. _____

Critical Thinking Exercises

1. Another medical assistant in the office criticizes a patient behind his or her back for wearing bizarre clothes. What would your response be? _____

   _____

2. Following are some questions that will help you do an interpersonal skill and professional attribute self-assessment. Read each of them carefully and try to answer them honestly. After you have completed them, identify and mark your strengths with an *S* and your weaknesses with a *W*. This will not only help you to know what areas you need to work on but also help you determine which type of job you may be best suited for.

   _____ a. Are you considerate of others?

   _____ b. Do you treat people with respect?

   _____ c. Do you have a kind, friendly, and good-natured manner?

   _____ d. Do you have the ability to be discreet and keep information confidential?

   _____ e. Do you have a positive attitude?

   _____ f. Can you smile easily?

   _____ g. Can you listen instead of talking all the time?

   _____ h. Are you polite?

   _____ i. Can you be sympathetic and empathetic and discern the difference?

   _____ j. Are you reliable and dependable?

   _____ k. Are you honest and trustworthy?

   _____ l. Can you accept responsibility?

   _____ m. Can you remain calm during an emergency?

_____ n. Are you well groomed, with a neat appearance?

_____ o. Are you a team player?

_____ p. Are you patient?

_____ q. Do you reserve judgment of others?

_____ r. Do you have good judgment?

_____ s. Are you willing to learn?

_____ t. Do you accept criticism?

_____ u. Are you sensitive to the feelings of others?

_____ v. Can you remain free from bias?

3. Answer "yes" or "no" to complete the following self-assessment to gain a better understanding of how to handle stress:

   a. Do you prefer to work alone rather than with coworkers? _____

   b. Do you give more than you receive in work relationships? _____

   c. Is it hard for you to establish warm relationships with your coworkers and peers? _____

   d. Do you have someone whom you can trust to discuss personal problems and keep the information confidential? _____

   e. Do you have a difficult time saying "no" and often overload yourself as a result? _____

   f. Do you guard yourself against talking, trusting, and feeling? _____

   g. Do you often get irritated, frustrated, or even angry when performing your regular work tasks?

   _____

   h. Do you often do things yourself rather than take the time to show someone else how to do them?

   _____

   i. Do you easily accept help from others? _____

   j. Do you place the needs of others before your own? _____

   k. Do you obtain your personal identity from your profession? _____

   l. Are most of your needs met by helping others? _____

   m. Do you feel guilty when you take a vacation or time to "play" or rest? _____

4. Role-play the following scenarios demonstrating empathy:

   a. A patient has been diagnosed with cancer and the prognosis looks very poor. You are left alone with the patient and his spouse. Demonstrate empathy as you interact with the patient and his family.

   b. Your coworker has just been told that she has had her hours cut and she is very angry. Respond with empathy.

5. Research organizations and support groups in the local community for the terminally ill. Make a list of available resources. _____

   _____

   _____

   _____

   _____

JOB SKILL 1-1
Interpret and Accurately Spell Medical Terms and Abbreviations

Name _____ Date _____ Score _____

Performance Objective

Task:	Decode abbreviations.
Conditions:	Need:
	• Pen or pencil
	Refer to:
	• *Textbook* Procedure 1-1 for step-by-step directions
Standards:	Complete all steps listed in this skill in _____ minutes with a minimum score of _____. (Time element and accuracy criteria may be given by instructor.)
Time:	**Start:** _____ **Completed:** _____ **Total:** _____ minutes
Scoring:	One point for each step performed satisfactorily unless otherwise listed or weighted by instructor.

Directions with Performance Evaluation Checklist

Read the patient's chart note and write the meanings for the abbreviations following the note. To decode any abbreviations you do not understand or that appear unfamiliar to you, refer to the list of abbreviations in Appendix B of this *Workbook*. Medical terms in the chart note are *italicized*; study them for spelling. Use your medical dictionary to look up their definitions. Your instructor may give a test for the spelling and definition of the words and abbreviations. Note: Although abbreviations are not presented in Chapter 1 of the textbook, they appear throughout the text, and a chart note with medical terms and abbreviations is presented at the beginning of each chapter of the *Workbook* entitled "Abbreviation and Spelling Review" to offer students the opportunity to learn these terms. Refer back to Procedure 1-1 in the *textbook* while doing these.

Bart J. Stephens

September 15, 20XX Routine PE. Ht 6 ft. Wt 163 lb. P 70. BP 130/70. Pt s̄ complaints. *Systemic* Ex neg. except for Grade I *pulmonic murmur*. EKG shows normal heart rhythm, CBC within normal limits, UA clear, & chest x-ray films indicate no lesions or fluid. IMP: No disease. Rx: *Tetanus toxoid* booster, 0.5 ml. Ret p.r.n.

Fran Practon, MD
Fran Practon, MD

1st Attempt	2nd Attempt	3rd Attempt	
_____	_____	_____	Gather materials (equipment and supplies) listed under *Conditions*.
_____	_____	_____	1. PE _____
_____	_____	_____	2. Ht _____
_____	_____	_____	3. ft _____
_____	_____	_____	4. wt _____
_____	_____	_____	5. lb _____
_____	_____	_____	6. P _____

JOB SKILL 1-1 (*continued*)

_____	_____	_____	7. BP	_____
_____	_____	_____	8. pt	_____
_____	_____	_____	9. $\bar{s}$	_____
_____	_____	_____	10. Ex	_____
_____	_____	_____	11. neg.	_____
_____	_____	_____	12. EKG	_____
_____	_____	_____	13. CBC	_____
_____	_____	_____	14. UA	_____
_____	_____	_____	15. IMP	_____
_____	_____	_____	16. Rx	_____
_____	_____	_____	17. ml	_____
_____	_____	_____	18. ret	_____
_____	_____	_____	19. p.r.n.	_____
_____	_____	_____	Complete within specified time.	

___/21   ___/21   ___/21   **Total points earned** (To obtain a percentage score, divide the total points earned by the number of points possible.)

Comments:

Evaluator's Signature: _____   **Need to Repeat:** _____

National Curriculum Competency: CAAHEP: Cognitive: V.C.10; Psychomotor: V.P.3	ABHES: 3. a, b, s, d

JOB SKILL 1-2
Use the Internet to Look Up Key Terms and Hear Pronunciation

Name _____ Date _____ Score _____

Performance Objective

Task: Use an Internet online dictionary to look up key terms and hear the words pronounced.

Conditions: Need:

           • Computer with Internet hookup

           Refer to:

           • *Textbook* key terms or abbreviations

Standards: Complete all steps listed in this job skill in _____ minutes with a minimum score of _____.
(Time element and accuracy criteria may be given by instructor.)

Time: **Start:** _____ **Completed:** _____ **Total:** _____ minutes

Scoring: One point for each step performed satisfactorily unless otherwise listed or weighted by
instructor.

Directions with Performance Evaluation Checklist

An online audio dictionary (e.g., Merriam-Webster) can be used to hear pronunciations for key terms in the
textbook. A "Thesaurus" can be selected for antonyms and synonyms. "English/Spanish" may be selected to
help translate from one language to the other. You may refer back to this Job Skill any time you need a pronunciation. Key terms are defined within each chapter as well as in the glossary at the end of the *textbook*.
Abbreviations are listed in various tables throughout the *textbook* and in Appendix B of this *Workbook*.

1st Attempt	2nd Attempt	3rd Attempt	
_____	_____	_____	Gather materials (equipment and supplies) listed under *Conditions*.
_____	_____	_____	1. Use a computer, obtain an Internet connection, and search: Online audio dictionary (e.g., Merriam-Webster).
_____	_____	_____	2. Type the term in the blank box that says, "Hello! What word would you like to learn today?" Type the first key term in Chapter 1, "accreditation."
_____	_____	_____	3. Click "Search." There will be a simple and full definition, parts of speech, and sentence examples.
____/2	____/2	____/2	4. The word will appear at the top of the page. Write the root for the term "accreditation." _____
____/2	____/2	____/2	5. The phonetic pronunciation guide will appear under the term. Click on the sound symbol next to the main entry as many times as necessary to learn how to pronounce the word. _____
____/2	____/2	____/2	6. Next, the "function" or part of speech will be listed (e.g., adjective, noun, verb, or abbreviation). List the part of speech. _____
____/3	____/3	____/3	7. The etymology will be listed next. Use the dictionary and type in the term "etymology" and write a simple definition. _____

JOB SKILL 1-2 (*continued*)

____/3   ____/3   ____/3   8. The term will then be used in a sentence. Write one sentence using the term "accreditation."

____/6   ____/6   ____/6   9. Select the "Thesaurus" and click on the term "accreditation." Write the synonyms. _____

_____

____/9   ____/9   ____/9   10. Write the "related words." _____

_____

_____

_____   _____   _____   Complete within specified time.

____/32   ____/32   ____/32   **Total points earned** (To obtain a percentage score, divide the total points earned by the number of points possible.)

Comments:

Evaluator's Signature: _____   **Need to Repeat:** _____

National Curriculum Competency: CAAHEP: Psychomotor: V.P.3 (Ch 1–20)	ABHES: 3.a–d (Ch 1–21)

JOB SKILL 1-3
Prioritize a Task List to Practice Time Management Skills

Name _____ Date _____ Score _____

Performance Objective

Task: Study each task listed and prioritize.

Condition: Need:
- Task list and paper
- Pen or pencil

Standards: Complete all steps listed in this skill in _____ minutes with a minimum score of _____.
(Time element and accuracy criteria may be given by instructor.)

Time: Start: _____ Completed: _____ Total: _____ minutes

Scoring: One point for each step performed satisfactorily unless otherwise listed or weighted by instructor.

Directions with Performance Evaluation Checklist

You are an administrative medical assistant who has arrived at work at 9:00 a.m. The office manager has opened the back door to let you in but only one other staff member has arrived who is a clinical medical assistant. She is running laboratory controls and getting the treatment rooms ready. The office manager says to you, "I received a telephone call from two coworkers. Due to an accident on the freeway they will not be arriving until approximately 9:30 a.m. Will you please cover the front until they arrive? The charts have already been pulled for today's patients and the telephone is still on the answering service. When you are able, please call them to pick up the messages and switch the telephone over to the office." Following are typical tasks that need to be done:

Task List

_____ Call the answering service and record all messages.

_____ Call your husband to let him know what time you will meet him for lunch.

_____ Go make coffee in the lunchroom.

_____ Turn on the lights in the front office and waiting room.

_____ Unlock the waiting room door.

_____ Print financial accounts or pull ledgers for patients who will be seen today.

_____ Straighten your desk in the back office.

_____ Look to see what is on your task list for today.

_____ Invite the patients who are waiting outside into the office.

_____ Open the drapes.

JOB SKILL 1-3 *(continued)*

Directions with Performance Evaluation Checklist

1st Attempt	2nd Attempt	3rd Attempt	
_____	_____	_____	Gather materials (equipment and supplies) listed under *Conditions*.
_____	_____	_____	1. Study each task to determine which is the most important, the next most important, and so forth down to the least important.
____/10	____/10	____/10	2. Mark the most important number 1, the next in priority number 2, and so forth, with number 10 being the least important; use commonsense.
____/10	____/10	____/10	3. List comments for the rationale you used to help you determine the order of priority.
_____	_____	_____	Complete within specified time.
____/23	____/23	____/23	**Total points earned** (To obtain a percentage score, divide the total points earned by the number of points possible.)

Comments:

Evaluator's Signature: _____   **Need to Repeat:** _____

National Curriculum Competency: ABHES: 1.d

JOB SKILL 1-4
Use the Internet to Obtain Information on Certification or Registration

Name _____ Date _____ Score _____

Performance Objective

Task: Research certification or registration via the Internet.

Conditions: Need:

   • Computer with Internet connection

   • *Textbook references* from Table 1-2

Standards: Complete all steps listed in this skill in _____ minutes with a minimum score of _____.
        (Time element and accuracy criteria may be given by instructor.)

Time: **Start:** _____ **Completed:** _____ **Total:** _____ minutes

Scoring: One point for each step performed satisfactorily unless otherwise listed or weighted by
        instructor.

Directions with Performance Evaluation Checklist

1st Attempt	2nd Attempt	3rd Attempt	
_____	_____	_____	Gather materials (equipment and supplies) listed under *Conditions*.
_____	_____	_____	1. Study Table 1-2 to determine what areas of certification or registration interest you.
_____	_____	_____	2. Access the Internet.
_____	_____	_____	3. Type in the name of the professional association in the "Search" box to find its website address.
_____	_____	_____	4. Select key terms ("certification," "registration," or "about" the program).
____/4	____/4	____/4	5. Print the information to read and share with your class, and label a file folder to keep it for future reference.
_____	_____	_____	Complete within specified time.
____/10	____/10	____/10	**Total points earned** (To obtain a percentage score, divide the total points earned by the number of points possible.)

Comments:

Evaluator's Signature: _____   **Need to Repeat:** _____

National Curriculum Competency: CAAHEP: Cognitive: X.C.5	ABHES: 1.c

JOB SKILL 1-5
Use the Internet to Test Your Knowledge of Anatomy and Physiology or Medical Terminology

Name _____ Date _____ Score _____

Performance Objective

Task: Test your knowledge of anatomy and physiology or medical terminology via the Internet. If you have not completed your course of study in anatomy and physiology or medical terminology, you may use this job skill to test your knowledge at a later time.

Conditions: Need:

• Computer with Internet connection

Standards: Complete all steps listed in this job skill in _____ minutes with a minimum score of _____. (Time element and accuracy criteria may be given by instructor.)

Time: **Start:** _____ **Completed:** _____ **Total:** _____ minutes

Scoring: One point for each step performed satisfactorily unless otherwise listed or weighted by instructor.

Directions with Performance Evaluation Checklist

1st Attempt	2nd Attempt	3rd Attempt	
_____	_____	_____	Gather materials (equipment and supplies) listed under *Conditions*.
_____	_____	_____	1. Access the Internet.
_____	_____	_____	2. Search for and type in the website address for the American Association of Medical Assistants (AAMA).
_____	_____	_____	3. Highlight "CMA (AAMA) Exam," then select "Study for the Exam."
_____	_____	_____	4. Under "Test Your Knowledge," select either "Anatomy and Physiology" or "Medical Terminology."
_____	_____	_____	5. Read the instructions and download, open, and print the answer form.
_____	_____	_____	6. Read each question and mark the answer.
___/50	___/50	___/50	7. Go to "answers" and compare your answers with the answer key; they are listed directly after the questions.
_____	_____	_____	8. Make note of the questions you need to study.
_____	_____	_____	Complete within specified time.
___/59	___/59	___/59	**Total points earned** (To obtain a percentage score, divide the total points earned by the number of points possible.)

JOB SKILL 1-5 (*continued*)

Comments:

Evaluator's Signature: _____   **Need to Repeat:** _____

National Curriculum Competency: CAAHEP: Cognitive: I.C.1–5	ABHES: 2.a; 3.a, b, c, d

JOB SKILL 1-6
Develop a Medical Practice Survey

Name _____ Date _____ Score _____

Performance Objective

Task: Design a patient satisfaction survey form.

Conditions: Need:

- White 8½" by 11" paper and pen or pencil
- Computer if available

Standards: Complete all steps listed in this skill in _____minutes with a minimum score of _____.
(Time element and accuracy criteria may be given by instructor.)

Time: Start: _____ Completed: _____ Total: _____ minutes

Scoring: One point for each step performed satisfactorily unless otherwise listed or weighted by instructor.

Directions with Performance Evaluation Checklist

Practon Medical Group is trying to incorporate customer service into all aspects of the practice. In serving the needs of Dr. Practon's patients, there may be areas that need improvement. Design a patient satisfaction survey that addresses this.

1st Attempt	2nd Attempt	3rd Attempt	
_____	_____	_____	Gather materials (equipment and supplies) listed under *Conditions*.
____/10	____/10	____/10	1. Design your own survey form using the reference material on Practon Medical Group, Inc., found in Appendix A of this *Workbook*.
____/25	____/25	____/25	2. Formulate at least five questions that address patient satisfaction.
_____	_____	_____	Complete within specified time.
____/37	____/37	____/37	**Total points earned** (To obtain a percentage score, divide the total points earned by the number of points possible.)

Comments:

Evaluator's Signature: _____ **Need to Repeat:** _____

National Curriculum Competency: CAAHEP: Cognitive: X.C.5

The Health Care Environment: Past, Present, and Future

STOP AND THINK CASE SCENARIOS

Refer to the end of Chapter 2 in the *textbook* for the following scenarios:

- Traditional Versus Managed Care
- Determination of Benefits
- Types of Medical Practice Settings

EXAM-STYLE REVIEW QUESTIONS

Refer to the end of Chapter 2 in the *textbook.*

Abbreviation and Spelling Review

Read the patient's chart note and write the meanings for the abbreviations following the note. To decode any abbreviations you do not understand or that appear unfamiliar to you, refer to the list of abbreviations in Appendix B of this *Workbook*. Step-by-step directions for this exercise are found in Procedure 1-1 of Chapter 1 in the *textbook*. Medical terms in the chart note are italicized; study them for spelling. Use your medical dictionary to look up their definitions. Your instructor may give a spelling and definition test that includes these words and abbreviations.

Troy Wenzlau

36-year-old W male seen as E for Fx L *humerus*. Pt DNS for re-exam last month as scheduled. Pt has been on SD X 3 mo for back pain and was determined P&S from a previous back injury last yr. Given I of *Demerol* 50 mg IM for pain, x-ray L arm ordered. Cast and return to ofc in 2 wks.

Gerald M. Practon, MD
Gerald M. Practon, MD

W _____   mo _____

E _____   P&S _____

Fx _____   yr _____

L _____   I _____

Pt _____   mg _____

DNS _____   IM _____

re-exam _____   ofc _____

SD _____   wks _____

X _____

Review Questions

Review the objectives, glossary, and chapter information before completing the following review questions.

1. Briefly describe the contribution of each of the following:

   a. Imhotep _____
   _____
   _____

   b. Edward Jenner _____
   _____
   _____

   c. Frederick Banting _____
   _____
   _____

   d. Anton van Leeuwenhoek _____
   _____

   e. Pierre and Marie Curie _____

   f. Paul Ehrlich _____
   _____
   _____

2. Match the pioneer in medicine in the left column with the appropriate item in the right column by writing the letters in the blanks.

_____ Ignaz Phillip Semmelweis		a. father of modern anatomy
_____ Joseph Lister		b. father of medicine
_____ Louis Pasteur		c. founder of nursing
_____ Jonas Edward Salk		d. discovered the x-ray
_____ Clara Barton		e. developed the first lens strong enough to see bacteria
_____ Asclepius		f. discovered how yellow fever is transmitted
_____ Ambroise Paré		g. father of bacteriology
_____ Walter Reed		h. discovered the vaccine against polio
_____ William Harvey		i. Greek god of healing
_____ Wilhem C. Roentgen		j. founded the American Red Cross
_____ Hippocrates		k. father of sterile surgery
_____ Andreas Vesalius		l. father of modern surgery
_____ James Marion Sims		m. fought against puerperal fever
_____ Florence Nightingale		n. demonstrated circulation of blood
_____ Alexander Fleming		o. invented the vaginal speculum
		p. discovered insulin
		q. discovered penicillin

3. Name several factors that contributed to the rise of health care costs as medicine advanced. _____

_____

4. List the benefits of using a managed care organization (MCO) and a traditional health care system as you compare and contrast their similarities and differences.

Traditional	Managed Care
a. _____	a. _____
b. _____	b. _____
c. _____	c. _____
d. _____	d. _____
e. _____	e. _____
f. _____	f. _____

5. In a health maintenance organization (HMO), what is a treating physician called? _____

_____

6. In a preferred provider organization (PPO), (a) what is the health care provider called and (b) what incentive is there for the patient to use this provider?

a. _____

b. _____

7. In an independent practice association (IPA), how is the physician paid? _____

_____

_____

8. Why is an exclusive provider organization (EPO) called *exclusive*? _____
_____
_____

9. What choice of care do patients have when belonging to a point-of-service plan? _____
_____
_____

10. Managed care plans pay the physician by _____.

11. Dr. Practon wants to know if Mrs. Snow's managed care plan covers a particular surgical procedure. This is a process known as _____.

12. Dr. Practon completes a form for preauthorization of a diagnostic test to be ordered for Lee Cho. This process may also be called _____ or _____.

13. Before scheduling elective surgery on Phyllis Horton, Dr. Practon wants to know the maximum amount the insurance plan will pay. This is a process known as _____
_____.

14. Name five popular types of managed care health plans and list their abbreviations.

    a. _____
    b. _____
    c. _____
    d. _____
    e. _____

15. A variety of specialists practicing medicine together is called: _____
_____
_____

16. List three services urgent care centers provide that most other practices do not offer.

    a. _____
    b. _____
    c. _____

17. Why should the medical assistant meet the hospital personnel where his or her physician is on staff?
_____

18. Name several types of nonprofit hospitals.

    a. _____
    b. _____
    c. _____
    d. _____
    e. _____

19. Name three important factors to consider when choosing a reliable laboratory.

   a. _____

   b. _____

   c. _____

Critical Thinking Exercises

1. Choose the type of health care *setting* you would like to work in and list the *reasons* for your choice.

   Setting: _____

   Reasons: _____

   _____

   _____

   _____

2. Debate the right of the physician to practice or not practice "concierge" medicine. _____

   _____

   _____

   _____

   _____

   _____

3. Determine the job duties of an administrative medical assistant working in a patient-centered medical home. _____

   _____

   _____

   _____

   _____

4. As a member of a multidisciplinary team, name several ways you, as an administrative medical assistant, can act as a patient advocate.

   a. _____

   b. _____

   c. _____

5. The following scenario is designed for students to role-play to gain experience interacting with insurance carriers and patients. Students should honor confidentiality, be courteous and demonstrate sensitivity, and display assertiveness and confidence while communicating with the provider and patient. Divide students into groups of three—one can play a medical assistant, the second the insurance company employee, and the third can be the patient.

   Dr. Gerald Practon has ordered a colonoscopy and has asked you to call the managed care company to see what policies and procedures are in place. The patient is waiting to see if the procedure can be scheduled immediately. Place a call to precertify benefits, predetermine the dollar amount allowed, and find out if preauthorization is needed; then notify the patient of your findings.

JOB SKILL 2-1
Use the Internet to Research and Write an Essay about a Medical Pioneer

Name _____ Date _____ Score _____

Performance Objective

Task: Use the Internet to look up information on a historical figure who contributed to medicine. Write a one-page essay describing their contribution. Note: If directed by instructor, this job skill may be done using library references.

Conditions: Need:

       • Computer with Internet connection

       • Printer and paper

Standards: Complete all steps listed in this job skill in _____ minutes with a minimum score of _____. (Time element and accuracy criteria may be given by instructor.)

Time: **Start: _____ Completed: _____ Total: _____** minutes

Scoring: One point for each step performed satisfactorily unless otherwise listed or weighted by instructor.

Directions with Performance Evaluation Checklist

Following are some famous medical pioneer names who are not already mentioned in the *textbook*. Select a name and research their discoveries or inventions: Frederick Banting; Vice Admiral Regina Benjamin; Herbert Boyer; Alexis Carrell; Stanley Cohen; Frank Colton; Peter Dunn; Robert Edwards; Peter Ellis; Gabriel Fahrenheit; Ray W. Fuller; Galen; John Gibbons; Claudius; Samuel Hahjnemann; Charles Hufnagel; Robert Jarvik; Willem Kolff; Rene Laennec; Walton C. Lillehei; Elias Metchnikoff; W. T. G. Morton; Daniel David Palmer; Trotula Platearius; Rhazes; Peter Safar; Albert Schatz; Ake Senning; Patrick Steptoe; Andrew Taylor; Nicholas Terrett; Ian Wilmut; Albert Wood; and Paul Zoll.

1st Attempt	2nd Attempt	3rd Attempt	
_____	_____	_____	Gather materials (equipment and supplies) listed under *Conditions*.
_____	_____	_____	1. Turn on computer and establish an Internet connection. Use a search engine such as Yahoo, Google, GoodSearch, or one of your favorites.
____/3	____/3	____/3	2. Select a famous medical pioneer not already mentioned in the *textbook* (see suggestions under "directions") or type in the key words "famous medical discoveries" or "inventor," then name a procedure or piece of medical equipment you would like to learn the history of, for example, "wheelchair inventor."
____/2	____/2	____/2	3. After selecting the pioneer or subject to write about, search for two more references containing information.
____/3	____/3	____/3	4. Print each of the references; read and study the material.
____/5	____/5	____/5	5. Type a one-page essay describing the historical figure or invention. Do not copy the text; use language at the level patients would understand if you were to read it to them.

JOB SKILL 2-1 (*continued*)

_____ _____ _____   6. Include a cover page with title.

___/3 ___/3 ___/3   7. Include a bibliography naming your references. To learn how Internet references are cited, search: "Columbia format for citing web research."

_____ _____ _____   Complete within specified time.

___/20 ___/20 ___/20   **Total points earned** (To obtain a percentage score, divide the total points earned by the number of points possible.)

Comments:

Evaluator's Signature: _____ **Need to Repeat:** _____

National Curriculum Competency: ABHES: 7h

JOB SKILL 2-2
Direct Patients to Specific Hospital Departments

Name _____ Date _____ Score _____

Performance Objective

Task: Make determinations to direct patients to specific hospital departments.

Conditions: Need:

- Pen or pencil

Refer to:

- *Textbook* Figure 2-7A and Figure 2-7B (hospital departments)
- *Textbook* Procedure 2-1 for step-by-step directions

Standards: Complete all steps listed in this skill in _____ minutes with a minimum score of _____. (Time element and accuracy criteria may be given by instructor.)

Time: Start: _____ Completed: _____ Total: _____ minutes

Scoring: One point for each step performed satisfactorily unless otherwise listed or weighted by instructor.

Directions with Performance Evaluation Checklist

In many situations, the administrative medical assistant will be interacting with the hospital. Knowledge of various hospital departments and the services they offer is helpful in order to expediently schedule tests, arrange surgery, obtain test results, and refer patients, "coaching" them along the right path. In the following scenario, you are the administrative assistant in Dr. Gerald Practon's office. A patient, Reiko Kimon, was discharged from the hospital last week and has various questions. List the correct hospital department you would direct the patient to.

1st Attempt	2nd Attempt	3rd Attempt	
_____	_____	_____	Gather materials (equipment and supplies) listed under *Conditions*.
_____	_____	_____	1. Where does she go to pick up a copy of her operative report?
_____	_____	_____	2. Where can she attend a nutritional education class?
_____	_____	_____	3. Where does she go for a urinalysis?
_____	_____	_____	4. She has a question about the medication that was given to her when she left the hospital.
_____	_____	_____	5. Should she use a bronchodilator before she goes to have a pulmonary function test?
_____	_____	_____	6. She would like to personally tell the hospital president how wonderfully she was cared for during her hospital stay.
_____	_____	_____	7. She would like to speak to the physician who admitted her when she first arrived by ambulance at the hospital.
_____	_____	_____	8. She would like to know whether anyone has found a convalescent hospital for her mother, who is an inpatient and soon to be discharged.
_____	_____	_____	9. She would like to schedule occupational therapy.
_____	_____	_____	10. She does not understand a hospital bill and would like it explained.
_____	_____	_____	11. She would like the name of the new OB-GYN doctor from San Francisco who is performing deliveries at the hospital.

JOB SKILL 2-2 *(continued)*

_____ _____ _____   12. She has a question regarding the contrast media that will be given to her before a bone scan.

_____ _____ _____   13. She would like to pick up a preparation kit for a barium enema.

_____ _____ _____   14. She has a question regarding an old refund that should have been sent to her by now.

_____ _____ _____   15. She would like to speak to the utilization review nurse who was assigned to her case.

_____ _____ _____   16. She would like to know if she can wear her wedding ring in the magnetic resonance imaging (MRI) machine.

_____ _____ _____   17. She would like to know how to dress for the treadmill test.

_____ _____ _____   18. She would like to know the preparation for a sigmoidoscopy that is scheduled.

_____ _____ _____   19. She would like to know what time to arrive for a blood transfusion.

_____ _____ _____   20. You are attentive, courteous, and diplomatic while demonstrating sensitivity when communicating with the patient and hospital personnel.

_____ _____ _____   Complete within specified time.

___/22 ___/22 ___/22   **Total points earned** (To obtain a percentage score, divide the total points earned by the number of points possible.)

Comments:

Evaluator's Signature: _____   **Need to Repeat:** _____

National Curriculum Competency: CAAHEP: Cognitive: V.C.6; Psychomotor: V.P.4

JOB SKILL 2-3
Refer Patients to the Correct Physician Specialist

Name _____ Date _____ Score _____

Performance Objective

Task: Match the correct specialist with the patient's complaint.

Conditions: Need:

- Pen or pencil

Refer to:

- *Textbook* Table 2-4 for a list of medical specialties with descriptions
- *Textbook* Procedure 2-2 for step-by-step directions

Standards: Complete all steps listed in this skill in _____ minutes with a minimum score of _____. (Time element and accuracy criteria may be given by instructor.)

Time: Start: _____ Completed: _____ Total: _____ minutes

Scoring: One point for each step performed satisfactorily unless otherwise listed or weighted by instructor.

Directions with Performance Evaluation Checklist

In many situations, administrative medical assistants deal with the authorization referral process. They may also handle patients being referred by primary care physicians to specialists. To enhance understanding of these processes, consider the patients' problems and match their complaints with the correct specialist, remembering to demonstrate empathy and using language skills that enable patients' understanding as you "coach" them along the right path according to their needs.

1st Attempt	2nd Attempt	3rd Attempt		
_____	_____	_____	Gather materials (equipment and supplies) listed under *Conditions*.	
_____	_____	_____	1. _____ Pregnant	A. Allergist
_____	_____	_____	2. _____ Operation	B. Dermatologist
_____	_____	_____	3. _____ Microbiology report	C. Neonatologist
_____	_____	_____	4. _____ Bladder and kidney problems	D. Neurologist
_____	_____	_____	5. _____ Chronic runny nose from dust	E. Nuclear medicine
_____	_____	_____	6. _____ Severe depression	F. Obstetrician
_____	_____	_____	7. _____ Face lift	G. Ophthalmologist
_____	_____	_____	8. _____ Premature infant	H. Orthopedic surgeon
_____	_____	_____	9. _____ Infant DPT (diphtheria, pertussis, and tetanus) injection	I. Otolaryngologist
_____	_____	_____	10. _____ Ear discharge	J. Pathologist
_____	_____	_____	11. _____ X-rays	K. Pediatrician
_____	_____	_____	12. _____ Fractured bone	L. Physiatrist
_____	_____	_____	13. _____ Rehabilitation for chronic back pain	M. Plastic surgeon
_____	_____	_____	14. _____ Multiple sclerosis (disease of nervous system)	N. Psychiatrist
				O. Radiologist

JOB SKILL 2-3 (*continued*)

_____ _____ _____ 15. _____ Glaucoma (increased pressure in eye)

P. Surgeon

Q. Urologist

_____ _____ _____ 16. _____ Severe case of skin psoriasis

_____ _____ _____ 17. _____ Bone scan (radionuclear)

_____ _____ _____ 18. Used empathy when communicating and language skills that enabled patients' understanding.

_____ _____ _____ Complete within specified time.

___/20 ___/20 ___/20 **Total points earned** (To obtain a percentage score, divide the total points earned by the number of points possible.)

Comments:

Evaluator's Signature: _____   **Need to Repeat:** _____

National Curriculum Competency: CAAHEP: Cognitive: V.C.6; Psychomotor: V.P.4   ABHES: 3.c, d

JOB SKILL 2-4
Define Abbreviations for Health Care Professionals

Name _____ Date _____ Score _____

Performance Objective

Task: Match terms for health care professionals with correct abbreviations.

Conditions: Need:

- Pen or pencil

Refer to:

- *Textbook* Table 2-5 for a list of physician specialists, health care professionals, and abbreviations
- *Textbook* Procedure 1-1 for step-by-step directions

Standards: Complete all steps listed in this skill in _____ minutes with a minimum score of _____. (Time element and accuracy criteria may be given by instructor.)

Time: Start: _____ Completed: _____ Total: _____ minutes

Scoring: One point for each step performed satisfactorily unless otherwise listed or weighted by instructor.

Directions with Performance Evaluation Checklist

Read the following scenario, decode the abbreviations for the appropriate physician specialists and health care professionals, and write the correct term on the line provided.

Laverne M. Stinowski   May 15, 20XX

Mrs. Stinowski was brought by ambulance to the hospital and was cared for by an EMT. In the emergency room she was treated by a DEM. During her hospital stay she was seen daily by the MD, who was also a FACS. After discharge, Mrs. Stinowski visited the physician's private office and was processed in by a CMA (AAMA). An LVN drew her blood and escorted her to the treatment room. The physician was out of the office, so an RNP saw Mrs. Stinowski. An order was given for her to see an RPT. The blood test was read in the laboratory by an MT (ASCP). The patient's record was keyed into the EMR by a CMT, and her insurance claim was processed by a CPC. The patient went home, and the PA-C was in charge of ordering the patient a VN for the following day.

Gerald M. Practon, MD
Gerald M. Practon, MD

1st Attempt	2nd Attempt	3rd Attempt	
_____	_____	_____	Gather materials (equipment and supplies) listed under *Conditions*.
_____	_____	_____	1. EMT _____
_____	_____	_____	2. DEM _____
_____	_____	_____	3. MD _____
_____	_____	_____	4. FACS _____
_____	_____	_____	5. CMA (AAMA) _____
_____	_____	_____	6. LVN _____
_____	_____	_____	7. RNP _____

JOB SKILL 2-4 (*continued*)

_____ _____ _____   8. RPT _____

_____ _____ _____   9. MT (ASCP) _____

_____ _____ _____   10. EMR _____

_____ _____ _____   11. CMT _____

_____ _____ _____   12. CPC _____

_____ _____ _____   13. PA-C _____

_____ _____ _____   14. VN _____

_____ _____ _____   Complete within specified time.

___/16 ___/16 ___/16   **Total points earned** (To obtain a percentage score, divide the total points earned by the number of points possible.)

Comments:

National Curriculum Competency: ABHES: 3.d

JOB SKILL 2-5
Determine Basic Skills Needed by the Administrative Medical Assistant

Name _____ Date _____ Score _____

Performance Objective

Task: Review job requirements and determine basic skills necessary for the administrative medical assistant.

Conditions: Need:

• Pen or pencil

Refer to:

• *Textbook* Table 2-4 for a list of medical specialties and administrative medical assistant job requirements.

Standards: Complete all steps listed in this skill in _____ minutes with a minimum score of _____. (Time element and accuracy criteria may be given by instructor.)

Time: Start: _____ Completed: _____ Total: _____ minutes

Scoring: One point for each step performed satisfactorily unless otherwise listed or weighted by instructor.

Directions with Performance Evaluation Checklist

Record some basic skills the administrative medical assistant needs. You will see these skills occurring repetitiously under the different specialties listed in *textbook* Table 2-4.

1st Attempt	2nd Attempt	3rd Attempt	
_____	_____	_____	Gather materials (equipment and supplies) listed under *Conditions*.
_____	_____	_____	1. _____
_____	_____	_____	2. _____
_____	_____	_____	3. _____
_____	_____	_____	4. _____
_____	_____	_____	5. _____
_____	_____	_____	6. _____
_____	_____	_____	7. _____
_____	_____	_____	8. _____
_____	_____	_____	Complete within specified time.
___/10	___/10	___/10	**Total points earned** (To obtain a percentage score, divide the total points earned by the number of points possible.)

JOB SKILL 2-5 *(continued)*

Comments:

National Curriculum Competency: CAAHEP: Cognitive: VI.C. Skills listed are found in the "Administrative Functions" section and throughout various competencies.
ABHES: 1.d

Medicolegal and Ethical Responsibilities

STOP AND THINK CASE SCENARIOS

Refer to the end of Chapter 3 in the *textbook* for the following scenarios:

- Ethics
- Bioethics
- Stem Cell Research

- Confidential Information
- HIPAA: Verbal Permission
- HIPAA: Written Permission

EXAM-STYLE REVIEW QUESTIONS

Refer to the end of Chapter 3 in the *textbook*.

Abbreviation and Spelling Review

Read the patient's chart note and write the meanings for the abbreviations following the note. To decide any abbreviations you do not understand or that appear unfamiliar to you, refer to the list of abbreviations in Appendix B of this *Workbook*. Step-by-step directions for this exercise are in Procedure 1-1 of Chapter 1 in the *textbook*. Medical terms in the chart note are italicized; study them for spelling. Use your medical dictionary to look up their definitions. Your instructor may give a spelling and definition test that includes these words and abbreviations.

David K. Chung

September 20, 20XX HX: *Diarrhea* 3 days. T 99°F. No A. Cough producing yellow *sputum*. *Wheezing* in lt base. Moderate PND. Rec *vaporizer* and *amoxicillin* 250 mg p.o. every .8h. Diag URI. Etiol. unknown. Ordered CXR, CBC, & UA. Retn 2 wks.

Gerald Practon, MD
Gerald Practon, MD

HX _____   h. _____

T _____   diag _____

F _____   URI _____

A _____   etiol. _____

lt _____   CXR _____

PND _____   CBC _____

rec _____   UA _____

mg _____   retn _____

p.o. _____   wks _____

Review Questions

Review the objectives, glossary, and chapter information before completing the following review questions.

1. Match the terms in the left column with the definitions in the right column by writing letters in the blanks.

   _____ Oath of Hippocrates

   _____ medical ethics

   _____ bioethics

   _____ privileged information

   _____ medical etiquette

   _____ Principles of Medical Ethics

   a. confidential information in a medical record

   b. code of conduct, courtesy, and manners customary in the medical profession

   c. moral principles and standards in the medical profession

   d. modern code of ethics

   e. branch of ethics concerning moral issues, questions, and problems that arise in the practice of medicine and in biomedical research

   f. first standards of medical conduct and ethics

2. HIPAA stands for _____.

3. According to Title II of HIPAA law, name several ways in which HIPAA affects a medical practice.

   a. _____

   b. _____

   c. _____

   d. _____

4. Information about a patient's past, present, or future health condition that contains personal identifying data is called _____.

5. What does the privacy rule provide?

   _____

   _____

   _____

6. State three key things you would tell a new employee about patient confidentiality.

   a. _____

   b. _____

   c. _____

7. What are the three items a voluntary signed consent form covers?

   a. _____

   b. _____

   c. _____

8. What form must be obtained for use and disclosure of protected health information (PHI)? _____

   _____

9. State the definition of a compliance plan. _____

   _____

   _____

10. What is the common term for litigation? _____

11. Another phrase used for medical malpractice is _____.

12. Name two types of medical professional liability insurance.

    a. _____

    b. _____

13. A physician is legally responsible for any act you perform while in his or her employ. The legal phrase

    used to describe this responsibility is _____,

    and it means _____.

14. Name three circumstances in which a minor may become emancipated.

    a. _____

    b. _____

    c. _____

15. Define *tort*. _____

    _____

16. Match the words in the left column with the definitions in the right column by writing the letters in the blanks.

    _____ malfeasance   a. carelessness or negligence by a professional person

    _____ misfeasance   b. lawful treatment done in the wrong way

    _____ nonfeasance   c. failure of the physician to do anything

    _____ malpractice   d. reckless disregard for the safety of another; being indifferent
                                             to an injury that could occur

    _____ criminal negligence   e. wrongful treatment of the patient

17. Name the three principal defenses in a malpractice lawsuit.

    a. _____

    b. _____

    c. _____

18. Name three types of bonding.

    a. _____

    b. _____

    c. _____

19. Name three alternatives to the litigation process.

    a. _____

    b. _____

    c. _____

Critical Thinking Exercises

1. A sales representative from the Hope Surgical Company brings a case of bourbon for your physician. Can your physician ethically accept this gift? Why or why not? _____

    _____

2. Betty Harper is given a booklet on the office policies that explains charges for missed appointments, telephone calls, and insurance form completion. She brings two insurance forms, and you bill her for this service. Is this ethical? _____ If so why?

    _____

    _____

3. You overhear Linda Mason telling another patient in the reception room that another physician is treating her for her stomach ulcer. You know Dr. Practon is also treating her for this same condition in addition to her high blood pressure. What should you do? _____

    _____

    _____

4. Margaret Silsbee, a patient of Fran Practon, MD, is seen on October 5 for a pelvic examination. She signed a consent form on her first visit. Although she has insurance, she pays cash for the visit and asks that you not bill the insurance company. The following month, her insurance company requests all of her medical records. State what you would do and why. _____

    _____

    _____

    _____

5. Gary Ryan has an outstanding bill of $200. You receive a signed authorization form for release of information from Dr. Homer's office requesting a copy of his progress notes since surgery. Can you ethically withhold this information until Mr. Ryan pays his bill? _____

    _____

6. An insurance company sends Dr. Practon a request for the records of Jerry Osborne. A signed authorization accompanies the request. The medical record indicates that the physician discussed HIV testing, and the patient refused the test. What would you do? _____

_____

_____

7. Martin P. Finley is examined, and the physician discovers a wart recurring on the patient's thumb.

Mr. Finley asks the physician to remove it. In this instance, what kind of contract exists? _____

_____

8. A tow truck has a head-on collision on a rural highway 25 miles out of town. Dr. O'Halloran is driving along and notices the accident. He stops, finds a victim of the accident bleeding profusely, and renders

first aid. Will he be held liable for any medical complication in aiding this victim? _____

_____

Name the law that governs this situation. _____

9. Candice Goodson, a 15-year-old, comes into the office and requests an examination for herself and her baby. Can the physician care for the infant and Candice without Candice's parents' consent?

_____ Why or why not? _____

_____

_____

10. Dr. Gerald Practon receives a request from a social worker for medical records on a minor who is a ward of the court. The minor has signed an authorization to release medical information. What would

you do? _____

_____

_____

11. Give two examples of tort law as it applies to the medical assistant. _____

a. _____

_____

b. _____

_____

12. Dr. Rodriguez examines Mr. Garcia and diagnoses a gallstone. He reports this to the patient and recommends surgery. The patient says he agrees to the surgery. Are all conditions of informed consent

present in this case? _____

If not, name any that might be missing. _____

_____

_____

13. A subpoena is served on Dr. Bradley in regard to patient Teri Sanchez. In this instance, is a patient

release-of-information form necessary? _____

14. Mrs. Marinacci states she wishes to donate her kidneys for transplant when she dies. How does she legally record her wishes? _____

_____

_____

15. Read the following scenarios and determine whether the information presented is protected health information (PHI). Indicate "yes" or "no" and a brief explanation on the line provided.

a. You are doing an externship in a large orthopedic office and a man comes in with multiple fractures of his femur. All the doctors gather to view his x-ray because this is quite unusual. After the physicians are gone, you take a picture of the x-ray with your cell phone and post it on Facebook so your classmates can view it. The enlarged x-ray shows the patient name and date of birth. Is this PHI? ____

_____

b. A patient suffered from schizophrenia and was hospitalized in a mental institution while in college. He is now 37 years old. Is information about his hospitalization still PHI? _____

_____

c. An operative report in which the patient's name and other identifiers have been removed is being shared by the office manager at a training session for insurance coders. Is this PHI? _____

_____

16. Mr. Smith saw Dr. Practon for an initial visit but never paid his bill. Does a physician-patient contract exist in this case (explain your answer)? _____

_____

_____

_____

_____

_____

_____

_____

_____

_____

_____

_____

_____

_____

JOB SKILL 3-1
List Personal Ethics and Set Professional Ethical Goals

Name _____ Date _____ Score _____

Performance Objective

Task: List your personal ethics that may affect professional ethics. Determine weak areas and set goals to become more professionally ethically centered for the future.

Conditions: Need:
- Quiet area for reflection
- Ethical partner to work with
- Paper and pen or pencil

Standards: Complete all steps listed in this job skill in _____ minutes with a minimum score of _____. (Time element and accuracy criteria may be given by instructor.)

Time: **Start:** _____ **Completed:** _____ **Total:** _____ minutes

Scoring: One point for each step performed satisfactorily unless otherwise listed or weighted by instructor.

Directions with Performance Evaluation Checklist

1st Attempt	2nd Attempt	3rd Attempt	
_____	_____	_____	Gather materials (equipment and supplies) listed under *Conditions*.
_____	_____	_____	1. Find a quiet area so you can reflect and think about the personal ethics you obtain and how they may influence your professional career as a medical assistant.
____/5	____/5	____/5	2. Write down five personal ethics that might affect your professional ethics as a medical assistant.

    a._____

    b._____

    c._____

    d._____

    e._____

| ____/2 | ____/2 | ____/2 | 3. State one situation where your personal ethics may interfere or contradict the professional ethics of a medical assistant. _____ |

_____

_____

| ____/2 | ____/2 | ____/2 | 4. Determine a situation where you need to separate personal from professional ethics (e.g., this could be how you feel about a bioethical situation). |

_____

_____

_____

JOB SKILL 3-1 *(continued)*

___/3   ___/3   ___/3   5. Determine three key goals to become more ethically centered for the future (you may determine more).

        a. _____

        b. _____

        c. _____

___/3   ___/3   ___/3   6. Pledge to make more time to achieve the goals by giving less priority or more priority to the following:

        a. _____

        b. _____

        c. _____

_____   _____   _____   7. Select a support person and together determine ways he or she can help you. This person's name is: _____

___/2   ___/2   ___/2   8. Select a method to maintain your momentum and record your weekly progress.

_____   _____   _____   9. Determine a reward for achieving your milestone and becoming a more professionally ethical person.

_____   _____   _____   Complete within specified time.

___/22   ___/22   ___/22   **Total points earned** (To obtain a percentage score, divide the total points earned by the number of points possible.)

Comments:

Evaluator's Signature: _____   **Need to Repeat:** _____

National Curriculum Competency: CAAHEP: Cognitive: XI.C.2, 2,5;	
Psychomotor: XI.P.1, 2; Affective: XI.A.1	ABHES: 4.g; 10.b

JOB SKILL 3-2
Complete an Authorization Form to Release Medical Records

Name _____ Date _____ Score _____

Performance Objective

Task: Apply HIPAA rules to protect patient privacy when completing an authorization form to release medical information.

Conditions: Need:
- Patient demographic information (found in the "scenario")
- Computer with Internet connection
- Online Form 1 (Authorization for Release of Information) located at www.cengagebrain.com
- Pen or pencil

Refer to:
- *Textbook* Figure 3-9 for an illustration
- *Textbook* Procedure 3-1 for step-by-step
- *Workbook*, Appendix A, Medical Practice Reference Material for physician and practice data

Standards: Complete all steps listed in this job skill in _____ minutes with a minimum score of _____. (Time element and accuracy criteria may be given by instructor.)

Time: Start: _____ Completed: _____ Total: _____ minutes

Scoring: One point for each step performed satisfactorily unless otherwise listed or weighted by instructor.

Directions with Performance Evaluation Checklist

Scenario: Patient Michele Ramsey (7796 Bluebird Street, Woodland Hills, XY 12345, telephone [555] 937-7102, DOB 04/08/1950, medical record #2078) comes into the office stating that the company she works for will be closing its local office and she is transferring to another city. She would like her medical records sent to her new physician (Margaret Birgelaitis, MD, 66948 Santa Clara Circle, Anytown, XY 12345-0000, telephone [555] 482-0010). Obtain and complete the correct authorization form to process this request. Ms. Ramsey was first seen on 02/13/2012 and last seen on 09/03/2016. Today's date is 10/10/2016 and the authorization will expire at the end of the calendar year.

1st Attempt	2nd Attempt	3rd Attempt	
_____	_____	_____	Gather materials (equipment and supplies) listed under *Conditions*.
___/10	___/10	___/10	1. Complete Section A of the form with the following: Patient identifying information, medical practice information, person receiving information, and the reason for and description of the request.
___/3	___/3	___/3	2. Complete Section B of the form and highlight the areas the patient needs to complete or initial.
___/6	___/6	___/6	3. Complete Section C of the form and highlight the areas the patient needs to complete or initial.
_____	_____	_____	Complete within specified time.
___/21	___/21	___/21	**Total points earned** (To obtain a percentage score, divide the total points earned by the number of points possible.)

JOB SKILL 3-2 (*continued*)

Comments:

Evaluator's Signature: _____ **Need to Repeat:** _____

| National Curriculum Competency: CAAHEP:; Psychomotor: X.P.2,; Affective: X.A.2 | ABHES: 4.b.1 |

JOB SKILL 3-3
Download State-Specific Scope of Practice Laws and Determine Parameters for a Medical Assistant

Name _____ Date _____ Score _____

Performance Objective

Task: Use the Internet to download Medical Assisting Scope of Practice Laws for the state in which you live. Review the laws, identify areas of practice, select a topic, and write a summary of what is included in your state.

Conditions: Need:

- Computer with Internet connection and printer
- Paper and pen or pencil

Standards: Complete all steps listed in this job skill in _____ minutes with a minimum score of _____. (Time element and accuracy criteria may be given by instructor.)

Time: **Start:** _____ **Completed:** _____ **Total:** _____ minutes

Scoring: One point for each step performed satisfactorily unless otherwise listed or weighted by instructor.

Directions with Performance Evaluation Checklist

Check with your instructor: You may want to do this job skill as a cooperative learning effort with several other students, depending on the state information available and the number of students in your class.

1st Attempt	2nd Attempt	3rd Attempt	
_____	_____	_____	Gather materials (equipment and supplies) listed under *Conditions*.
_____	_____	_____	1. Turn on the computer and obtain an Internet connection. Go to the website for the American Association of Medical Assistants: http://www.aama-ntl.org
_____	_____	_____	2. Click on "Employers," then "State Scope of Practice Laws."
_____	_____	_____	3. Select the state in which you live. If your state is not listed, click on "Questions Regarding Your State."
___/5	___/5	___/5	4. Select an area to research or frequently asked questions (FAQs) to report on. Print and read the material. Note: Your instructor may direct you to a specific topic, law, or medical task prohibition.
___/10	___/10	___/10	5. Write a paragraph on your findings.
___/2	___/2	___/2	6. What may be the consequences of not working within the legal scope of practice? _____ _____
_____	_____	_____	Complete within specified time.
___/22	___/22	___/22	**Total points earned** (To obtain a percentage score, divide the total points earned by the number of points possible.)

JOB SKILL 3-3 *(continued)*

Comments:

Evaluator's Signature: _____   **Need to Repeat:** _____

National Curriculum Competency: CAAHEP: Cognitive: X.C.1, 2; Psychomotor: X.P.1 | ABHES: 4.f.1, 2

JOB SKILL 3-4
Compose a Letter of Withdrawal

Name _____ Date _____ Score _____

Performance Objective

Task: Compose a letter of withdrawal from Dr. Gerald Practon to a patient who has failed to pay his medical bill.

Conditions: Need:

  • White paper (8½" by 11") and computer

  Refer to:

  • *Workbook*, Appendix A (letterhead reference information)

  • *Textbook* Figure 3-11 (illustration of a letter and sample wording)

Standards: Complete all steps listed in this skill in _____ minutes with a minimum score of _____.
  (Time element and accuracy criteria may be given by instructor.)

Time: **Start: _____ Completed: _____ Total: _____** minutes

Scoring: One point for each step performed satisfactorily unless otherwise listed or weighted by instructor.

Directions with Performance Evaluation Checklist

Patrick C. Pieper of 697 Williams Street, Woodland Hills, XY 12345 has received medical services amounting to $525. He provided insurance information at the time services were rendered but he is not eligible for medical coverage or benefits under the plan. He has received four statements and made two promises to pay over the telephone, which he has not kept. Dr. Gerald Practon would now like to send a letter of withdrawal and is allowing Mr. Pieper 30 days to locate another physician. He will be referred to the Ventura County Medical Society, (555) 676-5544, if he is unable to locate a new physician. Compose a personal letter of withdrawal on Dr. Practon's letterhead stating the above information.

1st Attempt	2nd Attempt	3rd Attempt	
_____	_____	_____	Gather materials (equipment and supplies) listed under *Conditions*.
____/5	____/5	____/5	1. Using a computer, prepare a letterhead that contains the Practon group name, street address, city, state, zip, and telephone number.
_____	_____	_____	2. Format the letter in block style (everything aligned to the left) or modified block style (as in Figure 3-11).
_____	_____	_____	3. Include the current date.
_____	_____	_____	4. Include the inside address.
_____	_____	_____	5. Include a salutation.
____/20	____/20	____/20	6. Compose a letter including the reason for withdrawing from the patient's care, number of days Dr. Practon will be available to attend to Mr. Pieper, referral source for finding a physician, and release of medical record information.
____/2	____/2	____/2	7. Apply ethical principles (honesty and integrity) in your choice of words as you compose this letter.
____/2	____/2	____/2	8. Include a closing and Dr. Practon's typed signature.

JOB SKILL 3-4 (*continued*)

_____	_____	_____	9. Include initials of the letter composer.
_____	_____	_____	10. Include a list of items that are enclosed with the letter.
_____	_____	_____	Complete within specified time.
___/37	___/37	___/37	**Total points earned** (To obtain a percentage score, divide the total points earned by the number of points possible.)

Comments:

Evaluator's Signature: _____ **Need to Repeat:** _____

National Curriculum Competency: ABHES: 4.c

JOB SKILL 3-5
View a MedWatch Online Form and Learn Submitting Requirements

Name _____ Date _____ Score _____

Performance Objective

Task: View a MedWatch Online Voluntary Reporting Form (3500) and note uses for areas for completion and submission requirements.

Conditions: Need:

- Computer with Internet connection
- Pen or pencil

Standards: Complete all steps listed in this job skill in _____ minutes with a minimum score of _____. (Time element and accuracy criteria may be given by instructor.)

Time: Start: _____ Completed: _____ Total: _____ minutes

Scoring: One point for each step performed satisfactorily unless otherwise listed or weighted by instructor.

Directions with Performance Evaluation Checklist

The U.S. Food and Drug Administration (FDA) states "the MedWatch online form is used to report serious adverse events for human medical products, including potential and actual product use errors and product quality problems."

1st Attempt	2nd Attempt	3rd Attempt	
_____	_____	_____	Gather materials (equipment and supplies) listed under *Conditions*.
____/2	____/2	____/2	1. Turn on the computer and obtain an Internet connection. Go to the U.S. FDA homepage.
____/2	____/2	____/2	2. Search "MedWatch HIPPA compliance page." Select "Reporting By Health Professionals," then click on "Complete voluntary Form FDA 3500 online" and answer the following questions:
____/7	____/7	____/7	3. What are the items listed to report to FDA MedWatch?

a. _____

b. _____

c. _____

d. _____

e. _____

f. _____

g. _____

| ____/6 | ____/6 | ____/6 | 4. List items NOT to be reported to MedWatch. |

a. _____

b. _____

c. _____

d. _____

e. _____

JOB SKILL 3-5 (*continued*)

5. Go back and download form "FDA 3500A" and "FDA 3500B," then answer the following questions:

a. The first section (A) contains _____

_____

b. The next section (B) asks you to:

B-1 _____

B-2 _____

B-3 _____

B-4 _____

B-5 _____

B-6 _____

B-7 _____

_____ _____ _____ Complete within specified time.

___/27 ___/27 ___/27 **Total points earned** (To obtain a percentage score, divide the total points earned by the number of points possible.)

Comments:

Evaluator's Signature: _____ **Need to Repeat:** _____

National Curriculum Competency: CAAHEP: Psychomotor: X.P.6	ABHES: 4.f

JOB SKILL 3-6
Print the *Patient Care Partnership* Online Brochure and Apply It to the Medical Office Setting

Name _____ Date _____ Score _____

Performance Objective

Task: View the *Patient Care Partnership* brochure (formerly the Patients' Bill of Rights) online and apply it to the medical office setting.

Conditions: Need:

- Computer with Internet connection
- Printer and paper
- Pen or pencil

Standards: Complete all steps listed in this job skill in _____ minutes with a minimum score of _____. (Time element and accuracy criteria may be given by instructor.)

Time: **Start:** _____ **Completed:** _____ **Total:** _____ minutes

Scoring: One point for each step performed satisfactorily unless otherwise listed or weighted by instructor.

Directions with Performance Evaluation Checklist

1st Attempt	2nd Attempt	3rd Attempt	
_____	_____	_____	Gather materials (equipment and supplies) listed under *Conditions*.
_____	_____	_____	1. Turn on the computer and obtain an Internet connection. Go to the American Hospital Association (AHA) homepage.
_____	_____	_____	2. Search: the "Patient Care Partnership brochure."
_____	_____	_____	3. Select your language (e.g., English). The file will download and the brochure may be printed. Note: This file may also be viewed online to obtain information.
___/6	___/6	___/6	4. Read the *Patient Care Partnership* and write the six areas this brochure addresses:

    a. _____

    b. _____

    c. _____

    d. _____

    e. _____

    f. _____

| ___/18 | ___/18 | ___/18 | 5. Relate each of these areas to the medical office and write a brief statement about the basic points: |

    a. **Example:** When you come to our medical facility, our first priority is to provide you with the care you need, when you need it, with skill, compassion, and respect.

    b. _____

    _____

    _____

JOB SKILL 3-6 *(continued)*

c. _____

_____

_____

d. _____

_____

_____

e. _____

_____

_____

f. _____

_____

_____

___/3   ___/3   ___/3   6. Circle the above items (a–f) that show sensitivity to patients' rights.

_____   _____   _____   Complete within specified time.

___/32   ___/32   ___/32   **Total points earned** (To obtain a percentage score, divide the total points earned by the number of points possible.)

Comments:

Evaluator's Signature: _____   **Need to Repeat:** _____

National Curriculum Competency: CAAHEP: Cognitive: X.C.4; Psychomotor: X.P.6; Affective: X.A.1	ABHES: 5g

JOB SKILL 3-7
Download and Compare State-Specific Advance Directives

Name _____ Date _____ Score _____

Performance Objective

Task:	Download your state-specific advance directive. Read and compare it to the example shown in the *textbook*.
Conditions:	Need:

     • Computer with Internet connection

     • Printer and paper

     • Pen or pencil

Standards: Complete all steps listed in this job skill in _____ minutes with a minimum score of _____. (Time element and accuracy criteria may be given by instructor.)

Time: **Start:** _____ **Completed:** _____ **Total:** _____ minutes

Scoring: One point for each step performed satisfactorily unless otherwise listed or weighted by instructor.

Directions with Performance Evaluation Checklist

Each state has an advance directive found on the Caring Connections website. Some are as long as 16 pages. Try to locate the unique features found in your state's directive.

1st Attempt	2nd Attempt	3rd Attempt	
_____	_____	_____	Gather materials (equipment and supplies) listed under *Conditions*.
_____	_____	_____	1. Turn on the computer and obtain an Internet connection. Go to the Caring Connections website: http://www.caringinfo.org/
_____	_____	_____	2. Click on "Download Your State Specific Advance Directive."
_____	_____	_____	3. Each state is listed. Click on your state.
_____	_____	_____	4. Print and read the advance directive.
_____	_____	_____	5. Now, look at the example in the *textbook* (Figure 3-17).
____/5	____/5	____/5	6. Write a one-page summary of your state's advance directive and list some of the choices given:

_____

_____

_____

_____

_____

_____

_____

_____

_____

_____

_____

JOB SKILL 3-7 (*continued*)

_____

_____

_____

_____

_____

_____ _____ _____   Complete within specified time.

___/12   ___/12   ___/12   **Total points earned** (To obtain a percentage score, divide the total points
earned by the number of points possible.)

Comments:

C H A P T E R **4**

The Art of Communication

STOP AND THINK CASE SCENARIOS

Refer to the end of Chapter 4 in the *textbook* for the following scenarios:
- Feedback
- Communication Challenges
- Socioeconomic Fairness
- Positive versus Negative Attitude

EXAM-STYLE REVIEW QUESTIONS

Refer to the end of Chapter 4 in the *textbook*.

ABBREVIATION AND SPELLING REVIEW

Read the patient's chart note and write the meanings for the abbreviations following the note. To decode any abbreviations you do not understand or that appear unfamiliar to you, refer to the list of abbreviations in Appendix B of this *Workbook*. Step-by-step directions for this exercise are found in Procedure 1-1 of Chapter 1 in the *textbook*. Medical terms in the chart note are italicized; study them for spelling. Use your medical dictionary to look up their definitions. Your instructor may give a spelling and definition test that includes these words and abbreviations.

Leslee Armstrong

32-year-old Cauc female came in for init visit CO chr pelvic pain, HA, and slt shortness of breath. No ALL. Performed H & P. PMH revealed FUO, PID and *chronic* UTI. Ordered lab work and M. Patient NYD. Pt to have re ch in approx 3 days. R/O STD.

Gerald Practon, MD
Gerald Practon, MD

Cauc	_____	PID	_____
Init	_____	UTI	_____
CO	_____	lab	_____
chr	_____	M	_____
HA	_____	NYD	_____
slt	_____	Pt	_____
ALL	_____	re ch	_____
H & P	_____	approx	_____
PMH	_____	R/O	_____
FUO	_____	STD	_____

Review Questions

Review the objectives, glossary, and chapter information before completing the following review questions.

1. Of all the professionals that make up a health care team, who has the most interaction with the patient?

   _____

2. Name the basic elements of the communication cycle.

   a. _____

   b. _____

   c. _____

   d. _____

   e. _____

3. List, in order of importance, the top three ways humans communicate messages.

   a. _____

   b. _____

   c. _____

4. Name four forms of communication, including the most productive.

   a. _____

   b. _____

   c. _____

   d. _____

5. When interviewing a patient, what is the key to obtaining accurate information and what should you avoid?

   a. key: _____

   b. avoid: _____

6. What is the number one reason for the failure of relationships? _____

7. When does trust begin to develop between the physician and the patient? _____

   _____

   _____

8. What is the term used when a patient refuses to follow the doctor's treatment plan? _____

_____

9. Describe defensive behavior._____

_____

_____

10. Name and briefly describe the five levels of needs according to Maslow's hierarchy theory.

a. _____

_____

b. _____

_____

c. _____

_____

d. _____

_____

e. _____

_____

11. How can the meaning of spoken words change? _____

_____

12. What is a "double message"? _____

_____

13. What is a "comfort zone" and why does it vary? _____

_____

14. Why do we all need to feel as if we are being listened to? _____

_____

15. What is the difference between active listening and reflective listening? _____

_____

16. When trying to encourage a patient to open up and talk, what type of feedback is recommended and

why? _____

_____

17. A silent pause may be used to:

a. _____

b. _____

c. _____

d. _____

e. _____

f. _____

g. _____

18. Why is a professional health care interpreter preferred over a family member when translation is needed?

_____

_____

_____

_____

19. Why is it important to keep an open mind when dealing with patients of varied ethnic backgrounds?

_____

_____

20. The following suggestions are made for patients with special needs. State the type of impairment that would match the recommendation listed.

   a. use verbal descriptions _____

   b. use simple words and short phrases, allowing plenty of time for the patient to digest what you have

      said _____

   c. eliminate background noises _____

   d. look directly at the patient when you are speaking _____

21. Name three of the "outward" signs of anxiety.

   a. _____

   b. _____

   c. _____

Critical Thinking Exercises

1. Name one or more common colloquialisms that may confuse a message. _____

_____

_____

2. Think about and describe one circumstance in which a person's body language did not match what he

   or she was saying. _____

_____

_____

3. The physician has asked you to convey the following message to a patient. Translate the message into layman's terms so it can be understood. Note: You may need to look up some terms in a medical dictionary. "*The patient's chronic diverticulosis has caused acute gastritis, which is resolving. The patient's cystitis and urethritis are unrelated and the ciprofloxacin will help clear that up.*"

_____

_____

_____

_____

_____

4. Convert the following "closed-ended" questions into "open-ended" questions or statements:

   a. Do you have pain? _____

   _____

   b. Does the pain feel worse at night? _____

   _____

   c. Did you take any medication to help with the pain? _____

   _____

   d. Is everything OK at home? _____

   _____

5. What are some environmental elements in your classroom that may interfere with active listening and communication? _____

   _____

6. Suggestions are listed in the *textbook* for how to deal with an angry patient. Can you think of a time when you were really angry and the person dealing with you:

   a. made the matter worse? Describe how. _____

   _____

   b. was able to help you dissipate your anger? Describe how. _____

   _____

7. In this chapter you read this powerful statement:

   > *In their research, psychologists have learned that the manner in which the medical staff interacts with a sick person can foster wellness or it can unintentionally aggravate a physical condition…that preserving the patient's mental state is often more important than performing expert medical skills.*

   What do you feel your responsibility is as a member of a health care team, and how does communication play a role in this?

   _____

   _____

   _____

   _____

   _____

   _____

8. Respond to the following situations:

   a. A patient, Mrs. Takuchi, stops at your desk on the way out, complaining that the physician wanted to give her an injection but she will not let anybody jab a needle into her and put something into her body. What would you say?

   _____

   _____

   _____

b. The clinical medical assistant, Susan Owens, complains that you did not order the supplies she had requested in time. What would your response be?

_____

_____

_____

JOB SKILL 4-1
Demonstrate Body Language

Name _____ Date _____ Score _____

Performance Objective

Task: Demonstrate positive and negative body language.

Conditions: Need:

    • Two or more persons

    • Props may be used

Standards: Complete all steps listed in this skill in _____ minutes with a minimum score of _____.
(Time element and accuracy criteria may be given by instructor.)

Time: **Start:** _____ **Completed:** _____ **Total:** _____ minutes

Scoring: One point for each step performed satisfactorily unless otherwise listed or weighted by
instructor.

Directions with Performance Evaluation Checklist

This exercise may be performed as a "role-playing" exercise by dividing the class into teams of two or more.
One person or team demonstrates the body language, and the other person or team guesses what feelings
the first is trying to display.

1st Attempt	2nd Attempt	3rd Attempt	
_____	_____	_____	Gather materials (equipment and supplies) listed under *Conditions*.
_____	_____	_____	1. Study the various types of body language described in the *textbook* under *Nonverbal Communication*.
___/10	___/10	___/10	2. Without speaking, use body language to convey the way you are feeling or may feel at times.
_____	_____	_____	Complete within specified time.
___/13	___/13	___/13	**Total points earned** (To obtain a percentage score, divide the total points earned by the number of points possible.)

Comments:

Evaluator's Signature: _____   **Need to Repeat:** _____

National Curriculum Competency: CAAHEP: Psychomotor: V.P.2; Affective: V.A.1   ABHES: 5.f

JOB SKILL 4-2
Use the Internet to Research Active Listening Skills and Write a Report

Name _____ Date _____ Score _____

Performance Objective

Task: Use the Internet to research active listening skills and write a short report.

Conditions: Need:

- Computer with Internet connection
- Printer and paper
- Pen or pencil

Refer to:

- *Textbook* section, *Active Listening*
- *Textbook* Procedure 4-1 for step-by-step directions

Standards: Complete all steps listed in this job skill in _____ minutes with a minimum score of _____.
(Time element and accuracy criteria may be given by instructor.)

Time: **Start:** _____ **Completed:** _____ **Total:** _____ minutes

Scoring: One point for each step performed satisfactorily unless otherwise listed or weighted by instructor.

Directions with Performance Evaluation Checklist

You will be writing a one-page essay on listening skills. Optional: This report may be presented orally, depending on instructor directions.

1st Attempt	2nd Attempt	3rd Attempt	
_____	_____	_____	Gather materials (equipment and supplies) listed under *Conditions*.
____/5	____/5	____/5	1. Read the *Active Listening* section in the *textbook* and Procedure 4-1 and note key points.
_____	_____	_____	2. Turn on the computer and obtain an Internet connection. Go to your favorite search engine (e.g., Google, GoodSearch, or Yahoo).
____/5	____/5	____/5	3. Key one of the following to begin your search: "Active Listening," "Effective Listening," "Good Listening Skills," or "Improving Listening Skills," and look for information or articles about listening.
____/5	____/5	____/5	4. Take notes on ways to improve your listening that are not already mentioned in the *textbook*.
____/10	____/10	____/10	5. Write a short one-page essay on listening skills and include five things that you are going to do to improve in this area.
_____	_____	_____	Complete within specified time.
____/28	____/28	____/28	**Total points earned** (To obtain a percentage score, divide the total points earned by the number of points possible.)

JOB SKILL 4-2 (*continued*)

Comments:

Evaluator's Signature: _____   **Need to Repeat:** _____

National Curriculum Competency: CAAHEP: Affective: V.A.1

INSTRUCTOR: Job Skills 4-3, 4-4, and 4-6 through 4-13 involve communication role-playing. Two or three students are needed to complete each job skill and you may want to assign one or more job skills to each group. Job Skill 4-12 (Communicate with a Patient and His or Her Family Members and Friends via Role-Playing) is the most comprehensive and if time were limited it would be the best choice to satisfy all of the CAAHEP or ABHES competencies.

JOB SKILL 4-3
Communicate with a Child via Role-Playing

Name _____ Date _____ Score _____

Performance Objective

Task:	Role-play to learn how to communicate with a child.
Conditions:	Need:
	• Three students who will role-play a communication scenario
	Refer to:
	• *Textbook* Procedure 4-2 for step-by-step directions
Standards:	Complete all steps listed in this job skill in _____ minutes with a minimum score of _____. (Time element and accuracy criteria may be given by instructor.)
Time:	**Start:** _____ **Completed:** _____ **Total:** _____ minutes
Scoring:	One point for each step performed satisfactorily unless otherwise listed or weighted by instructor.

Directions with Performance Evaluation Checklist

Scenario: A father comes into the office with Kara, his 6-year-old daughter. He says she has been pulling her left ear and complaining of pain. She appears bashful, is clinging to her father, and is crying softly. Role-play the communication between the administrative medical assistant, father, and child as you prepare her to be taken to the treatment room for the examination.

1st Attempt	2nd Attempt	3rd Attempt	
_____	_____	_____	Gather materials (equipment and supplies) listed under *Conditions*.
____/2	____/2	____/2	1. Position yourself at the child's eye level.
____/2	____/2	____/2	2. Talk at a level the child understands.
____/2	____/2	____/2	3. Speak with a soft, low-pitched voice, consoling the child.
____/2	____/2	____/2	4. Ask simple questions making sure they are understood.
____/2	____/2	____/2	5. Allow the child to be involved.
____/2	____/2	____/2	6. Offer a toy or prop to gain attention and cooperation.
____/2	____/2	____/2	7. Allow the child to express fear and cry.
____/2	____/2	____/2	8. Recognize that the child may be stressed and accept the child's behavior, showing sensitivity and empathy.
____/2	____/2	____/2	9. Encourage feedback making sure the message is understood.
_____	_____	_____	Complete within specified time.
____/20	____/20	____/20	**Total points earned** (To obtain a percentage score, divide the total points earned by the number of points possible.)

JOB SKILL 4-3 (*continued*)

Comments:

Evaluator's Signature: _____ **Need to Repeat:** _____

National Curriculum Competency: CAAHEP: Psychomotor: V.P.1, 5; Affective: V.A.3   ABHES: 5.f

JOB SKILL 4-4
Communicate with an Older Adult via Role-Playing

Name _____ Date _____ Score _____

Performance Objective

Task: Role-play to learn how to communicate with an older adult.

Conditions: Need:

• Three students who will role-play a communication scenario

Refer to:

• *Textbook* Procedure 4-3 for step-by-step directions

Standards: Complete all steps listed in this job skill in _____ minutes with a minimum score of _____. (Time element and accuracy criteria may be given by instructor.)

Time: Start: _____ Completed: _____ Total: _____ minutes

Scoring: One point for each step performed satisfactorily unless otherwise listed or weighted by instructor.

Directions with Performance Evaluation Checklist

Scenario: A 93-year-old man comes into the office with his daughter. She says he has urinary frequency. He seems a little confused and the daughter keeps trying to manipulate the conversation when the administrative medical assistant is attempting to talk to him. Role-play the communication between the administrative medical assistant, the older adult, and the daughter.

1st Attempt	2nd Attempt	3rd Attempt	
_____	_____	_____	Gather materials (equipment and supplies) listed under *Conditions*.
____/2	____/2	____/2	1. Approach the patient in a friendly manner and look directly at him while speaking; do not prejudge.
____/2	____/2	____/2	2. Speak clearly and slowly; offer simple explanations.
____/2	____/2	____/2	3. Form short sentences and ask brief questions.
____/2	____/2	____/2	4. Analyze communication and encourage responses and feedback.
____/2	____/2	____/2	5. Rephrase statements or questions as necessary.
____/2	____/2	____/2	6. React calmly if or when the patient seemed confused or forgetful.
____/2	____/2	____/2	7. Do not make excuses for the patient.
____/2	____/2	____/2	8. Tell the patient when you did not understand him; ask the patient to repeat what was said.
____/2	____/2	____/2	9. Be gentle but honest and truthful when communicating; do not mislead the patient.
____/2	____/2	____/2	10. Offer written instructions.
_____	_____	_____	Complete within specified time.
____/22	____/22	____/22	**Total points earned** (To obtain a percentage score, divide the total points earned by the number of points possible.)

JOB SKILL 4-4 (*continued*)

Comments:

Evaluator's Signature: _____ **Need to Repeat:** _____

National Curriculum Competency: CAAHEP: Psychomotor: V.P.1, 5; Affective: V.A.3   ABHES: 5.f

JOB SKILL 4-5
Name Unique Qualities of Other Cultures

Name _____ Date _____ Score _____

Performance Objective

Task: Research and discover unique qualities of other cultures in order to help you understand and
            serve patients in your geographical area; write a brief report

Conditions: Need:

            • This will vary according to region but could include library and Internet research or personal
              interviews

            Refer to:

            • *Textbook "Resources" at the end of Chapter 4*

Standards: Complete all steps listed in this skill in _____ minutes with a minimum score of _____.
            (Time element and accuracy criteria may be given by instructor.)

Time: **Start:** _____ **Completed:** _____ **Total:** _____ minutes

Scoring: One point for each step performed satisfactorily unless otherwise listed or weighted by
            instructor.

Directions with Performance Evaluation Checklist

1st Attempt	2nd Attempt	3rd Attempt	
_____	_____	_____	Gather materials (equipment and supplies) listed under *Conditions*.
_____	_____	_____	1. Determine which culture you will be researching and what method you will use to discover unique qualities. If you live in an area where there is little ethnic diversity, you may want to look at the migration statistics for your state.
_____	_____	_____	2. Determine which unique features would have an impact on communication.
_____	_____	_____	3. Determine which unique features would have an impact on the delivery of health care.
_____	_____	_____	4. Select one quality that you admire from a culture that is different from yours.
___/10	___/10	___/10	5. Write a one-page summary of unique qualities and be prepared to present it orally to your class.
_____	_____	_____	Complete within specified time.
___/16	___/16	___/16	**Total points earned** (To obtain a percentage score, divide the total points earned by the number of points possible.)

JOB SKILL 4-5 (*continued*)

Comments:

National Curriculum Competency: CAAHEP: Psychomotor: V.P.5; Affective: V.A.3, XI.A.3   ABHES: 3.i

JOB SKILL 4-6
Communicate with a Hearing-Impaired Patient via Role-Playing

Name _____ Date _____ Score _____

Performance Objective

Task: Role-play to learn how to communicate with a hearing-impaired patient.

Conditions: Need:

   • Two students who will role-play a communication scenario

   Refer to:

   • *Textbook* Procedure 4-4 for step-by-step directions

Standards: Complete all steps listed in this job skill in _____ minutes with a minimum score of _____.
   (Time element and accuracy criteria may be given by instructor.)

Time: **Start:** _____ **Completed:** _____ **Total:** _____ minutes

Scoring: One point for each step performed satisfactorily unless otherwise listed or weighted by
   instructor.

Directions with Performance Evaluation Checklist

Scenario: Mr. Osborn, a 60-year-old man, comes into the office with a large hearing device on his right ear. He is there for a physical examination, and it has been several years since his last appointment. You are responsible for obtaining a new history form and updating his registration information. Role-play the communication between the administrative medical assistant and the patient.

1st Attempt	2nd Attempt	3rd Attempt	
_____	_____	_____	Gather materials (equipment and supplies) listed under *Conditions*.
____/2	____/2	____/2	1. Select a quiet place to communicate, and give the patient your complete attention.
____/2	____/2	____/2	2. Eliminate distractions or background noises.
____/2	____/2	____/2	3. Choose a good seating arrangement, sitting on the side of the patient's good ear.
____/2	____/2	____/2	4. Face the patient in an area of good light.
____/2	____/2	____/2	5. Touch the patient lightly, as necessary, to gain his attention.
____/2	____/2	____/2	6. Speak in a natural tone, slowly, and distinctly, enunciate clearly, and use a low-pitched voice.
____/2	____/2	____/2	7. Use short, simple sentences and repeat or rephrase as necessary.
____/2	____/2	____/2	8. Use gestures as needed.
____/2	____/2	____/2	9. Write down words or phrases that you have difficulty communicating.
____/2	____/2	____/2	10. Practice active listening techniques and get feedback by asking questions to verify understanding.
_____	_____	_____	Complete within specified time.
____/22	____/22	____/22	**Total points earned** (To obtain a percentage score, divide the total points earned by the number of points possible.)

JOB SKILL 4-6 (*continued*)

Comments:

Evaluator's Signature: _____   **Need to Repeat:** _____

National Curriculum Competency: CAAHEP: Cognitive: V.C.3; Psychomotor: V.P.5; Affective: V.A.3	ABHES: 5.f

JOB SKILL 4-7
Communicate with a Visually Impaired Patient via Role-Playing

Name _____ Date _____ Score _____

Performance Objective

Task: Role-play to learn how to communicate with a visually impaired patient.

Conditions: Need:

                 • Two students who will role-play a communication scenario

                 Refer to:

                 • *Textbook* Procedure 4-5 for step-by-step directions

Standards: Complete all steps listed in this job skill in _____ minutes with a minimum score of _____.
                 (Time element and accuracy criteria may be given by instructor.)

Time: **Start:** _____ **Completed:** _____ **Total:** _____ minutes

Scoring: One point for each step performed satisfactorily unless otherwise listed or weighted by
                 instructor.

Directions with Performance Evaluation Checklist

Scenario: Mrs. Gretna, a 50-year-old legally blind patient, comes into the office to have her back checked. She is complaining of lumbar pain. The physician has asked you to escort Mrs. Gretna to his office where he would like to obtain information before the clinical medical assistant escorts her into an examination room. Role-play the communication between the administrative medical assistant and the patient.

1st Attempt	2nd Attempt	3rd Attempt	
_____	_____	_____	Gather materials (equipment and supplies) listed under *Conditions*.
____/2	____/2	____/2	1. Approach the patient cheerfully and identify yourself by name.
____/2	____/2	____/2	2. Look directly at the patient, greet her by name and speak clearly in a normal tone and speed.
____/2	____/2	____/2	3. Inform the patient of others who are in the same room or area.
____/2	____/2	____/2	4. Let the patient know exactly what you will be doing.
____/2	____/2	____/2	5. Ask the patient if you could take her hand to show her the surroundings.
____/2	____/2	____/2	6. Escort the patient to the physician's office, look for obstacles along the way, and provide verbal cues.
____/2	____/2	____/2	7. Inform the patient of the location and tell her when you leave the room; knock before reentering, even if the door was left open.
____/2	____/2	____/2	8. Explain the sounds of unusual noises and office machines.
____/2	____/2	____/2	9. Use large-print material when available.
_____	_____	_____	Complete within specified time.
____/20	____/20	____/20	**Total points earned** (To obtain a percentage score, divide the total points earned by the number of points possible.)

JOB SKILL 4-7 (*continued*)

Comments:

Evaluator's Signature: _____ **Need to Repeat:** _____

National Curriculum Competency: CAAHEP: Cognitive: V.C.3; Psychomotor: V.P.5; Affective: V.A.3	ABHES: 5.f

JOB SKILL 4-8
Communicate with a Speech-Impaired Patient via Role-Playing

Name _____ Date _____ Score _____

Performance Objective

Task:	Role-play to learn how to communicate with a speech-impaired patient.
Conditions:	Need:
	• Two or three students who will role-play a communication scenario
	Refer to:
	• *Textbook* Procedure 4-6 for step-by-step directions
Standards:	Complete all steps listed in this job skill in _____ minutes with a minimum score of _____. (Time element and accuracy criteria may be given by instructor.)
Time:	**Start:** _____ **Completed:** _____ **Total:** _____ minutes
Scoring:	One point for each step performed satisfactorily unless otherwise listed or weighted by instructor.

Directions with Performance Evaluation Checklist

Scenario: Michelle Kunup, a 40-year-old woman, comes into the office to see the neurologist for a consultation and is escorted by her husband. She has just had a major stroke and was released from the hospital last week. She is walking fine and has full use of her arms and so forth but her speech has been affected. Role-play the communication between the administrative medical assistant and the patient.

1st Attempt	2nd Attempt	3rd Attempt	
_____	_____	_____	Gather materials (equipment and supplies) listed under *Conditions*.
____/2	____/2	____/2	1. Look directly at the patient without making her feel self-conscious.
____/2	____/2	____/2	2. Allow the patient time to think through what she is going to say; give her time to speak.
____/2	____/2	____/2	3. Do not speak for the patient or rush the conversation.
____/2	____/2	____/2	4. Do not pretend to understand; ask her to repeat as necessary.
____/2	____/2	____/2	5. Act in a courteous manner and do not shout; show sensitivity.
____/2	____/2	____/2	6. Offer a notepad as necessary.
_____	_____	_____	Complete within specified time.
____/14	____/14	____/14	**Total points earned** (To obtain a percentage score, divide the total points earned by the number of points possible.)

JOB SKILL 4-8 (*continued*)

Comments:

Evaluator's Signature: _____   **Need to Repeat:** _____

National Curriculum Competency: CAAHEP: Cognitive: V.C.3; Psychomotor; V.P.5 Affective: V.A.3   ABHES: 5.f

JOB SKILL 4-9
Communicate with a Patient Who Has an Impaired Level of Understanding via Role-Playing

Name _____ Date _____ Score _____

Performance Objective

Task: Role-play to learn how to communicate with a patient who has an impaired level of understanding.

Conditions: Need:
- Three students who will role-play a communication scenario

Refer to:
- *Textbook* Procedure 4-7 for step-by-step directions

Standards: Complete all steps listed in this job skill in _____ minutes with a minimum score of _____. (Time element and accuracy criteria may be given by instructor.)

Time: Start: _____ Completed: _____ Total: _____ minutes

Scoring: One point for each step performed satisfactorily unless otherwise listed or weighted by instructor.

Directions with Performance Evaluation Checklist

Scenario: Pricilla Longfellow, a 30-year-old woman, comes into Dr. Fran Practon's office with her mother. She is having an ingrown toenail looked at today to see if surgery is needed. She has experienced traumatic brain injury from an automobile accident that occurred when she was 18 years old. She has difficulty speaking and has a level of understanding somewhere between that of a 5- and a 7-year-old. You will be greeting her at the reception desk and collecting a copayment. The patient is emphatic about wanting to see the physician herself and tells her mother, "I can do it by myself, I don't need you." Role-play the communication between the administrative medical assistant, the patient, and her mother.

1st Attempt	2nd Attempt	3rd Attempt	
_____	_____	_____	Gather materials (equipment and supplies) listed under *Conditions*.
____/2	____/2	____/2	1. Greet the patient warmly; address the patient by name.
____/2	____/2	____/2	2. Act professionally and keep the conversation focused.
____/2	____/2	____/2	3. Speak slowly and in a calm manner.
____/2	____/2	____/2	4. Select simple words and short phrases.
____/2	____/2	____/2	5. Use verbal and nonverbal cues.
____/2	____/2	____/2	6. Use tone of voice to express concern; do not raise your voice.
____/2	____/2	____/2	7. Repeat and rephrase the message as necessary.
____/2	____/2	____/2	8. Use demonstration when appropriate to reinforce the message.
____/2	____/2	____/2	9. Allow more time than usual.
____/2	____/2	____/2	10. Reassure the patient and do not overload her with information.
____/2	____/2	____/2	11. Inform the patient of what to expect prior to it happening.
____/2	____/2	____/2	12. Exhibit tolerance and sensitivity; do not force answers.
____/2	____/2	____/2	13. Remind the patient why she is at the physician's office; orient her to reality.

JOB SKILL 4-9 (*continued*)

_____ _____ _____   Complete within specified time.

___/28 ___/28 ___/28   **Total points earned** (To obtain a percentage score, divide the total points
earned by the number of points possible.)

Comments:

Evaluator's Signature: _____ **Need to Repeat:** _____

National Curriculum Competency: CAAHEP: Cognitive: V.C.3; Psychomotor: V.P.5; Affective: V.A.3	ABHES: 5.f

JOB SKILL 4-10
Communicate with an Anxious Patient via Role-Playing

Name _____ Date _____ Score _____

Performance Objective

Task: Role-play to learn how to communicate with an anxious patient.

Conditions: Need:

              • Two students who will role-play a communication scenario

              Refer to:

              • *Textbook* Procedure 4-8 for step-by-step directions

Standards: Complete all steps listed in this job skill in _____ minutes with a minimum score of _____.
              (Time element and accuracy criteria may be given by instructor.)

Time: **Start:** _____ **Completed:** _____ **Total:** _____ minutes

Scoring: One point for each step performed satisfactorily unless otherwise listed or weighted by
              instructor.

Directions with Performance Evaluation Checklist

Scenario: Jessica McMullin, a 20-year-old woman, presents as a new patient. She looks frightened and is shaking when she fills out the paperwork. You later find out that she has a lump in her breast, and her aunt died of breast cancer. Role-play the communication between the administrative medical assistant and the patient.

1st Attempt	2nd Attempt	3rd Attempt	
_____	_____	_____	Gather materials (equipment and supplies) listed under *Conditions*.
____/2	____/2	____/2	1. Recognize the signs of anxiety and acknowledge them.
____/2	____/2	____/2	2. Pinpoint possible sources of anxiety.
____/2	____/2	____/2	3. Make the patient feel as comfortable as possible.
____/2	____/2	____/2	4. Give the patient personal space.
____/2	____/2	____/2	5. Demonstrate a warm and caring attitude.
____/2	____/2	____/2	6. Speak with confidence and calmness; ask the patient to describe what is causing her anxiety. Allow her to describe her feelings and thoughts.
____/2	____/2	____/2	7. Listen attentively without interruption.
____/2	____/2	____/2	8. Maintain eye contact and keep an open posture.
____/2	____/2	____/2	9. Accept the patient's thoughts and feelings; demonstrate empathy.
____/2	____/2	____/2	10. Help the patient recognize the anxiety and cope with it by providing information and suggesting relaxation techniques.
_____	_____	_____	Complete within specified time.
____/22	____/22	____/22	**Total points earned** (To obtain a percentage score, divide the total points earned by the number of points possible.)

JOB SKILL 4-10 (*continued*)

Comments:

_____

_____

Evaluator's Signature: _____ **Need to Repeat:** _____

National Curriculum Competency: CAAHEP: Cognitive: V.C.3; Psychomotor: V.P.5; Affective: V.A.1   ABHES: 5.f

JOB SKILL 4-11
Communicate with an Angry Patient via Role-Playing

Name _____ Date _____ Score _____

Performance Objective

Task: Role-play to learn how to communicate with an angry patient.

Conditions: Need:

 • Two students who will role-play a communication scenario

 Refer to:

 • *Textbook* Procedure 4-9 for step-by-step directions

Standards: Complete all steps listed in this job skill in _____ minutes with a minimum score of _____. (Time element and accuracy criteria may be given by instructor.)

Time: Start: _____ Completed: _____ Total: _____ minutes

Scoring: One point for each step performed satisfactorily unless otherwise listed or weighted by instructor.

Directions with Performance Evaluation Checklist

Scenario: Mr. Murray VanNelson, a retired male patient, comes into the office and checks in at the window. He seems agitated and sits down in a full waiting room and stares at the receptionist with a nasty look on his face. It is almost as if steam is coming out of his ears. You later find out that he is mad because he feels he always has to wait for the doctor and no one respects the time he takes out of his day each time an appointment is necessary. Role-play the communication between the administrative medical assistant and the patient.

1st Attempt	2nd Attempt	3rd Attempt	
_____	_____	_____	Gather materials (equipment and supplies) listed under *Conditions*.
____/2	____/2	____/2	1. Recognize that the patient is angry; do not ignore him.
____/2	____/2	____/2	2. Honor the patient's personal space.
____/2	____/2	____/2	3. Keep an open posture, maintain eye contact, and position yourself at the patient's eye level.
____/2	____/2	____/2	4. Remain calm showing that you care about his feelings; demonstrate positive body language and respect.
____/2	____/2	____/2	5. Focus on why the patient is there.
____/2	____/2	____/2	6. Listen attentively with an open mind and ask the patient to describe the cause of his anger and how it makes him feel. Let him vent openly.
____/2	____/2	____/2	7. Do not take a defensive attitude or try to talk the patient out of being angry.
____/2	____/2	____/2	8. Allow the patient time alone.
____/2	____/2	____/2	9. Determine a time frame to get back to the patient with a solution.
_____	_____	_____	Complete within specified time.
____/20	____/20	____/20	**Total points earned** (To obtain a percentage score, divide the total points earned by the number of points possible.)

JOB SKILL 4-11 (*continued*)

Comments:

Evaluator's Signature: _____ **Need to Repeat:** _____

National Curriculum Competency: CAAHEP: Cognitive: V.C.3; Psychomotor: V.P.5; Affective: V.A.1   ABHES: 5.f

JOB SKILL 4-12
Communicate with a Patient and His or Her Family Members and Friends via Role-Playing

Name _____ Date _____ Score _____

Performance Objective

Task: Role-play to learn how to communicate with a patient and his or her family and friends.

Conditions: Need:

              • Two students who will role-play a communication scenario

              Refer to:

              • *Textbook* Procedure 4-10 for step-by-step directions

Standards: Complete all steps listed in this job skill in _____ minutes with a minimum score of _____.
              (Time element and accuracy criteria may be given by instructor.)

Time: Start: _____ Completed: _____ Total: _____ minutes

Scoring: One point for each step performed satisfactorily unless otherwise listed or weighted by
              instructor.

Directions with Performance Evaluation Checklist

Scenario: You are an administrative medial assistant and the office manager has asked you to speak to Mrs. Madelyn Wilson when she comes in today about charges that were denied by Medicare. She just moved into the area in March 2016 and had a 24-hour Holter monitor put on in your office on April 2, 2016. The results were positive, showing that the patient goes in and out of a bigeminal rhythm. However, she had this same service done in January 2016 by a physician where she used to live; the results were negative. Medicare pays for one Holter monitor every 6 months. When she received these services you had her sign an Advance Beneficiary Notice (ABN) and advised her that Medicare might not pay for the services. You can legally bill her and expect to receive payment; however, you have done so and she has not paid. It is June 10, 2016.

After your conversation, she pays the bill in full. Optional: You may role-play a family member or friend who is accompanying the patient to the office to expand this exercise (*three students will be needed*).

1st Attempt	2nd Attempt	3rd Attempt	
_____	_____	_____	Gather materials (equipment and supplies) listed under *Conditions*.
____/2	____/2	____/2	1. Pay attention to your personal appearance, knowing that it will affect the patient's responses.
____/2	____/2	____/2	2. Warmly greet the patient and offer her a seat in a private, comfortable area.
____/2	____/2	____/2	3. Introduce yourself and explain why you would like to have a conversation with her.
____/2	____/2	____/2	4. Use a genuine approach and respect her comfort zone.
____/2	____/2	____/2	5. Display a positive attitude and focus on the patient with your undivided attention.
____/2	____/2	____/2	6. Demonstrate confidence while communicating accurately and succinctly.
____/2	____/2	____/2	7. Display sensitivity and empathy while putting the patient at ease and acknowledging any sources of anxiety.
____/2	____/2	____/2	8. Listen carefully to comments and allow time for questions.
____/2	____/2	____/2	9. Answer questions honestly.

JOB SKILL 4-12 (*continued*)

___/2	___/2	___/2	10.	Obtain feedback so you are sure that the message has been received correctly.
___/2	___/2	___/2	11.	Offer support and guidance; reward the patient's compliance with praise.
_____	_____	_____		Complete within specified time.
___/24	___/24	___/24		**Total points earned** (To obtain a percentage score, divide the total points earned by the number of points possible.)

Comments:

___

Evaluator's Signature: _____   **Need to Repeat:** _____

National Curriculum Competency: CAAHEP: Psychomotor: IV.P.5; Affective: V.A.1, 3	ABHES: 5.f

JOB SKILL 4-13

Communicate with a Coworker on the Health Care Team via Role-Playing

Name _____ Date _____ Score _____

Performance Objective

Task: Role-play to learn how to communicate with a coworker on the health care team.

Conditions: Need:

• Two students who will role-play a communication scenario

Refer to:

• *Textbook* Procedure 4-11 for step-by-step directions

Standards: Complete all steps listed in this job skill in _____ minutes with a minimum score of _____. (Time element and accuracy criteria may be given by instructor.)

Time: Start: _____ Completed: _____ Total: _____ minutes

Scoring: One point for each step performed satisfactorily unless otherwise listed or weighted by instructor.

Directions with Performance Evaluation Checklist

Scenario: You are the receptionist and have just opened the office and switched all calls from the answering service. Patients have been waiting at the door and now come into the office wanting to check in. Sheryl, a coworker, is trying to tell you about her weekend, but you do not have time to listen to her. How can you respond without hurting her feelings and be able to give your full attention to your job? Role-play the communication between the administrative medical assistant and the coworker.

1st Attempt	2nd Attempt	3rd Attempt	
_____	_____	_____	Gather materials (equipment and supplies) listed under *Conditions*.
____/2	____/2	____/2	1. Be polite and cheerful, use a friendly approach.
____/2	____/2	____/2	2. Use correct names and titles.
____/2	____/2	____/2	3. Use tack and diplomacy when attempting to resolve the problem.
____/2	____/2	____/2	4. Speak calmly and respectfully; do not become angry or defensive.
____/2	____/2	____/2	5. Use proper channels of communication. Try to work out the problem.
____/2	____/2	____/2	6. Do not judge; instead practice empathy.
____/2	____/2	____/2	7. Have a positive attitude.
____/2	____/2	____/2	8. Bring the issue that bothered you to the forefront.
____/2	____/2	____/2	9. Perform all your duties and responsibilities cheerfully.
____/2	____/2	____/2	10. Avoid gossip, arguments, and uncomplimentary statements.
____/2	____/2	____/2	11. Do not complain; instead be a problem solver.
_____	_____	_____	Complete within specified time.
____/24	____/24	____/24	**Total points earned** (To obtain a percentage score, divide the total points earned by the number of points possible.)

JOB SKILL 4-13 (*continued*)

Comments:

National Curriculum Competency: CAAHEP: Psychomotor: V.P.5; Affective: V.A.1   ABHES: 5.f

Receptionist and the Medical Office Environment

STOP AND THINK CASE SCENARIOS

Refer to the end of Chapter 5 in the *textbook* for the following scenarios:
- Privacy Protection
- First Impression
- HIPAA Violation versus Incidental Disclosure
- Signs, Symbols, and Labels

EXAM-STYLE REVIEW QUESTIONS

Refer to the end of Chapter 5 in the *textbook*.

Abbreviation and Spelling Review

Read the patients' chart notes and write the meanings for the abbreviations following the note. To decode any abbreviations you do not understand or that appear unfamiliar to you, refer to the list of abbreviations in Appendix B of this *Workbook*. Step-by-step directions for this exercise are found in Procedure 1-1 of Chapter 1 in the *textbook*. Medical terms in the chart note are italicized; study them for spelling. Use your medical dictionary to look up their definitions. Your instructor may give a spelling and definition test that includes these words and abbreviations.

DATE	PROGRESS
10/1/20XX	**Maria D. Gomez**, well-developed Hispanic ♀ fell on sharp object at 9 a.m. *Laceration* of L lower lip 0.5 cm. Tr.: cleaned, *sutured*, & drained. DTaP inj. Retn in 5 days.
	Fran Practon, MD
	Fran Practon, MD

♀ _____   Tr. _____

a.m. _____   DTaP _____

L _____   inj. _____

cm _____   Retn _____

DATE	PROGRESS
10/1/20XX	**Barry K. Wesson** This white ♂ had severe pain Ⓛ sternoclavicular area. Chest clear to P&A, EKG, ō. AP&L chest XR-N. Demerol 75mg for pain Dx neuralgia.
	Fran Practon, MD
	Fran Practon, MD

♂ _____   AP&L _____

Ⓛ _____   XR _____

P&A _____   N _____

EKG _____   mg _____

ō _____   Dx _____

Review Questions

Review the objectives, glossary, and chapter information before completing the following review questions.

1. Why are first impressions so important in a medical setting? _____

    _____

2. What benefits are attained by patients and the physician when the receptionist is attentive to the

    patients' needs? _____

    _____

3. Name several things that are necessary for a person to be successful when performing multiple tasks.

    a. _____

    b. _____

    c. _____

    d. _____

4. If you are asked in the evening to pull the records of all patients who will be seen the following day, in

    what order should they be organized? _____

    _____

    _____

5. What should you check for in each medical record, or chart, to be sure it is complete and ready for the physician prior to the patient's arrival? _____

_____

_____

6. What safeguard can be taken against the mispronunciation of a patient's name? _____

_____

_____

7. When greeting patients, what is the easiest way to customize requests and comments to prevent sounding like a broken record? _____

_____

8. Is calling out a patient's name who is seated in the reception area a violation of HIPAA? Why or why not? _____

_____

_____

9. When addressing patients, when should surnames be used? _____

_____

_____

10. List alternatives to using a standard patient sign-in log so patient names and "reason for visit" are not viewed by others.

    a. _____

    b. _____

    c. _____

    d. _____

    e. _____

11. What is the leading nonviolent crime in the United States?

    a. burglary

    b. drug violations

    c. car theft

    d. identity theft

    e. embezzlement

12. The "Red Flags Rule" offers:

    a. a disaster preparedness plan mandated.

    b. guidelines for a written prevention and detection program for identity theft.

    c. fire alert symbols.

    d. hazard warning labels.

    e. rules for medical offices regarding patients with disabilities.

13. List typical ways patients can be registered or preregistered in a medical office.

    a. _____

    b. _____

    c. _____

    d. _____

14. Does a primary care physician with a managed care plan need an authorization prior to seeing a new patient? _____

15. What steps need to be taken before releasing PHI to a patient's family member? _____

    _____

    _____

16. You are the receptionist and have just found out the doctor will be an hour late. Name three options that can be given to waiting patients.

    a. _____

    b. _____

    c. _____

17. List six special considerations that the office staff can provide a disabled or geriatric patient.

    a. _____

    b. _____

    c. _____

    d. _____

    e. _____

    f. _____

18. List five community resources that can be of value to patients. Note: These need not be on the list from the *textbook*.

    a. _____

    b. _____

    c. _____

    d. _____

    e. _____

19. If your office has an open reception area, what are the three things you need to take into consideration on a daily basis to protect patient confidentiality?

    a. _____

    b. _____

    c. _____

20. When you visit a physician's office, what are some things that favorably impress you in the reception area?

_____

_____

_____

_____

_____

21. Write the "general duty" clause from the Occupational Safety and Health Act, which is the basis of compliance mandated by OSHA. _____

_____

_____

_____

_____

22. True or False. PPE shall be provided by the employer at no cost to the employee. _____

23. Define the term *ergonomics*: _____

_____

_____

24. Medical offices may be the target of theft because of _____

_____; therefore, the medical assistant needs to be aware of how to help keep the office secure.

25. What are the three common causes of major injury in the workplace? _____

_____

_____

26. List 10 electrical-related items, areas, or situations to check to prevent an electrical fire and keep from receiving an electrical burn or shock.

a. _____

b. _____

c. _____

d. _____

e. _____

f. _____

g. _____

h. _____

i. _____

j. _____

27. Three sources needed to start a fire are _____, _____, and _____.

28. When starting a fire, common sources of ignition are:

    a. electrical equipment and machinery.

    b. hot surfaces.

    c. matches and open flames.

    d. smoking.

    e. all of the above.

29. Explain what Material Safety Data Sheets are and their use in the medical office. _____
    _____
    _____
    _____

30. State what the acronym RACER stands for.

    R. _____

    A. _____

    C. _____

    E. _____

    R. _____

31. Name the type of fire extinguisher listed and the type of burning material it is used on.

    a. Class A: _____ Used on: _____

    b. Class B: _____ Used on: _____

    c. Class C: _____ Used on: _____

    d. Class D: _____ Used on: _____

32. Define *disaster response plan*: _____
    _____
    _____
    _____

33. Name the four colors used on a hazardous material label and state what type of hazard the color represents.

    a. Color: _____ Represents: _____

    b. Color: _____ Represents: _____

    c. Color: _____ Represents: _____

    d. Color: _____ Represents: _____

34. The medical receptionist needs to maintain a _____ attitude, react _____, and

    follow _____

    in a situation that demands immediate attention, such as an office medical emergency.

Critical Thinking Exercises

Study the office situations. Use critical thinking skills, tact, and consideration to determine and record your responses. Indicate the situations you have difficulty handling by circling the corresponding numbers in red and bringing them to class for discussion.

1. An impatient Mr. Griffin complains about being kept waiting. How would you respond? _____

   _____

   _____

   _____

   _____

   _____

2. A patient, Mr. Avery, invites you to have lunch with him. What would you do? _____

   _____

   _____

   _____

   _____

   _____

   _____

   _____

3. Despite a "No Smoking" sign, a patient in the waiting room, Mrs. Wilson, lights a cigarette. What would

   you do or say? _____

   _____

   _____

   _____

   _____

   _____

   _____

4. An overtalkative patient, Mrs. Crowe, is bothering you while you are trying to complete a number of

   tasks before the next patient arrives. What would you do? _____

   _____

   _____

   _____

   _____

   _____

   _____

5. A patient, Mr. Mendez, comes into the reception room, arrives at your desk or window, and asks your advice about some medication he has seen advertised. What would be your response? _____

_____

_____

_____

_____

6. A patient, Mrs. Jeffers, asks you when she will be through with her treatment. She has just finished seeing the physician and comes to your desk to make her return appointment. What would be your response?

_____

_____

_____

_____

_____

_____

_____

7. Mrs. Jones comes up to your desk and asks you if you think cigarette smoking is harmful. What would you say? _____

_____

_____

_____

8. A friend of yours stops in to see you at the office and wants to "visit." She remains at your desk for 15 minutes talking. The reception room is full of patients. What would you say? _____

_____

_____

_____

_____

_____

9. Mr. Carson, a blind patient, comes to your office for medical care. How would you handle this patient during his visit? _____

_____

_____

_____

_____

_____

10. A patient, Mrs. Jesse Bacon, has just had an appointment and thinks that the physician is withholding information from her. She stops by your desk and inquires, "What do you think the chances are of my returning to work on Monday?" How would you respond? _____

_____

_____

_____

_____

_____

11. An elderly female patient, accompanied by her husband, has arrived for an emergency appointment. She seems to be in pain and is barely able to walk. What should be your immediate response? _____

_____

_____

_____

_____

_____

_____

JOB SKILL 5-1
Prepare a Patient Registration Form

Name _____ Date _____ Score _____

Performance Objective

Task: Become familiar with questions on a patient registration form.

Conditions: Need:

- Computer with Internet connection
- Online Form 2 (Patient Registration Information) located at www.cengagebrain.com with student resources
- Pen

Refer to:

- *Textbook* Figure 5-5 for an illustration
- *Textbook* Procedure 5-2 for step-by-step directions

Standards: Complete all steps listed in this skill in _____ minutes with a minimum score of _____.
(Time element and accuracy criteria may be given by instructor.)

Time: Start: _____ Completed: _____ Total: _____ minutes

Scoring: One point for each step performed satisfactorily unless otherwise listed or weighted by instructor.

Directions with Performance Evaluation Checklist

Ask a classmate, friend, or family member to write the information requested on the form as one would when visiting a medical office for the first time. Ask for an insurance card and photocopy it if possible. Proofread the form after completion and make corrections or additions to verify that all information is complete. Keep the information secure and confidential.

1st Attempt	2nd Attempt	3rd Attempt	
_____	_____	_____	Gather materials (equipment and supplies) listed under *Conditions*.
_____	_____	_____	1. Select a classmate, friend, or family member to interview.
____/2	____/2	____/2	2. Direct the person to fill out all areas on the Patient Registration form and put NA (not applicable) in areas that do not apply.
_____	_____	_____	3. Obtain and photocopy insurance card(s) for the file (if possible).
_____	_____	_____	4. Proofread the form for legibility.
____/7	____/7	____/7	5. Verify that the header information (date, account number, insurance number, copayment, work injury, auto accident, and date of injury) at the top of the form was completed.
____/20	____/20	____/20	6. Verify that the patient's personal information section is completed and all nonapplicable blanks are marked NA.
____/20	____/20	____/20	7. Verify that the patient's responsible party information section is completed and all nonapplicable blanks are marked NA.
____/20	____/20	____/20	8. Verify that the patient's insurance information section is completed and all nonapplicable blanks are marked NA.
____/3	____/3	____/3	9. Verify that the patient's referral information section is completed and all nonapplicable blanks are marked NA.

JOB SKILL 5-1 (*continued*)

_____/5 _____/5 _____/5   10. Verify that the emergency contact section is completed and all nonapplicable blanks are marked NA.

_____/4 _____/4 _____/4   11. Verify that the assignment of benefits name is filled in, the financial agreement is dated and signed, and method of payment is indicated.

_____ _____ _____   12. Keep the information secure and confidential.

_____ _____ _____   Complete within specified time.

_____/86 _____/86 _____/86   **Total points earned** (To obtain a percentage score, divide the total points earned by the number of points possible.)

Comments:

Evaluator's Signature: _____ **Need to Repeat:** _____

National Curriculum Competency: CAAHEP: Cognitive: VI.C.3, 4; Psychomotor: VI.P.3; Affective: X.A.1, 2

JOB SKILL 5-2
Prepare an Application Form for a Disabled Person Placard

Name _____ Date _____ Score _____

Performance Objective

Task: 1. Ask a student, family member, or friend to complete an application form for a disabled person placard, making up a medical condition that is either permanent or temporary; review and verify its completion.

             2. Complete the physician portion for physician review and signature.

Conditions: Need:

- Computer with Internet connection
- Online Form 3 (Disabled Person Parking Placard Application) located at www.cengagebrain.com with student resources
- *Workbook* (Appendix A), Medical Practice Reference Material
- Pen

Refer to:

- *Textbook* Figure 5-8 for an illustration
- *Textbook* Procedure 5-3 for step-by-step directions

Standards: Complete all steps listed in this skill in _____ minutes with a minimum score of _____.
(Time element and accuracy criteria may be given by instructor.)

Time: **Start:** _____ **Completed:** _____ **Total:** _____ minutes

Scoring: One point for each step performed satisfactorily unless otherwise listed or weighted by instructor.

Directions with Performance Evaluation Checklist

1st Attempt	2nd Attempt	3rd Attempt	
_____	_____	_____	Gather materials (equipment and supplies) listed under *Conditions*.
_____	_____	_____	1. Check to see that the correct box was marked at the top of the form.
___/10	___/10	___/10	2. Complete the applicant's information.
___/2	___/2	___/2	3. Verify that the applicant signed and dated the form.
_____	_____	_____	4. Indicate the reason the patient is applying (1 through 7).
_____	_____	_____	5. Complete the type of disability (temporary, moderate, or permanent).
___/7	___/7	___/7	6. Complete the physician's information.
_____	_____	_____	7. Proofread the document before physician review and signature.
_____	_____	_____	Complete within specified time.
___/25	___/25	___/25	**Total points earned** (To obtain a percentage score, divide the total points earned by the number of points possible.)

Comments:

Evaluator's Signature: _____ **Need to Repeat:** _____

> National Curriculum Competency: CAAHEP: Cognitive: V.C.6

JOB SKILL 5-3
Research Community Resources for Patient Referrals and Patient Education

Name _____ Date _____ Score _____

Performance Objective

Task: Use the Internet to research and determine what materials are available for patient referrals or patient education; order sample items to share with the class and determine how you would direct or navigate patients to resource material.

Conditions: Need:

- Computer with Internet connection
- Printer and paper

Refer to:

- *Textbook* Procedures 5-4 and 5-5 for step-by-step directions

Standards: Complete all steps listed in this skill in _____ minutes with a minimum score of _____. (Time element and accuracy criteria may be given by instructor.)

Time: **Start:** _____ **Completed:** _____ **Total:** _____ minutes

Scoring: One point for each step performed satisfactorily unless otherwise listed or weighted by instructor.

Directions with Performance Evaluation Checklist

1st Attempt	2nd Attempt	3rd Attempt	
_____	_____	_____	Gather materials (equipment and supplies) listed under *Conditions*.
____/2	____/2	____/2	1. Read the resources list at the end of the chapter in the *textbook*.
____/2	____/2	____/2	2. Determine if you would like to research community resources for office referrals or patient education and select a specific topic.
____/6	____/6	____/6	3. Look up the appropriate topic on the Internet and determine what resources are available.
____/1	____/1	____/1	4. Request a sample of the item(s) selected.
____/2	____/2	____/2	5. Determine how you would navigate patients to community resources and encourage or coach them to take advantage of the materials. _____
			_____
			_____
			_____
_____	_____	_____	Complete within specified time.
___/15	___/15	___/15	**Total points earned** (To obtain a percentage score, divide the total points earned by the number of points possible.)

Comments:

Evaluator's Signature: _____ **Need to Repeat:** _____

National Curriculum Competency: CAAHEP: Cognitive: V.C.6; Psychomotor: V.P.9, 10

JOB SKILL 5-4
Assess and Use Proper Body Mechanics

Name _____ Date _____ Score _____

Performance Objective

Task: List body positions used on the job or in a school setting (i.e., sitting, standing, bending, stooping, and lifting) and any repetitive motions used (e.g., computer work). Then assess yourself, naming areas that need changing to comply with ergonomic standards.

Conditions: Need:
- Work or school environment
- Computer with printer
- Paper, pen or pencil

Refer to:
- *Textbook* section, "Ergonomics"
- *Textbook* Procedure 5-6 for step-by-step directions
- *Textbook* Figure 5-13 through Figure 5-16 for visual examples

Standards: Complete all steps listed in this skill in _____ minutes with a minimum score of _____. (Time element and accuracy criteria may be given by instructor.)

Time: Start: _____ Completed: _____ Total: _____ minutes

Scoring: One point for each step performed satisfactorily unless otherwise listed or weighted by instructor.

Directions with Performance Evaluation Checklist

1st Attempt	2nd Attempt	3rd Attempt	
_____	_____	_____	Gather materials (equipment and supplies) listed under *Conditions*.
____/3	____/3	____/3	1. Mentally walk yourself through a work or school day and list all the body positions used.
			_____
			_____
____/5	____/5	____/5	2. Name any repetitive motions you perform.
			_____
____/5	____/5	____/5	3. Compare the information with the ergonomic standards mentioned or shown in the *textbook*.
____/5	____/5	____/5	4. List areas you need to change to comply with ergonomic standards.
			_____
			_____
			_____

JOB SKILL 5-4 (*continued*)

___/3   ___/3   ___/3   5. Determine goals for improving these areas and list ways to remind yourself
of ergonomic standards.

_____

_____

_____

_____   _____   _____   Complete within specified time.

___/23   ___/23   ___/23   **Total points earned** (To obtain a percentage score, divide the total points
earned by the number of points possible.)

Comments:

Evaluator's Signature: _____   **Need to Repeat:** _____

National Curriculum Competency: CAAHEP: Cognitive: V.C.7; Psychomotor: V.P.3

JOB SKILL 5-5
Evaluate the Work or School Environment and Develop a Safety Plan

Name _____ Date _____ Score _____

Performance Objective

Task: Evaluate the work or school environment to identify safe and unsafe working conditions, then apply risk management as you develop a plan that provides a safe environment for employees /students and patients.

Conditions: Need:

- Work or school environment
- Computer with printer
- Paper, pen or pencil

Refer to:

- *Textbook* sections, Safe Working Environment ("Slips, Trips, and Falls" and "Electrical Safety").

Standards: Complete all steps listed in this job skill in _____ minutes with a minimum score of _____. (Time element and accuracy criteria may be given by instructor.)

Time: Start: _____ Completed: _____ Total: _____ minutes

Scoring: One point for each step performed satisfactorily unless otherwise listed or weighted by instructor.

Directions with Performance Evaluation Checklist

1st Attempt	2nd Attempt	3rd Attempt	
_____	_____	_____	Gather materials (equipment and supplies) listed under *Conditions*.
____/5	____/5	____/5	1. Perform a walk-through in the office or school setting and look for various areas or objects that could cause an accident.
____/5	____/5	____/5	2. List the dangerous areas or objects that were identified. _____ _____ _____
____/13	____/13	____/13	3. Develop a plan to correct these "risk areas" by naming each area or object and stating what changes need to be made to make the environment safe for workers or students and patients of all ages.
_____	_____	_____	Complete within specified time.
____/25	____/25	____/25	**Total points earned** (To obtain a percentage score, divide the total points earned by the number of points possible.)

Comments:

Evaluator's Signature: _____ **Need to Repeat:** _____

National Curriculum Competency: CAAHEP: Cognitive: X.C.7; Psychomotor: XII.P.5   ABHES: 8.g

JOB SKILL 5-6
Take Steps to Prevent and Prepare for Fires in a Health Care Setting

Name _____ Date _____ Score _____

Performance Objective

Task: Follow step-by-step procedures to prevent and prepare for fires in a health care setting.

Conditions: Need:

- Home, work, or school environment
- Computer with printer
- Paper, pen or pencil

Refer to:

- *Textbook* Procedure 5-7 for step-by-step directions

Standards: Complete all steps listed in this job skill in _____ minutes with a minimum score of _____. (Time element and accuracy criteria may be given by instructor.)

Time: Start: _____ Completed: _____ Total: _____ minutes

Scoring: One point for each step performed satisfactorily unless otherwise listed or weighted by instructor.

Directions with Performance Evaluation Checklist

This job skill may be performed in students' homes rather than in a workplace or school setting. If using a school setting, it may be a collaborative assignment.

1st Attempt	2nd Attempt	3rd Attempt	
_____	_____	_____	Gather materials (equipment and supplies) listed under *Conditions*.
____/2	____/2	____/2	1. Conduct a walk-through in your home, workplace, or school setting.
____/2	____/2	____/2	2. Look for and note sources of ignition that contribute to the starting of a fire.
			_____
			_____
			_____
			_____
____/2	____/2	____/2	3. Look for and note sources of fuel that contribute to the starting of a fire.
			_____
			_____
			_____
			_____
____/2	____/2	____/2	4. Look for and note sources of oxygen that contribute to the starting of a fire.
			_____
			_____
			_____

JOB SKILL 5-6 (*continued*)

___/22   ___/22   ___/22   5. Use the following items listed in Procedure 5-7 as a checklist to prepare for a fire. Indicate a checkmark (✓) when you have completed each of the following (2 points each). Write NA if it does not apply.

_____ a. Posted the fire department telephone number.

_____ b. Became familiar with the location and operation of fire alarms.

_____ c. Learned the location and operation of all fire extinguishers.

_____ d. Tested smoke detectors and sprinkler systems.

_____ e. Developed a floor plan marking the location of fire alarms, fire extinguishers, smoke detectors, stairwells, and routes out of the home, office, or school.

_____ f. Memorized and posted evacuation routes.

_____ g. Determined evacuation procedures for patients with special needs.

_____ h. Ensured good housekeeping practices.

_____ i. Trained or received training and practiced fire drills.

_____ j. Memorized the path between your bed (in a home setting), workstation, or desk and the nearest exit route.

_____ k. Established a meeting place for family members, employees, or students in the event of an evacuation.

_____ _____ _____   Complete within specified time.

___/32   ___/32   ___/32   **Total points earned** (To obtain a percentage score, divide the total points earned by the number of points possible.)

Comments:

Evaluator's Signature: _____   **Need to Repeat:** _____

National Curriculum Competency: CAAHEP: Cognitive: XII.C.3	ABHES: 8.g

JOB SKILL 5-7
Demonstrate Proper Use of a Fire Extinguisher

Name _____ Date _____ Score _____

Performance Objective

Task: Demonstrate proper use of a fire extinguisher.

Conditions: Need:
- Fire extinguisher (can simulate)
- Computer with printer
- Paper, pen or pencil

Refer to:
- *Textbook* Procedure 5-8 for step-by-step directions

Standards: Complete all steps listed in this job skill in _____ minutes with a minimum score of _____. (Time element and accuracy criteria may be given by instructor.)

Time: Start: _____ Completed: _____ Total: _____ minutes

Scoring: One point for each step performed satisfactorily unless otherwise listed or weighted by instructor.

Directions with Performance Evaluation Checklist

Scenario: A patient threw a cigarette in a wastebasket in the waiting room of the medical office where you are working. You are the receptionist and saw smoke coming from the basket. You left your desk and by the time you got there a small fire had started. You have several fire extinguishers in the hallway near the waiting room.

1st Attempt	2nd Attempt	3rd Attempt	
_____	_____	_____	Gather materials (equipment and supplies) listed under *Conditions*.
____/2	____/2	____/2	1. Select and note the classification of the proper fire extinguisher. _____ _____
____/6	____/6	____/6	2. Get a _____ and successfully demonstrate the steps to put out the fire (you can talk your way through the demonstration indicating what you are doing).
____/2	____/2	____/2	3. Stand _____ feet from the fire.
____/2	____/2	____/2	4. Face the fire with your back to the _____.
____/2	____/2	____/2	5. Release the locking mechanism by _____.
____/2	____/2	____/2	6. Aim the nozzle at _____.
____/2	____/2	____/2	7. Use a _____ motion until the fire is completely out.
_____	_____	_____	Complete within specified time.
____/20	____/20	____/20	**Total points earned** (To obtain a percentage score, divide the total points earned by the number of points possible.)

JOB SKILL 5-7 (*continued*)

Comments:

Evaluator's Signature: _____   **Need to Repeat:** _____

National Curriculum Competency: CAAHEP: Psychomotor: XII.P.2	ABHES: 8.g

JOB SKILL 5-8
Determine Potential Disaster Hazards in Your Local Community

Name _____ Date _____ Score _____

Performance Objective

Task: Evaluate your local community to determine potential hazards and name associated risks.

Conditions: Need:

- Computer with Internet connection
- Printer and paper
- Pen or pencil

Refer to:

- *Textbook* Procedure 5-9 for specific guidance
- *Textbook* Table 5-2 for a listing of potential disasters

Standards: Complete all steps listed in this job skill in _____ minutes with a minimum score of _____. (Time element and accuracy criteria may be given by instructor.)

Time: **Start:** _____ **Completed:** _____ **Total:** _____ minutes

Scoring: One point for each step performed satisfactorily unless otherwise listed or weighted by instructor.

Directions with Performance Evaluation Checklist

1st Attempt	2nd Attempt	3rd Attempt	
_____	_____	_____	Gather materials (equipment and supplies) listed under *Conditions*.
____/3	____/3	____/3	1. Use the list in *textbook* Table 5-2 to explore potential disasters in your local community (e.g., earthquakes and tornadoes).
____/5	____/5	____/5	2. Refer to the *textbook* "*Resources*" section at the end of Chapter 5 to search for various Internet sites that help determine what risks your region may be exposed to.
____/5	____/5	____/5	3. Use your favorite search engine to look for more information regarding hazards in your area.
____/5	____/5	____/5	4. List all potential hazards found.

_____

_____

_____

1st Attempt	2nd Attempt	3rd Attempt	
_____	_____	_____	Complete within specified time.
___/20	___/20	___/20	**Total points earned** (To obtain a percentage score, divide the total points earned by the number of points possible.)

Comments:

Evaluator's Signature: _____ **Need to Repeat:** _____

National Curriculum Competency: CAAHEP: Cognitive: XII.C.8;	ABHES: 8.g

JOB SKILL 5-9
Develop an Emergency Response Template with an Evacuation Plan

Name _____ Date _____ Score _____

Performance Objective

Task: To develop an emergency response template that can be used with various hazards and determine an evacuation plan, including drawing a diagram of the medical office or school with escape routes.

Conditions: Need:
- Computer with printer
- Paper and pen or pencil

Refer to:
- *Textbook* Procedure 5-9 for step-by-step directions

Standards: Complete all steps listed in this job skill in _____ minutes with a minimum score of _____. (Time element and accuracy criteria may be given by instructor.)

Time: Start: _____ Completed: _____ Total: _____ minutes

Scoring: One point for each step performed satisfactorily unless otherwise listed or weighted by instructor.

Directions with Performance Evaluation Checklist

In Steps 1 through 10 you will be developing a generic emergency response template that can be used with various types of emergencies. In step 11, this job skill can be coupled with Job Skill 5-8 in order to develop actions tailored to the specific risks discovered in your region. This step is optional so completion points have not been assigned.

1st Attempt	2nd Attempt	3rd Attempt	
_____	_____	_____	Gather materials (equipment and supplies) listed under *Conditions*.
_____	_____	_____	1. Determine what facility you will use for this exercise (i.e., office or school).
___/18	___/18	___/18	2. Refer to Procedure 5-9 and list the following:

    a. Capacity of facility:_____

    b. Safe places inside and outside facility: _____

    _____

    _____

    c. Alternative site for operation: _____

    _____

    d. Services most likely used during an emergency: _____

    _____

    _____

    e. Location of quarantine housing: _____

    _____

    _____

JOB SKILL 5-9 (*continued*)

f. Procedures for closing facility: _____

_____

_____

___/20 ___/20 ___/20   3. State emergencies that may require partial or full evacuation, then draw a diagram of the medical office or school with fire alarms and extinguishers, exits, and escape routes clearly marked (attach).

___/5 ___/5 ___/5   4. Name emergency supplies needed in the facility. _____

_____

_____

___/5 ___/5 ___/5   5. Identify the role of employees involved in evacuating patients and visitors and define expectations. _____

_____

_____

_____

___/2 ___/2 ___/2   6. State where the command post is and who is in command. _____

_____

___/2 ___/2 ___/2   7. What lines of communication will be used? _____

_____

___/5 ___/5 ___/5   8. Write a script for the telephone answering machine. _____

_____

_____

_____

___/3 ___/3 ___/3   9. State criteria for calling an end to the emergency and reopening the facility. _____

_____

___/2 ___/2 ___/2   10. Identify relevant physical, psychological, and emotional issues that may be experienced by persons involved in an emergency situation. _____

_____

_____

Optional: Instructor assigns points   11. Develop an Emergency Operations Plan (EOP) for all potential disasters identified in Table 5-2 and used in Job Skill 5-8. Tailor each plan according to specific needs (attach plan).

___ ___ ___   Complete within specified time.

___/65 ___/65 ___/65   **Total points earned** (To obtain a percentage score, divide the total points earned by the number of points possible.)

JOB SKILL 5-9 *(continued)*

Comments:

.

National Curriculum Competency: CAAHEP: Cognitive: XII.C.8; Psychomotor: XII.P.4; Affective: XII.A.1, 2   ABHES: 8.g

Telephone Procedures

STOP AND THINK CASE SCENARIOS

Refer to the end of Chapter 6 in the *textbook* for the following scenarios:

- Respond to Personal Call from Friend
- Evaluate Telephone Equipment
- Compose Outgoing Voice Mail Message
- Prioritize Incoming Telephone Calls

EXAM-STYLE REVIEW QUESTIONS

Refer to the end of Chapter 6 in the *textbook*.

Abbreviation and Spelling Review

Read the patient's chart note and write the meanings for the abbreviations following the note. To decode any abbreviations you do not understand or that appear unfamiliar to you, refer to the list of abbreviations in Appendix B of this *Workbook*. Step-by-step directions for this exercise are found in Procedure 1-1 of Chapter 1 in the *textbook*. Medical terms in the chart note are italicized; study them for spelling. Use your medical dictionary to look up their definitions. Your instructor may give a spelling and definition test that includes these words and abbreviations.

John F. Mason

October 15, 20XX. Pt comes in PO complaining of *anorexia, nausea, & stomatitis*. CBC reveals RBC 80–90, WBC 60–80, Hgb 17 g/100 ml. Applied AgNO$_3$. Wound healing well. Cont. med. Ordered BUN. Retn 3 days. RO *uremia*.

Gerald Practon, MD
Gerald Practon, MD

Pt	_____	ml	_____
PO	_____	AgNO$_3$	_____
CBC	_____	Cont.	_____
RBC	_____	med.	_____
WBC	_____	BUN	_____
Hgb	_____	retn	_____
g	_____	RO	_____

Review Questions

Review the objectives, glossary, and chapter information before completing the following review questions.

1. What are the three voice components to consider when practicing telephone technique and cultivating a cheerful and calm voice?

    a. _____

    b. _____

    c. _____

2. What are the two basic things to consider when choosing a telephone system?

    a. _____

    b. _____

3. Give four reasons the physician might choose to use a cellular telephone.

    a. _____

    b. _____

    c. _____

    d. _____

4. All incoming calls should be answered before the _____ ring.

5. When speaking to an elderly caller, you should be prepared to _____
    _____

6. When placing outgoing calls, you should always plan your conversation and _____
    _____

7. Name five ways to ensure confidentiality when leaving a message in a voice mail system.

    a. _____

    b. _____

    c. _____

    d. _____

    e. _____

8. How does an answering service assist the medical office? _____
    _____

9. Name and define two types of critical situations requiring medical care.

   a. _____

   _____

   b. _____

   _____

10. List five telephone procedures that might be discussed in an information booklet presented to a patient on his or her first visit to the office.

   a. _____

   b. _____

   c. _____

   d. _____

   e. _____

11. When telephone lines are busy and calls have to be placed on hold, list several things to consider and actions to take.

   a. _____

   b. _____

   c. _____

   d. _____

   e. _____

   f. _____

   g. _____

12. Name five things that should be included when recording information on a telephone message slip.

   a. _____

   b. _____

   c. _____

   d. _____

   e. _____

13. If no action has been taken on a patient call during the day, what should you do so that the call will not be overlooked in a telephone log? _____

14. Define *conference call* and discuss the procedures for setting up this type of call. _____

   _____

   _____

   _____

Critical Thinking Exercises

1. Dr. Practon reproaches you for having forgotten to make a telephone call he asked you to make. What would you say? _____

_____

_____

_____

2. A patient, Mrs. Braun, wishes to use the physician's telephone. You know she is a talkative person. How would you handle this situation? _____

_____

_____

_____

_____

3. You are the administrative medical assistant for Drs. Fran and Gerald Practon. Simulate using a telephone to role-play the following scenarios:

   a. Dr. Gerald Practon has asked you to call Marilyn Macy to let her know that her thyroid tests came back normal. She is not home and you reach her answering machine. Leave a message following voice mail guidelines.

   b. Later, Marilyn Macy calls the office and asks to speak with you. Answer the telephone and tell her the results of her lab work.

   c. You receive a telephone call from Dr. Fran Practon's patient Samantha Delong. She would like to book an appointment for next week; however, before you can schedule her, the telephone rings again and it is Dr. Armstrong, who wants to speak to Dr. Gerald Practon immediately.

   d. You receive a call from a prospective patient wanting to know about Practon Medical Group. She said that a friend told her about Drs. Fran and Gerald Practon. Answer the call and determine how you would proceed with the conversation. Note: Details about Practon Medical Group, Inc. can be found in Appendix A of the *Workbook*.

   e. Andréa calls from College Hospital Laboratory and says he has the urine culture results for patient Nolan Vanpelt.

   f. Margo, a managed care plan coordinator, calls and wants to speak to someone regarding contract renewal.

   g. Quinn Ortiz, a workers' compensation adjuster, calls saying she received a call from someone in the insurance department but couldn't understand the name.

   h. Gincy Clark, an established patient, calls saying she has scheduled her yearly physical for next week but never received a requisition slip for the laboratory work that Dr. Practon usually orders.

   i. A medical sales supply person calls saying he would like to schedule an appointment to talk to the office manager about sales items.

   j. Hal, the pharmacist at College Pharmacy, calls saying he has a question about a triplicate prescription that Dr. Gerald Practon's patient Ariel Kessler brought in; she is waiting for it to be filled.

   k. You receive a call from the office manager's mother, who seems frantic to speak to her.

l. Dr. Palmer, an orthopedic surgeon, calls. Dr. Fran Practon had referred patient Austin Westerfield to him for a total hip replacement. He now wants to refer the patient back to Dr. Practon for full medical clearance.

m. Reagan, an operating room nurse at College Hospital, calls regarding patient Cody Lowe, who is scheduled for surgery tomorrow. Dr. Palmer Winstrom is the primary surgeon but Reagan cannot reach him, and since Dr. Gerald Practon will be the assistant surgeon, she would like to speak to him regarding the patient.

JOB SKILL 6-1
Screen Incoming Telephone Calls

Name _____ Date _____ Score _____

Performance Objective

Task:	Screen incoming telephone calls and determine the person or persons the calls should be transferred to.
Conditions:	Need:
	• Pen or pencil
	Refer to:
	• *Textbook* Table 6-1 for examples
	• *Textbook* Procedure 6-5 for step-by-step directions
Standards:	Complete all steps listed in this skill in _____ minutes with a minimum score of _____. (Time element and accuracy criteria may be given by instructor.)
Time:	**Start:** _____ **Completed:** _____ **Total:** _____ minutes
Scoring:	One point for each step performed satisfactorily unless otherwise listed or weighted by instructor.

Directions with Performance Evaluation Checklist

Refer to the *Telephone Routing Decision Grid* (Table 6-1) in the *textbook* to aid in determining how the receptionist would screen and transfer incoming telephone calls. Members of the staff are the physician (MD [doctor of medicine]), nurse practitioner (NP), office manager (OM), clinical personnel (RN [registered nurse], LPN [licensed practical nurse], or MA [medical assistant]), insurance supervisor (INS), and bookkeeper (BK). Write the abbreviations of all those who would be appropriate to receive each telephone call in the space provided. If a message slip would be appropriate, place a check mark on the line (✓). If a return call would be appropriate, place a hash mark on the line (#).

1st Attempt	2nd Attempt	3rd Attempt			
			Transfer Call to		**Telephone Call Description**
			MD OM Clinical Personnel (RN LPN MA) INS BK		
_____	_____	_____	Gather materials (equipment and supplies) listed under *Conditions*.		
_____	_____	_____	1. _____		Daughter wants to talk to her father, the physician, and he is with a patient.
_____	_____	_____	2. _____		Doctor is on another line when a nurse at the hospital telephones regarding a patient. After determining urgency, to whom should the call be directed?
_____	_____	_____	3. _____		New patient, ill, wants to speak to physician about recently prescribed medication.
_____	_____	_____	4. _____		Patient requests laboratory test results.
_____	_____	_____	5. _____		Insurance carrier requests patient information.
_____	_____	_____	6. _____		Doctor's wife calls to inquire about time of medical association dinner, and doctor is involved with an emergency situation.
_____	_____	_____	7. _____		Patient telephones about a recent bill.
_____	_____	_____	8. _____		Pharmacy telephones regarding a new prescription.

JOB SKILL 6-1 (*continued*)

_____ _____ _____ 9. _____ Attorney telephones physician regarding malpractice matter.

_____ _____ _____ 10. _____ Professional society member calls for physician.

_____ _____ _____ 11. _____ A mother calls about a child who has sunburn.

_____ _____ _____ 12. _____ Pharmacy requests Rx refill for patient.

_____ _____ _____ 13. _____ Family member asks for information about a child who is under the doctor's care.

_____ _____ _____ 14. _____ Patient requests telephone consultation with physician, who is out of the office.

_____ _____ _____ 15. _____ Pharmaceutical representative asks to make an appointment with physician for sales presentation.

_____ _____ _____ 16. _____ Another doctor desires to talk to physician, who is available.

_____ _____ _____ 17. _____ Occupational Safety and Health Administration (OSHA) representative calls about making visit to do inspection.

_____ _____ _____ 18. _____ Established patient asks to talk to physician, who is unable to take the call.

_____ _____ _____ 19. _____ Accountant telephones regarding tax records.

_____ _____ _____ 20. _____ Established patient requests Rx refill.

_____ _____ _____ 21. _____ Established patient calls to report chest pain.

_____ _____ _____ 22. _____ Nurse at convalescent home calls regarding a patient refusing all medications.

_____ _____ _____ 23. _____ Telephone referral request is received from another physician, and your doctor is with a patient.

_____ _____ _____ 24. _____ Dentist calls to ask if doctor's patient is taking a new drug.

_____ _____ _____ 25. _____ Former office employee telephones to request a recommendation for a job.

___/5 ___/5 ___/5 26. _____ Put check mark by those needing message slips.

_____ _____ _____ Complete within specified time.

___/32 ___/32 ___/32 **Total points earned** (To obtain a percentage score, divide the total points earned by the number of points possible.)

Comments:

Evaluator's Signature: _____ **Need to Repeat:** _____

National Curriculum Competency: CAAHEP: Psychomotor: I.P.3; V.P.6   ABHES: 7.g; 8.b

JOB SKILL 6-2
Prepare Telephone Message Forms

Name _____ Date _____ Score _____

Performance Objective

Task: Evaluate the following incoming telephone calls and determine action to be taken on each call. Complete message forms for all calls that require the transfer of information to message slips.

Conditions: Need:

• Computer with Internet connection

• Online Form 4 through 7 (telephone message slips) located at www.cengagebrain.com with student resources

• Pen or pencil

Refer to:

• *Textbook* Figure 6-5 for a visual illustration

Standards: Complete all steps listed in this skill in _____ minutes with a minimum score of _____. (Time element and accuracy criteria may be given by instructor.)

Time: **Start:** _____ **Completed:** _____ **Total:** _____ minutes

Scoring: One point for each step performed satisfactorily unless otherwise listed or weighted by instructor.

Directions with Performance Evaluation Checklist

It is the morning of Tuesday, November 6, (current year), and both physicians (Fran Practon, MD, and Gerald Practon, MD) are at the hospital and will not be in the office until 1 p.m. Determine which calls may be taken care of immediately (e.g., by making an appointment) and which calls need information transferred to a message slip. Then, indicate what action has been taken on each telephone call and write it on the line following the call (e.g., message F.P., made appt., or other action). If a message should be taken, record the necessary information (name of patient and caller, telephone number, if chart is attached, and so forth) on the left portion of the form. Be sure to indicate the date and time of the call and your initials.

On the right portion of the form, record to whom the message is for (i.e., G.P. or F.P.) and compose the message in a complete but brief statement or question. Refer to call no. 0 for an example:

EXAMPLE

0. (9:15) Marguerite Houston (Mrs. C. F. Houston) calls and sounds upset. She wants to ask Dr. Gerald Practon if she can discontinue the medication he prescribed Friday because she thinks she is allergic to it; she now has a rash on her face. She is due to take her next dose tomorrow morning. You have told her that the doctor is not in the office and that you will ask him to call her (678-7892) as soon as he comes in. You check her chart and see that she has no known allergies listed.

JOB SKILL 6-2 *(continued)*

EXAMPLE

	Name of Caller	Tel. #	Reason for Call	Action Taken
Call No. 0	*Marguerite Houston*	*678-7892*	*Can she discontinue medication? Rash on face.*	*Message GP*

PRIORITY ☐		TELEPHONE RECORD ☎
PATIENT Marguerite Houston AGE	**MESSAGE** G.P.	
CALLER	Rash on face - possibly allergic to newly	
TELEPHONE 678-7892	prescribed medication - call asap.	
REFERRED TO		**TEMP**	**ALLERGIES** NKA
CHART #	**RESPONSE**	
CHART ATTACHED ☒ YES ☐ NO		
DATE Nov. 6, 20XX **TIME** 9:15 **REC'D BY** B.C.		
Copyright © 1978 Bibbero Systems, Inc. Printed in the U.S.A.	**PHY/RN INITIALS**	**DATE** / /	**TIME**	**HANDLED BY**

FIGURE 6-1

1st Attempt	2nd Attempt	3rd Attempt	
_____	_____	_____	Gather materials (equipment and supplies) listed under *Conditions*.
___/10	___/10	___/10	1. (9:35) Donald Eggert (765-3145) asks to speak to Dr. Fran Practon. He wants to make an appointment for an injection next week.
___/10	___/10	___/10	2. (9:40) A person calls and refuses to identify himself. He requests information on a patient, Marilyn Turner.
___/10	___/10	___/10	3. (9:55) A patient, Bruce Jeffers (486-2468), calls to cancel his appointment with Dr. Gerald Practon that is scheduled for this afternoon because he needs to get ready to leave on a flight to New York tomorrow (N.Y. phone: 542-671-0121). He will make another appointment upon his return late next week. He would like to know what to do about the series of daily injections he has been receiving from Dr. Practon.
___/10	___/10	___/10	4. (9:58) Phyllis Sperry (678-1162) wants to know the results of the Pap test taken last week by Dr. Fran Practon. (You can find these results in the file and they are normal.)
___/10	___/10	___/10	5. (10:15) Mr. G. W. Witte (678-5478) represents the General Surgical Supply Company and wants to show the doctors a new instrument. You have suggested he call the next day when you will let him know whether either of the physicians will be able to talk to him or schedule an appointment.

JOB SKILL 6-2 (continued)

___/10 ___/10 ___/10   6. (10:20) Midway Pharmacy (649-3762) calls Dr. Fran Practon and wants to know if a refill is allowed on Philip Stevenson Jr.'s prescription for sleeping pills, No. 8711342.

_____

___/10 ___/10 ___/10   7. (10:25) Sylvia Cone (411-8215) calls and asks to speak to Dr. Gerald Practon. She refuses to leave a message and says that it is urgent.

_____

___/10 ___/10 ___/10   8. (10:55) Charles Jones (487-6650) calls to ask if the Practons can recommend an eye, ear, and nose specialist. (There is a reference sheet near the telephone.)

_____

___/10 ___/10 ___/10   9. (11:00) Mary Lu Practon, the Practons' 14-year-old daughter, calls to report that she is going to Disneyland with the Cone family for the day. She will return home about 9:00 p.m. (Cones' cell phone: 555-678-9000).

_____

___/10 ___/10 ___/10 10. (11:05) Betty Knott (678-0076) calls to ask if Dr. Gerald Practon will donate time to give flu injections next Sunday from either 9 to 12 or 1 to 3. She needs to know as soon as possible. She is calling from the Reseda Red Cross office on Sepulveda Boulevard, where the injections are to be given.

_____

___/10 ___/10 ___/10 11. (11:18) Alan Becker (486-9993) calls and is upset about the bill he received today from Dr. Fran Practon. He thinks the amount is exorbitant, and he asks to speak to Dr. Practon or someone with authority.

_____

___/10 ___/10 ___/10 12. (11:20) Patricia Papakostikus (687-4512) calls the office to make an appointment. She is having daily headaches.

_____

___/10 ___/10 ___/10 13. (11:30) Dr. Martin Laird (643-1108) calls to ask if Dr. Gerald Practon would like a ride to the American Medical Association (AMA) meeting tonight. Dr. Practon should let Dr. Laird know before 4:00 p.m.

_____

___/10 ___/10 ___/10 14. (11:45) Elizabeth Montague (411-0068) calls to ask if she should continue her medication. She feels fine now. Dr. Gerald Practon is her physician.

_____

___/10 ___/10 ___/10 15. (11:50) Alyson Pierce (Mrs. D. M.) (765-9077) calls to ask if Dr. Fran Practon can stop by on her way home tonight at 562 Lynnbrook Avenue, Agoura, to look at her little girl, Courtney, age 3, who has a high fever (103°F). Alyson has no means of transportation. You tell her you will check with the physician as soon as possible and will let her know if this home visit can be worked out.

_____

JOB SKILL 6-2 (continued)

___/10 ___/10 ___/10   16. Wrote message forms legibly.

_____ _____ _____   Completed within specified time.

___/162 ___/162 ___/162   **Total points earned** (To obtain a percentage score, divide the total points earned by the number of points possible.)

Comments:

Evaluator's Signature: _____   **Need to Repeat:** _____

National Curriculum Competency: CAAHEP: Psychomotor: V.P.7, 11   ABHES: 7.a, g

JOB SKILL 6-3
Document Telephone Messages and Physician Responses

Name _____ Date _____ Score _____

Performance Objective

Task: Document telephone messages and physician responses on telephone message slips. Separate slips and attach to file page for insertion in medical record.

Conditions: Need:

- One sheet of colored paper
- Computer with Internet connection
- Online Forms 8 and 9 (telephone message forms) located at www.cengagebrain.com with student resources
- Scissors
- Cellophane adhesive tape or glue
- Pen or pencil

Refer to:

- *Textbook* Figures 6-4 and 6-6 for visual illustrations

Standards: Complete all steps listed in this skill in _____ minutes with a minimum score of _____. (Time element and accuracy criteria may be given by instructor.)

Time: **Start:** _____ **Completed:** _____ **Total:** _____ minutes

Scoring: One point for each step performed satisfactorily unless otherwise listed or weighted by instructor.

Directions with Performance Evaluation Checklist

This exercise is for patient Krista Lee Carlisle, Record Number 1181. You will be preparing her chart in Chapter 9 (*Medical Records*). On a sheet of colored paper, key or type "Telephone Messages" in the upper left corner and the patient's name and record number in the upper right corner. Insert the following data on the telephone message slips. When completed, cut apart the message forms and tape or glue them to the sheet of colored paper; retain it for future use.

1st Attempt	2nd Attempt	3rd Attempt	
_____	_____	_____	Gather materials (equipment and supplies) listed under *Conditions*.
___/15	___/15	___/15	1. On February 28, 20XX, at 3:00 p.m., Mrs. Robyn Carlisle called Dr. Gerald Practon stating Krista Lee, age 17, is in bed with flu symptoms. She cancelled her appointment for 3/1/XX. Patient's telephone number is 849-7730. Dr. Practon telephoned Mrs. Carlisle at 4:40 p.m. to recommend that Krista Lee drink plenty of fluids; he will prescribe medication if flu symptoms worsen.
___/15	___/15	___/15	2. On March 2, 20XX, at 3:10 p.m., Robyn Carlisle called Dr. Gerald Practon about her daughter, Krista Lee, who has a temperature of 100.2°F. She said Krista is having chest congestion and a persistent dry cough. She asked for a prescription of cough syrup. The family pharmacy is Long's Drug Store (phone: 849-2221). Dr. Practon asks you to fax an order to the pharmacy for Robitussin-PE, 2 teaspoons, every 4 hours. You ordered the medication from the pharmacy and called Mrs. Carlisle at 4:05 p.m. to give her the information.

JOB SKILL 6-3 *(continued)*

___/15 ___/15 ___/15   3. On March 3, 20XX, at 9 a.m., you receive another call from Robyn Carlisle about Krista Lee. She says she thinks Krista has a possible allergy to the medication because she has a rash on her chest; she is continuing to cough and her temperature is 100°F.

     Dr. Practon returns the call at 11:15 a.m. He tells Robyn to discontinue the Robitussin and suggests an appointment be made for the next day, March 4.

___/15 ___/15 ___/15   4. Krista Lee sees Dr. Practon on March 4, 20XX, and he prescribes a different cough medication. Dr. Practon asks Mrs. Carlisle to report back in a day or two regarding the rash and cough. Robyn Carlisle calls on March 6, 20XX, at 3:30 p.m., saying Krista's rash has disappeared but she still has a cough, which is now producing discolored phlegm, and has a temperature of 100.3°F.

     Dr. Practon returns her call at 4:15 p.m. and orders a chest x-ray at College Hospital the following morning and a return appointment the afternoon of March 7. Krista Lee's chart is updated to indicate that she is allergic to codeine.

___/4 ___/4 ___/4   Wrote message forms legibly.

_____ _____ _____   Complete within specified time.

___/66 ___/66 ___/66   **Total points earned** (To obtain a percentage score, divide the total points earned by the number of points possible.)

Comments:

Evaluator's Signature: _____ **Need to Repeat:** _____

National Curriculum Competency: CAAHEP: Psychomotor: V.P.7, 11	ABHES: 7.a, g

JOB SKILL 6-4
Role-Play Emergency Telephone Scenario(s)

Name _____ Date _____ Score _____

Performance Objective

Task: Role-play a telephone scenario to gain practical experience in telephone technique and critical thinking when determining and managing an emergency call.

Conditions: Need:

- Pen or pencil
- Telephone (can simulate)
- Scenario(s)

Refer to:

- *Textbook* Procedure 6-6 for step-by-step directions

Standards: Complete all steps listed in this job skill in _____ minutes with a minimum score of _____. (Time element and accuracy criteria may be given by instructor.)

Time: **Start:** _____ **Completed:** _____ **Total:** _____ minutes

Scoring: One point for each step performed satisfactorily unless otherwise listed or weighted by instructor.

Directions with Performance Evaluation Checklist

This scenario is most realistically role-played with two students: one playing the caller and the other playing the medical assistant.

Scenario: Mrs. Ruby Pristine telephones Dr. Practon's office; she is upset and crying. She says that her husband (Mr. Clarence Pristine) fell and she cannot get him up. The student role-playing Mrs. Pristine can "ad lib" Mr. Pristine's condition, thereby making this scenario available to be role-played by different pairs of students who each demonstrate critical thinking skills and telephone technique for a variety of outcomes.

1st Attempt	2nd Attempt	3rd Attempt	
_____	_____	_____	Gather materials (equipment and supplies) listed under *Conditions*.
____/2	____/2	____/2	1. Allow the caller to state the problem without interruptions.
____/5	____/5	____/5	2. Ask appropriate questions to determine if the call is an urgent or emergent situation.
____/2	____/2	____/2	3. Maintain a calm, even, low-pitched tone of voice and take deep breaths as necessary to remain composed.
____/2	____/2	____/2	4. Use the caller's and patient's names when asking specific questions.
____/2	____/2	____/2	5. Ask whether the patient has experienced this same problem at a prior time.
____/2	____/2	____/2	6. Ask what is being done, or what the caller had tried to do for the patient.
____/5	____/5	____/5	7. Request that a coworker bring up the patient's medical record in the computer system or get the patient's chart while obtaining details about the patient's symptoms, accident description, current status, and any treatment administered.
____/10	____/10	____/10	8. Take action according to the severity of the patient's condition as explained.

JOB SKILL 6-4 (continued)

_____ _____ _____ Complete within specified time.

___/32 ___/32 ___/32 **Total points earned** (To obtain a percentage score, divide the total points earned by the number of points possible.)

Comments:

Evaluator's Signature: _____ **Need to Repeat:** _____

National Curriculum Competency: CAAHEP: Psychomotor: V.P.6; Affective: I.A.I, XII.A.1   ABHES: 7.g, 8.g

CHAPTER 7

Appointments

STOP AND THINK CASE SCENARIOS

Refer to the end of Chapter 7 in the *textbook* for the following scenarios:

- Handle a Patient with an Unverified Appointment
- Determine a Routine, Urgent, or Emergency Appointment

- Explain Office Policy for Urgent and Emergent Appointments
- Reasons Physicians Refuse to Accept and Treat Patients

EXAM-STYLE REVIEW QUESTIONS

Refer to the end of Chapter 7 in the *textbook*.

Abbreviation and Spelling Review

Read the patient's chart note and write the meanings for the abbreviations following the note. To decode any abbreviations you do not understand or that appear unfamiliar to you, refer to the list of abbreviations in Appendix B of this *Workbook*. Step-by-step directions for this exercise are in Procedure 1-1 of Chapter 1 in the *textbook*. Medical terms in the chart note are italicized; study them for spelling. Use your medical dictionary to look up their definitions. Your instructor may give a spelling and definition test that includes these words and abbreviations.

Dan F. Goodson

September 3, 20XX IV *chemotherapy* started in hospital. Daily hosp PO exams. See op. report giving dx: *superficially infiltrating transitional* cell Ca Class III. Pt DC from hosp 11-1-20XX. Retn for OV 3 p.m. Friday. PT to be started in 1 mo.

Gerald Practon, MD
Gerald Practon, MD

IV	_____	DC	_____
hosp	_____	retn	_____
PO	_____	OV	_____
op.	_____	p.m.	_____
dx	_____	PT	_____
Ca	_____	mo	_____
Pt	_____		

Review Questions

Review the objectives, glossary, and chapter information before completing the following review questions.

1. Describe an appointment template. _____

   _____

2. State the definition of a "new patient." _____

   _____

   _____

3. In a typical office, what time intervals are usually assigned for the following types of patients? Initial

   visits: _____ Follow-up examinations: _____

4. What is the name of the sheet used to track the number of patients seen daily for various types of

   appointments in order to determine a scheduling system? _____

   _____

5. What five factors should be taken into consideration when an appointment book is being selected?

   a. _____   d. _____

   b. _____   e. _____

   c. _____

6. What is one of the most valuable and time-saving tools an electronic scheduling system offers? _____

   _____

7. Using appointment software, name several places a patient's appointment can be automatically
   recorded.

8. Why is it advantageous to schedule patient appointments one right after the other?

   _____

   _____

9. What is the benefit of having a medical assistant make confirmation telephone calls to patients sched-

   uled to be seen within 1 or 2 days? _____

10. Which patient flow technique do most physicians' offices use? _____

11. Describe true wave scheduling. _____

    _____

    _____

12. What are long wait times equated with? _____

13. List four actions the medical assistant might take when an emergency telephone call indicates an immediate response.

   a. _____

   b. _____

   c. _____

   d. _____

14. When might an appointment be scheduled for a patient who is habitually late? _____

_____

15. Besides having a written record of all appointments, why is it important to keep accurate and permanent

   information? _____

16. What systems or devices might a physician use to keep track of out-of-office appointments? _____

_____

17. When a patient "no shows" an appointment, name what action should be taken. _____

_____

_____

_____

_____

18. Who should the medical assistant call when scheduling a hospital surgery? _____

_____

19. Name what interval the physician should visit a (a) convalescent hospital patient and a (b) hospital patient.

   a. _____

   b. _____

20. Why should postcards not be sent to remind patients of upcoming appointments?

_____

21. Explain what an appointment reference sheet is and what purpose it serves.

_____

✖ Critical Thinking Exercises

1. Mrs. Bettle, who has arrived for her appointment 1 hour early, is sure that she has come at the right

   time. What would you say to her? _____

_____

_____

_____

_____

_____

2. After seeing the physician, Mrs. Hall stops at your desk for a new appointment. What do you say to her?

_____

_____

_____

3. Andy Gage walks into the office saying a friend has spoken highly of Dr. Gerald Practon and he would like to make an appointment as a new patient; he has Medicaid insurance. Dr. Practon advised you last month that he and his wife (Dr. Fran) are not accepting any new Medicaid patients. He has contacted the Centers for Medicare and Medicaid Services and posted a notice to this effect. How would you

respond? _____

_____

_____

4. It is Monday afternoon and a drug detail representative walks into the office and would like to see both physicians. Dr. Fran Practon is out of the office and Dr. Gerald Practon is behind schedule, and there

are no available appointments that week. How would you respond? _____

_____

_____

_____

5. An established patient, Mrs. Barker, is in the waiting room and the physician is running behind schedule. You had called her prior to her leaving her house and advised her that the physician had an emergency and had not returned to the office. You asked her if she wanted to reschedule; she choose to come at her scheduled time. After she waited for about 10 minutes she started complaining, and after another 10 minutes you approached her and asked if she would like to run an errand and then return, remain and wait, or reschedule. She insisted on staying but has become very loud as she complains

about the office always running behind schedule. How would you handle this situation? _____

_____

_____

_____

_____

_____

_____

JOB SKILL 7-1
Set Up Appointment Matrix

Name _____ Date _____ Score _____

Performance Objective

Task: Prepare an appointment matrix for three days, labeling each page and blocking segments of time.

Conditions: Need:

- Computer with Internet connection
- Online Forms 10, 11, and 12 (three appointment records) located at www.cengagebrain.com with student resources
- Pen or pencil

Refer to:

- *Textbook* Procedure 7-1 and 7-2 for step-by-step directions

Standards: Complete all steps listed in this skill in _____ minutes with a minimum score of _____. (Time element and accuracy criteria may be given by instructor.)

Time: **Start:** _____ **Completed:** _____ **Total:** _____ minutes

Scoring: One point for each step performed satisfactorily unless otherwise listed or weighted by instructor.

Directions with Performance Evaluation Checklist

1st Attempt	2nd Attempt	3rd Attempt	
_____	_____	_____	Gather materials (equipment and supplies) listed under *Conditions*.
____/6	____/6	____/6	1. Set up three appointment sheets for Dr. Gerald Practon (left column) and Dr. Fran Practon (right column).
____/2	____/2	____/2	2. Label the first sheet Monday, October 27, 20XX.
____/2	____/2	____/2	3. Label the second sheet Tuesday, October 28, 20XX.
____/2	____/2	____/2	4. Label the third sheet Wednesday, October 29, 20XX.
____/6	____/6	____/6	5. Refer to the Office Hours section of Office Policies in Appendix A of this *Workbook* to determine when the physicians are in the office. Circle the opening and closing hours of the office for each day.
____/9	____/9	____/9	6. Block off all periods when the physicians are not in the office, that is, lunch hours, afternoons off, and surgery/hospital responsibility time.
____/2	____/2	____/2	7. Record Dr. G. Practon's plans to visit Donald Pierce at the hospital at 9:00 a.m. on Tuesday morning and at noon on Wednesday.
____/2	____/2	____/2	8. Record Dr. F. Practon's 1-hour dental appointment with Dr. Bryce Crowe at 2:30 p.m. on Wednesday. She will need to leave the office at 2:15 p.m.
____/9	____/9	____/9	9. Indicate which appointment times are reserved for unscheduled patients (work-ins, emergencies, and so forth).
_____	_____	_____	Complete within specified time.
____/42	____/42	____/42	**Total points earned** (To obtain a percentage score, divide the total points earned by the number of points possible.)

JOB SKILL 7-1 (*continued*)

Comments:

Evaluator's Signature: _____   **Need to Repeat:** _____

National Curriculum Competency: CAAHEP: Psychomotor: VI.P.1   ABHES: 7.e

JOB SKILL 7-2
Schedule Appointments

Name _____ Date _____ Score _____

Performance Objective

Task: Record patient appointments accurately using acceptable abbreviations on appointment sheets. Adjust to individual patient preferences, medical needs, and unexpected changes.

Conditions: Need:

- Computer with Internet connection
- Online Forms 10, 11, and 12 from Job Skill 7-1 (three appointment scheduling sheets) located at www.cengagebrain.com with student resources
- Pen and pencil

Refer to:

- *Workbook* Table 7-1 for patient list and appointment reference information
- *Textbook* Table 7-1 to decode abbreviations (also found in Appendix B of *Workbook*)
- *Workbook* Appendix A for office and appointment policies
- *Textbook* Procedure 7-3 for step-by-step directions

Standards: Complete all steps listed in this skill in _____ minutes with a minimum score of _____. (Time element and accuracy criteria may be given by instructor.)

Time: Start: _____ **Completed:** _____ **Total:** _____ minutes

Scoring: One point for each step performed satisfactorily unless otherwise listed or weighted by instructor.

Directions with Performance Evaluation Checklist

All patients are established unless otherwise indicated. An asterisk (*) by a patient's name indicates a patient of Dr. Fran Practon; all others are patients of Dr. Gerald Practon. Refer to the Appointment section of Office Policies to determine the amount of time for each appointment. Schedule an appointment for each patient appearing in this exercise. It may help to use a ruler as you go down the list of names in *Workbook* Table 7-1 and check them off as you schedule.

1st Attempt	2nd Attempt	3rd Attempt	
_____	_____	_____	Gather materials (equipment and supplies) listed under *Conditions*.
____/5	____/5	____/5	1. Schedule an appointment for *Melissa Jones.
____/5	____/5	____/5	2. Schedule an appointment for *Marsha MacFadden.
____/5	____/5	____/5	3. Schedule an appointment for Wendy Snow.
____/5	____/5	____/5	4. Schedule an appointment for Phyllis Dayton.
____/5	____/5	____/5	5. Schedule an appointment for *Rebecca Martinez.
____/5	____/5	____/5	6. Schedule an appointment for Jane Call.
____/5	____/5	____/5	7. Schedule an appointment for *Mary Fay Jeffers.
____/5	____/5	____/5	8. Schedule an appointment for *Philip Stevenson Jr.
____/5	____/5	____/5	9. Schedule an appointment for *Shirley Van Alystine.
____/5	____/5	____/5	10. Schedule an appointment for Courtney Pierce.
____/5	____/5	____/5	11. Schedule an appointment for Paul Stone.

JOB SKILL 7-2 (*continued*)

____/5 ____/5 ____/5 12. Schedule an appointment for *Alan Becker.

____/5 ____/5 ____/5 13. Schedule an appointment for *Marguerite Houston.

____/5 ____/5 ____/5 14. Schedule an appointment for *Paul Frenzel.

____/5 ____/5 ____/5 15. Schedule an appointment for Elizabeth Montgomery, RN.

____/5 ____/5 ____/5 16. Schedule an appointment for Lu Chung.

____/5 ____/5 ____/5 17. Schedule an appointment for Jerry Calhoun.

____/5 ____/5 ____/5 18. Schedule an appointment for Cathy Martinez.

____/5 ____/5 ____/5 19. Schedule an appointment for Lloyd Wix.

____/5 ____/5 ____/5 20. Schedule an appointment for Bruce Jeffers.

____/5 ____/5 ____/5 21. Schedule an appointment for *Ashley Jones.

____/5 ____/5 ____/5 22. Schedule an appointment for *David Martinez.

____/5 ____/5 ____/5 23. Schedule an appointment for Carl Freeburg.

____/5 ____/5 ____/5 24. Schedule an appointment for *Anne Rule.

____/5 ____/5 ____/5 25. Schedule an appointment for Charles Jones.

____/5 ____/5 ____/5 26. Schedule an appointment for Robert LaRue.

____/5 ____/5 ____/5 27. Schedule an appointment for *Phyllis Sperry.

____/5 ____/5 ____/5 28. Schedule an appointment for Sylvia Cone.

____/5 ____/5 ____/5 29. Schedule an appointment for *Pat Wochesky.

____/5 ____/5 ____/5 30. Schedule an appointment for Sheila Haley.

____/5 ____/5 ____/5 31. Schedule an appointment for Frank Elder.

____/5 ____/5 ____/5 32. Schedule an appointment for *Donald Eggert.

____ ____ Complete within specified time.

___/162 ___/162 ___/162 **Total points earned** (To obtain a percentage score, divide the total points earned by the number of points possible.)

JOB SKILL 7-2 (*continued*)

TABLE 7-1
Patient List and Appointment Reference Information
*Drs. Fran T. Practon and Gerald M. Practon

Name	Phone Number	Complaint or Procedure	Appointment Preference
*Melissa Jones	487–6650	Pap, estrogen inj.	Tues. p.m.
*Marsha MacFadden	487–0027	ECG, ltd. OV	Tues. a.m.
Wendy Snow	765–6626	Cast ck, leg	Mon.
Phyllis Dayton	411–2244	Pap, limited exam	Mon.
*Rebecca Martinez	765–0008	Measles inj.	Wed.
Jane Call	678–0134	Smallpox vac.	Wed.
*Mary Fay Jeffers	486–2468	MMR	Mon. after school
*Philip Stevenson Jr.	457–1133	BP, UA ltd. exam	Mon.
*Shirley Van Alystine	678–4421	IUD, BP	Tues.
Courtney Pierce	765–9077	Fever, cough	Tues. p.m.
Paul Stone	411–7206	F/U	Late Tues.
*Alan Becker	486–9993	Face infection, ltd. exam	Mon.
*Marguerite Houston	678–7892	Inj. for allergy	Tues. around 3:00 p.m.
*Paul Frenzel	765–8897	Dressing change	Early Wed. a.m.
Elizabeth Montgomery, RN	411–0068	BP	Tues. a.m. (see F. P.?)
Lu Chung	678–4455	Allergy complaint	Mon.
Jerry Calhoun	678–8771	N/P, CPX, CBC	Late as possible Tues.
Cathy Martinez	765–0008	Excise lesion on back	Wed.
Lloyd Wix	678–5529	Consult	Tues. 10:30 a.m.—must see G. P. (Wed.?)
Bruce Jeffers	486–2468	Remove glass from eye	Early Wed.
*Ashley Jones	487–6650	Suture removal	Mon. after 2:30 p.m.
*David Martinez	765–0008	Remove splinter from leg	Wed. a.m.
Carl Freeburg	486–0011	Aspirate left elbow	Late Wed.
*Anne Rule	457–9001	N/P, CPX	Mon. a.m.
Charles Jones	487–6650	Audiogram, ear lavage	Mon. p.m.
Robert LaRue	487–3355	Brief OV, VDRL	Must have Tues. a.m. (see F. P.?)
*Phyllis Sperry	678–1162	N/P, CPX	Tues. p.m.
Sylvia Cone	411–8215	HA, N/P	Wed. after lunch
*Pat Wochesky	765–3446	New OB	Wed. a.m.
Sheila Haley	678–6669	Tetanus	Wed. a.m.
Frank Elder	486–0918	N/P, pain in side, BUN, CBC	Mon.
*Donald Eggert	765–3145	Sore elbow, ltd. exam	Early Mon. p.m.

*Asterisks indicate Dr. Fran T. Practon's patients.

Comments:

Evaluator's Signature: _____   **Need to Repeat:** _____

National Curriculum Competency: CAAHEP: Psychomotor: VI.P.1	ABHES: 7.e

JOB SKILL 7-3
Prepare an Appointment Reference Sheet

Name _____ Date _____ Score _____

Performance Objective

Task: Key the names of patients who are to be seen by the physician on a given day for a reference sheet. Make a photocopy of the appointment sheet for comparison or to use as an alternative reference.

Conditions: Need:

- One sheet of white paper
- Computer
- Printer
- Photocopy machine

Refer to:

- Dr. Gerald Practon's completed appointment page for 10/29/20XX, from Job Skill 7-2

Standards: Complete all steps listed in this skill in _____ minutes with a minimum score of _____. (Time element and accuracy criteria may be given by instructor.)

Time: **Start:** _____ **Completed:** _____ **Total:** _____ minutes

Scoring: One point for each step performed satisfactorily unless otherwise listed or weighted by instructor.

Directions with Performance Evaluation Checklist

1st Attempt	2nd Attempt	3rd Attempt	
_____	_____	_____	Gather materials (equipment and supplies) listed under *Conditions*.
_____	_____	_____	1. Locate information from Dr. Gerald Practon's schedule for Day 3 listed in Job Skill 7-2.
____/3	____/3	____/3	2. Center and boldface the following information as the title for the appointment reference sheet: Dr. Gerald Practon, Wednesday, October 29, 20XX.
____/3	____/3	____/3	3. Make three columns and title them in capital letters: TIME, NAME, REASON FOR VISIT.
____/15	____/15	____/15	4. Abstract information and key a single-spaced list of appointment times, patient names (last name first), and reason for visit to let Dr. G. Practon know who is expected the morning of Wednesday, October 29, 20XX.
_____	_____	_____	5. Photocopy the appointment page for Wednesday, October 29, 20XX, and compare it with the typed list. Additional copies would generally be made for office staff.
_____	_____	_____	Complete within specified time.
____/25	____/25	____/25	**Total points earned** (To obtain a percentage score, divide the total points earned by the number of points possible.)

JOB SKILL 7-3 (continued)

Comments:

Evaluator's Signature: _____   **Need to Repeat:** _____

National Curriculum Competency: CAAHEP: Psychomotor: VI.P.1	ABHES: 7.e

JOB SKILL 7-4
Complete Appointment Cards

Name _____ Date _____ Score _____

Performance Objective

Task: Write accurate and legible appointment cards.

Conditions: Need:
- Computer with Internet connection
- Online Form 13 (appointment cards) located at www.cengagebrain.com with student resources
- Pen or pencil

Standards: Complete all steps listed in this skill in _____ minutes with a minimum score of _____. (Time element and accuracy criteria may be given by instructor.)

Time: Start: _____ Completed: _____ Total: _____ minutes

Scoring: One point for each step performed satisfactorily unless otherwise listed or weighted by instructor.

Directions with Performance Evaluation Checklist

Write the patient's name at the top of the card, check the correct physician, circle the day of the week, and write the appointment date and time for the following patients. *Indicates patient of Fran Practon, MD.

1st Attempt	2nd Attempt	3rd Attempt	
_____	_____	_____	Gather materials (equipment and supplies) listed under *Conditions*.
____/5	____/5	____/5	1. Charles Jones, Wednesday, October 29, at 2:00 p.m.
____/5	____/5	____/5	2. *Marguerite Houston, Tuesday, November 12, at 3:00 p.m.
____/5	____/5	____/5	3. Carl Freeburg, Wednesday, November 6, at 2:45 p.m.
____/5	____/5	____/5	4. *Pat Wochesky, Monday, December 2, at 9:00 a.m.
_____	_____	_____	Complete within specified time.
____/22	____/22	____/22	**Total points earned** (To obtain a percentage score, divide the total points earned by the number of points possible.)

Comments:

Evaluator's Signature: _____ **Need to Repeat:** _____

National Curriculum Competency: CAAHEP: Psychomotor: VI.P.1   ABHES: 7.e

JOB SKILL 7-5
Abstract Information and Complete a Hospital/Surgery Scheduling Form

Name _____ Date _____ Score _____

Performance Objective

Task: Review a patient's medical record, and then abstract and key the required information on the hospital/surgery scheduling form.

Conditions: Need:
- *Workbook* Figure 7-1 (Wayne G. Weather's patient information)
- Computer with Internet connection
- Online Form 14 (Hospital/Surgery scheduling form) located at www.cengagebrain.com with student resources
- Pen or pencil

Refer to:
- *Textbook* Procedure 7-6 for step-by-step directions

Standards: Complete all steps listed in this skill in _____ minutes with a minimum score of _____. (Time element and accuracy criteria may be given by instructor.)

Time: **Start:** _____ **Completed:** _____ **Total:** _____ minutes

Scoring: One point for each step performed satisfactorily unless otherwise listed or weighted by instructor.

Directions with Performance Evaluation Checklist

Using Mr. Weather's "Patient Information for Medical Records" found in *Workbook* Figure 7-1, abstract data to complete the hospital/surgical scheduling form. Use the following additional information: Mr. Weather was referred to Dr. Gerald Practon by Dr. Mary Hill and is to be admitted to College Hospital for a 3-day stay on Tuesday, October 28, 20XX, at 5:30 a.m. His diagnosis is lumbar herniated nucleus pulposus, and a second opinion is not required. His preadmission testing of complete blood count (CBC), electrocardiogram (EKG), and chest x-ray was performed on October 27, 20XX. He has not been previously hospitalized. Mr. Weather is a smoker and prefers a ward room. The elective lumbar (L4-L5) laminectomy is scheduled for Tuesday, October 28, 20XX, at 7:30 a.m. Preadmission operation instructions as well as insurance and financial arrangements have been discussed.

Dr. Clarence Cutler will be the assistant surgeon and Dr. Harold Barker will give general anesthesia. The surgery, scheduled by hospital employee Robert Slye, should take approximately 1 hour to complete. Kevin Raye of Aetna Casualty & Security Company provided the authorization number, 8036981, and the scheduling was completed and reported to the patient on October 24. Susan Smith at the referring physician's office has been notified, and all arrangements have been posted in the appointment book.

1st Attempt	2nd Attempt	3rd Attempt	
_____	_____	_____	Gather materials (equipment and supplies) listed under *Conditions*.
_____	_____	_____	1. Section 1: Indicate patient name.
_____	_____	_____	2. Section 1: Indicate procedure.
_____	_____	_____	3. Section 1: Indicate status of surgery.
_____	_____	_____	4. Section 1: Indicate diagnosis.
_____	_____	_____	5. Section 1: Indicate facility.
_____	_____	_____	6. Section 1: Indicate admitting status.
_____	_____	_____	7. Section 1: Indicate preferred assistant surgeon.

JOB SKILL 7-5 (*continued*)

_____	_____	_____	8.	Section 1: Indicate preferred anesthesiologist.
_____	_____	_____	9.	Section 1: Indicate referring physician.
_____/3	_____/3	_____/3	10.	Section 2: Indicate patient's age, date of birth, and smoking status.
_____	_____	_____	11.	Section 2: Indicate type of room preferred.
_____/2	_____/2	_____/2	12.	Section 2: Indicate telephone numbers.
_____/2	_____/2	_____/2	13.	Section 2: Indicate insurance information.
_____	_____	_____	14.	Section 2: Indicate second opinion requirements.
_____/3	_____/3	_____/3	15.	Section 2: Indicate emergency contact.
_____	_____	_____	16.	Section 2: Indicate previous admitting information.
_____/3	_____/3	_____/3	17.	Section 2: Indicate preadmission testing.
_____	_____	_____	18.	Section 2: Indicate admission procedures reported.
_____	_____	_____	19.	Section 2: Indicate instructions given to patient.
_____	_____	_____	20.	Section 2: Indicate insurance/financial discussion.
_____/2	_____/2	_____/2	21.	Section 3: Indicate operating room reservation.
_____	_____	_____	22.	Section 3: Indicate hospital surgical scheduling person.
_____	_____	_____	23.	Section 3: Indicate assistant surgeon notified.
_____	_____	_____	24.	Section 3: Indicate anesthesiologist notified.
_____	_____	_____	25.	Section 3: Indicate referring physician notified.
_____	_____	_____	26.	Section 3: Indicate admission and preadmission tests confirmed.
_____	_____	_____	27.	Section 3: Indicate prior authorization obtained.
_____	_____	_____	28.	Section 3: Indicate appointment book data posted.
_____	_____	_____	29.	Section 3: Indicate patient advised.
_____	_____	_____	30.	Section 3: Indicate H&P done.
_____/2	_____/2	_____/2	31.	Section 3: Indicate name of office scheduler and date scheduled.
_____	_____	_____		Complete within specified time.
_____/43	_____/43	_____/43		**Total points earned** (To obtain a percentage score, divide the total points earned by the number of points possible.)

Comments:

JOB SKILL 7-5 *(continued)*

Insurance cards copied ☐	**Patient Registration**	Account # : _____
Date: __10/24/XX__	**Information**	Insurance # : _____
		Co-Payment: $ _____

Please PRINT AND complete ALL sections below!

Is your condition a result of a work injury? YES (NO)   An auto accident? YES (NO)   Date of injury: ___N/A___

PATIENT'S PERSONAL INFORMATION Marital Status: ☐ Single ☑ Married ☐ Divorced ☐ Widowed Sex: ☑ Male ☐ Female

Name: _____Weather_____ (last name) _____Wayne_____ (first name) _____G_____ (initial)

Street address: __6304 Fracture Road__ (Apt #____) City: __Woodland Hills__ State: __XY__ Zip: __12345__

Home phone: (555) 965-2110   Work phone: (555) 861-0122   Social Security # __XXX__ - __XX__ - __5334__

Date of Birth: __1__ / __6__ / __43__ (month/day/year) Driver's License: (State & Numebr) __G-0073-121__

Employer / Name of School __Bu. T. Floor Coverings__   ☐ Full Time ☐ Part Time

Spouse's Name: __Weather__ (last name) __Nancy__ (first name) __B__ (initial) Spouse's Work phone: (555) 761-0811

How do you wish to be addressed? _____ Social Security # _____ - _____ - _____

PATIENT'S / RESPONSIBLE PARTY INFORMATION

Responsible party: _____ Date of Birth: _____

Relationship to Patient: ☐ Self ☐ Spouse ☐ Other _____ Social Security # _____ - _____ - _____

Responsible party's home phone: (____) _____ Work phone: (____) _____

  Address: _____ (Apt # ____) City: _____ State: _____ Zip: _____

Employer's name: _____ Phone number: (____) _____

  Address: _____ City: _____ State: _____ Zip: _____

  Your occupation: _____

Spouse's Employer's name: _____ Spouse's Work phone: (____) _____

  Address: _____ City: _____ State: _____ Zip: _____

PATIENT'S INSURANCE INFORMATION Please present insurance cards to receptionist.

PRIMARY insurance company's name: __Aetna Casualty and Security Co.__

Insurance address: __2412 Wilshire Blvd.__ City: __Woodland Hills__ State: __XY__ Zip: __12345-0000__

Name of insured: _____ Date of Birth: _____ Relationship to insured: ☐ Self ☐ Spouse ☐ Other ☐ Child

Insurance ID number: __3201__ Group number: _____

SECONDARY insurance company's name: _____

Insurance address: _____ City: _____ State: _____ Zip: _____

Name of insured: _____ Date of Birth: _____ Relationship to insured: ☐ Self ☐ Spouse ☐ Other ☐ Child

Insurance ID number: _____ Group number: _____

Check if appropriate: ☐ Medigap policy ☐ Retiree coverage

PATIENT'S REFERRAL INFORMATION   (please circle one)

Referred by: _____ If referred by a friend, may we thank her or him? YES NO

Name(s) of other physician(s) who care for you: _____

_____

EMERGENCY CONTACT

Name of person not living with you: __Jolly B. Rosen__ Relationship: __stepbrother__

Address: __3641 Hope St__ City: __Woodland Hills__ State: __XY__ Zip: __12345__

Phone number (home): (555) 876-6025   Phone number (work): (____) _____

Assignment of Benefits • Financial Agreement

I hereby give lifetime authorization for payment of insurance benefits to be made directly to __Gerald Practon__ , and any assisting physicians for services rendered. I understand that I am financially responsible for all charges whether or not they are covered by insurance. In the event of default, I agree to pay all costs of collection, and reasonable attorney's fees. I hereby authorize this healthcare provider to release all information necessary to secure the payment of benefits.

I further agree that a photocopy of this agreement shall be as valid as the original.

Date: __10/24/XX__ Your Signature: __Wayne G. Weather__

Method of Payment: ☐ Cash ☐ Check ☐ Credit Card

FORM # 58-8424 • BIBBERO SYSTEMS, INC. • PETALUMA, CA. • TO ORDER CALL TOLL FREE : 800-BIBBERO (800-242-2376) • FAX (800) 242-9330 © 7/94

PATIENT REGISTRATION

FIGURE 7-1

JOB SKILL 7-5 (*continued*)

National Curriculum Competency: CAAHEP: Cognitive: VI.C.3; Psychomotor VI.P.2   ABHES: 7.e

JOB SKILL 7-6
Transfer Surgery Scheduling Information to a Form Letter

Name _____ Date _____ Score _____

Performance Objective

Task: Use surgical scheduling information and fill in a form letter to be mailed to persons involved in the procedure.

Conditions: Need:
- Computer with Internet connection
- Online Form 15 (surgical form letter) located at www.cengagebrain.com with student resources
- Photocopy machine

Refer to:
- Online Form 14 (Hospital/Surgery scheduling form) used in Job Skill 7-5

Standards: Complete all steps listed in this skill in _____ minutes with a minimum score of _____. (Time element and accuracy criteria may be given by instructor.)

Time: **Start:** _____ **Completed:** _____ **Total:** _____ minutes

Scoring: One point for each step performed satisfactorily unless otherwise listed or weighted by instructor.

Directions with Performance Evaluation Checklist

October 24, 20XX: You have completed all the surgical scheduling arrangements for Mr. Wayne Weather. The next step is to complete the surgical form letter and photocopy it. One copy will be sent to the patient and one will be retained in Dr. Practon's files.

1st Attempt	2nd Attempt	3rd Attempt	
_____	_____	_____	Gather materials (equipment and supplies) listed under *Conditions*.
_____	_____	_____	1. Read the surgical scheduling form letter to determine what information needs to be abstracted from the hospital/surgery scheduling form used in Job Skill 7-5.
____/4	____/4	____/4	2. Fill in the date and complete the inside address.
____/10	____/10	____/10	3. Fill in the information in the body of the letter.
____/4	____/4	____/4	4. Sign the letter and fill in the information for the physicians involved.
_____	_____	_____	Complete within specified time.
____/21	____/21	____/21	**Total points earned** (To obtain a percentage score, divide the total points earned by the number of points possible.)

Comments:

Evaluator's Signature: _____ **Need to Repeat:** _____

National Curriculum Competency: CAAHEP: Cognitive: V.C.7, VI.C.3   ABHES: 7.e

JOB SKILL 7-7
Complete Requisition Forms to Schedule Outpatient Diagnostic Tests

Name _____ Date _____ Score _____

Performance Objective

Task: Handwrite information on requisition forms to be given to patients when scheduling outpatient diagnostic tests.

Conditions: Need:

- Computer with Internet connection
- Online Form 16 (Laboratory Requisition) located at www.cengagebrain.com with student resources
- Online Form 17 (X-Ray Request) located at www.cengagebrain.com with student resources
- Pen

Refer to:

- *Textbook* Procedure 7-7 for step-by-step directions
- *Workbook* Appendix A (Medical Practice Reference Material) for physician data

Standards: Complete all steps listed in this skill in _____ minutes with a minimum score of _____. (Time element and accuracy criteria may be given by instructor.)

Time: Start: _____ Completed: _____ Total: _____ minutes

Scoring: One point for each step performed satisfactorily unless otherwise listed or weighted by instructor.

Directions with Performance Evaluation Checklist

Read the following case scenario, abstract information, and complete two requisition forms.

Scenario: An HMO patient, Ted N. Thatcher, comes to the office complaining of neck and right shoulder pain. After an examination, Dr. Fran Practon orders fasting laboratory tests (arthritis profile, uric acid, and urinalysis). Diagnosis is acute cervical arthritis (*ICD-10-CM* code M47.892[*]).

Comprehensive cervical spine x-rays and a complete shoulder series are scheduled for March 4, 20XX, at 11:00 a.m. Diagnosis is acute cervical arthritis and shoulder pain (*ICD-10-CM* code M25.511). Patient to return in 1 week.

Mr. Thatcher is 30 years old, born 5/8/XX. His medical record number is THA1234, Social Security number: XXX-XX-9509; new address: 870 N. Seacrest St., Woodland Hills, XY 12345-0846; telephone number: (555) 987-4589; insurance: HMO Net, 4390 Main Street, Woodland Hills, XY 12345-0846, policy no. 459-0987-0. For this particular managed care plan, the outside services that Dr. Practon ordered do not require preauthorization. Today's date: February 28, 20XX.

1st Attempt	2nd Attempt	3rd Attempt	
_____	_____	_____	Gather materials (equipment and supplies) listed under *Conditions*.
_____	_____	_____	1. Highlight on each form what type of diagnostic tests are to be performed. _____
_____	_____	_____	2. Note the date the patient has agreed upon. _____
_____	_____	_____	3. Write the name of the insurance carrier. _____
_____	_____	_____	4. Telephone the diagnostic facility (ABC Radiology) and schedule the tests. Note the time the tests are scheduled. _____

[*]2017 *International Classification of Diseases, 10th Edition, Clinical Modification*, Professional for Physicians, Optum™ 2016

JOB SKILL 7-7 (*continued*)

___/20   ___/20   ___/20   5. Abstract information from the case scenario and fill in the Laboratory Requisition form; hand the form to the patient and record the information in the medical record.

___/15   ___/15   ___/15   6. Abstract information from the case scenario and fill in the X-Ray Request form; hand to the patient and record information in the medical record.

_____ _____ _____   Complete within specified time.

___/41   ___/41   ___/41   **Total points earned** (To obtain a percentage score, divide the total points earned by the number of points possible.)

Comments:

Evaluator's Signature: _____   **Need to Repeat:** _____

National Curriculum Competency: CAAHEP: Psychomotor:	VI.P.2 ABHES: 7.e

C H A P T E R **8**

Filing Procedures

STOP AND THINK CASE SCENARIOS

Refer to the end of Chapter 8 in the *textbook* for the following scenarios:

- Locate a Mission Record
- Determine Document Types and Filing Systems

EXAM-STYLE REVIEW QUESTIONS

Refer to the end of Chapter 8 in the *textbook*.

Abbreviation and Spelling Review

Read the patient's chart note and write the meanings for the abbreviations following the note. To decode any abbreviations you do not understand or that appear unfamiliar to you, refer to the list of abbreviations in Appendix B of this *Workbook*. Step-by-step directions for this exercise are found in Procedure 1-1 of Chapter 1 in the *textbook*. Medical terms in the chart note are italicized; study them for spelling. Use your medical dictionary to look up their definitions. Your instructor may give a spelling and definition test that includes these words and abbreviations.

DATE	PROGRESS
12-3-20XX	Doris A. Waxman, PC: *occipital* headaches PX: HEENT No *diplopia*, no *tinnitus*. See PI TPR neg. CV: no chest pain, *palpitation*, *orthopnea*, *dyspnea* or exertion, or *hemoptysis*. GI: one episode of *emesis* last night. Some belching & intolerance to fried foods. RUQ abdom pain; no *hematemesis* or *melena*. GU: no frequency or *dysuria*. GYN: no abnormal bleeding. Ordered *oral cholecystography*. Dx: rule out GB disease.
	Fran Practon, MD
	Fran Practon, MD

PC _____   GI _____

PX _____   RUQ _____

HEENT _____   abdom _____

PI _____   GU _____

TPR _____   GYN _____

neg. _____   Dx _____

CV _____   GB _____

Review Questions

Review the objectives, glossary, and chapter information before completing the following review questions.

1. Why is it important for all members of the office staff to follow a general office filing system and obey filing rules? _____

2. When choosing a medical filing system, what must be considered?

   a. _____

   b. _____

   c. _____

   d. _____

   e. _____

   f. _____

   g. _____

3. A collection of electronic files stored on the computer's hard drive or on the Internet is referred to as a _____.

4. What machine is used to create electronic documents from paper copy? _____.

5. What is the HIPAA rule called that safeguards both the physical and technical aspects of electronic security? _____ _____.

6. Name three advantages of using an alphabetical color-coded file system.

   a. _____

   b. _____

   c. _____

7. Name several types of information that may be filed in a subject file.

   a. _____

   b. _____

   c. _____

   d. _____

8. Why is numerical filing considered an indirect method? _____

   _____

   _____

9. Where are numerical filing systems primarily used? _____

_____

10. In a chronological filing system, numbers are used based on _____.

11. Managing files so that information is not lost in a computerized system requires _____.

12. What is the purpose of a tickler file? _____

13. A person's first name is also called the _____ and the last name is the

_____.

14. A married woman may legally write her name in three different ways. Give three examples of the way a name can be written.

    a. _____

    b. _____

    c. _____

15. What considerations should be made when selecting filing equipment?

    a. _____

    b. _____

    c. _____

    d. _____

    e. _____

16. Name the two purposes served by file guides.

    a. _____

    b. _____

17. What steps would you take when a patient's chart cannot be located?

    a. _____

    b. _____

    c. _____

    d. _____

    e. _____

    f. _____

    g. _____

    h. _____

18. To purge files, what two procedures can solve the problem of determining when to transfer patient files from active to inactive status?

    a. _____

    b. _____

19. What electronic technology is used today to convert paper documents into electronic documents for

    storage? _____

Critical Thinking Exercises

State at least two circumstances that might require cross-referencing of names in alphabetical files.

a. _____

b. _____

JOB SKILL 8-1
Determine Filing Units

Name _____ Date _____ Score _____

Performance Objective

Task: Demonstrate knowledge of standard alphabetizing rules as you assemble 50 names and designate filing units.

Conditions: Need:

- Names found in the following exercise
- Pen or pencil

Refer to:

- *Textbook* "Alphabetical Filing Rules" used for indexing
- *Textbook* Procedure 8-4 for step-by-step directions

Standards: Complete all steps listed in this skill in _____ minutes with a minimum score of _____.
(Time element and accuracy criteria may be given by instructor.)

Time: Start: _____ **Completed:** _____ **Total:** _____ minutes

Scoring: One point for each step performed satisfactorily unless otherwise listed or weighted by instructor.

Directions with Performance Evaluation Checklist

Study each name and designate units, numbering each unit 1, 2, 3, and so forth. Use number one for the first unit, number two for the second unit, number three for the third unit, and number four for the fourth unit. Office preference for Practon Medical Group is to file "St." as written and not spell it out, and to file all names of businesses as written. Study the following example before beginning.

EXAMPLE

1st Attempt	2nd Attempt	3rd Attempt	
			Number each unit of name A. Marsha Moore: A. (2) Marsha (3) Moore (1)
_____	_____	_____	Gather materials (equipment and supplies) listed under *Conditions*.
_____	_____	_____	1. Number each unit of name: Rebecca ( ) Rodene ( ) Rochester ( ).
_____	_____	_____	2. Number each unit of name: Wm. ( ) John ( ) Taylor ( ) Kelly ( ).
_____	_____	_____	3. Number each unit of name: Jamie ( ) Trethorn ( ).
_____	_____	_____	4. Number each unit of name: Dan ( ) A. ( ) DeLeon ( ).
_____	_____	_____	5. Number each unit of name: E. ( ) Mary ( ) LeVan ( ).
_____	_____	_____	6. Number each unit of name: Amy ( ) Kay ( ) M'Oeters ( ).
_____	_____	_____	7. Number each unit of name: Shelby ( ) C. ( ) St. John ( ).
_____	_____	_____	8. Number each unit of name: Robert ( ) F. ( ) MacGregor ( ).
_____	_____	_____	9. Number each unit of name: S. ( ) J. ( ) VanderLinder ( ).
_____	_____	_____	10. Number each unit of name: Kelly ( ) Saint ( ) Thomas ( ).
_____	_____	_____	11. Number each unit of name: Priscilla ( ) Ruby ( ) DuMont ( ).
_____	_____	_____	12. Number each unit of name: Peter ( ) deWinter ( ).
_____	_____	_____	13. Number each unit of name: Sister ( ) Mary ( ) Beth ( ).

JOB SKILL 8-1 (*continued*)

_____ _____ _____ 14. Number each unit of name: Mayor ( ) Bill ( ) A. ( ) King ( ).

_____ _____ _____ 15. Number each unit of name: Dr. ( ) John ( ) J. ( ) Jackson ( ).

_____ _____ _____ 16. Number each unit of name: Mary-Kay ( ) deVille ( ).

_____ _____ _____ 17. Number each unit of name: Sji ( ) Mulzono ( ).

_____ _____ _____ 18. Number each unit of name: Mark ( ) Philip-DeGeer ( ).

_____ _____ _____ 19. Number each unit of name: Pope ( ) John ( ) Paul ( ).

_____ _____ _____ 20. Number each unit of name: Maj. ( ) Steve ( ) Royal ( ) Smith ( ).

_____ _____ _____ 21. Number each unit of name: Mrs. ( ) Noreen ( ) J. ( ) Cline ( ).

_____ _____ _____ 22. Number each unit of name: Charles ( ) T. ( ) Lloyd ( ) Jr. ( )

_____ _____ _____ 23. Number each unit of name: Charles ( ) T. ( ) Lloyd ( ) II ( ).

_____ _____ _____ 24. Number each unit of name: Peter ( ) L. ( ) Morrison, ( ) MD ( ).

_____ _____ _____ 25. Number each unit of name: Sarah ( ) May ( ) Dennis-Brit ( ).

_____ _____ _____ 26. Number each unit of name: C. ( ) Ngyume ( ).

_____ _____ _____ 27. Number each unit of name: Paul ( ) Wm. ( ) SeValle ( ).

_____ _____ _____ 28. Number each unit of name: Foster ( ) Memorial ( ) Community ( ) Hospital ( ).

_____ _____ _____ 29. Number each unit of name: Ft. ( ) Benning ( ) Convalescent ( ) Home ( ).

_____ _____ _____ 30. Number each unit of name: A-1 ( ) Pharmacy ( ).

_____ _____ _____ 31. Number each unit of name: American ( ) Medical ( ) Corp ( ).

_____ _____ _____ 32. Number each unit of name: Dr. ( ) Spock's ( ) Clinic ( ).

_____ _____ _____ 33. Number each unit of name: St. ( ) Jude's ( ) Hospital ( ).

_____ _____ _____ 34. Number each unit of name: Russ ( ) Wilder ( ) Ambulance ( ) Service ( ).

_____ _____ _____ 35. Number each unit of name: Mt. ( ) Blanc ( ) Druggist ( ).

_____ _____ _____ 36. Number each unit of name: Century ( ) 21 ( ) Medical ( ) Supply ( ).

_____ _____ _____ 37. Number each unit of name: College ( ) of St. ( ) Catherine ( ).

_____ _____ _____ 38. Number each unit of name: Washington ( ) School, ( ) St. ( ) Paul, ( ) MN ( ).

_____ _____ _____ 39. Number each unit of name: Mary ( ) Cain Pharmacy, ( ) Waco, ( ) TX ( ).

_____ _____ _____ 40. Number each unit of name: Mary ( ) Cain ( ) Pharmacy, ( ) Inc ( ).

_____ _____ _____ 41. Number each unit of name: Riverside ( ) County ( ) Public ( ) Library ( ).

_____ _____ _____ 42. Number each unit of name: St. ( ) Joseph's ( ) Community ( ) Hospital, ( ) Austin, ( ) TX ( ).

_____ _____ _____ 43. Number each unit of name: University ( ) of ( ) California– ( ) Los ( ) Angeles ( ).

_____ _____ _____ 44. Number each unit of name: University ( ) of ( ) California– ( ) Davis ( ).

_____ _____ _____ 45. Number each unit of name: St. ( ) Louis ( ) Publications ( ).

_____ _____ _____ 46. Number each unit of name: Father ( ) Buechner ( ).

_____ _____ _____ 47. Number each unit of name: Sister ( ) Sue ( ) Ellen ( ).

JOB SKILL 8-1 *(continued)*

_____ _____ _____ 48. Number each unit of name: C. ( ) R. ( ) Toll ( ).

_____ _____ _____ 49. Number each unit of name: Rebecca ( ) Toll ( ) (Mrs. John) ( ).

_____ _____ _____ 50. Number each unit of name: Mrs. ( ) John ( ) A. ( ) Peterson ( ).

_____ _____ _____ Complete within specified time.

___/52 ___/52 ___/52 **Total points earned** (To obtain a percentage score, divide the total points earned by the number of points possible.)

Comments:

Evaluator's Signature: _____ **Need to Repeat:** _____

National Curriculum Competency: CAAHEP: Cognitive: VI.C.7; Psychomotor: VI.P.5	ABHES: 7.a

JOB SKILL 8-2
Index and File Names Alphabetically

Name _____ Date _____ Score _____

Performance Objective

Task: Demonstrate knowledge of standardized alphabetizing rules to competently file and retrieve medical records; apply this knowledge as you alphabetize names for class discussion.

Conditions: Need:

- Eighteen groups of names found in the following exercise
- Pen or pencil

Refer to:

- *Textbook* "Alphabetical Filing Rules" used for indexing
- *Textbook* Procedure 8-4 for step-by-step directions

Standards: Complete all steps listed in this skill in _____ minutes with a minimum score of _____. (Time element and accuracy criteria may be given by instructor.)

Time: Start: _____ **Completed:** _____ **Total:** _____ minutes

Scoring: One point for each step performed satisfactorily unless otherwise listed or weighted by instructor.

Directions with Performance Evaluation Checklist

Underline the first, second, and third units of each name to show proper indexing order, placing one line under the surname, two lines under the given name, and three lines under the third name or initial. Then, alphabetize each group of three names in the correct filing order, writing the corresponding letters—in order—in the answer column.

EXAMPLE

Units underlined:	(a) J. T. Jefferson (b) John Thompson (c) Mrs. T. T. Brown (Marsha)
Units in correct order:	(a) Jefferson, J. T. (b) Thompson, John (c) Brown, Marsha (Mrs. T. J.)
Correct filing order: c a b	(c) Brown, Marsha (Mrs. T. J.) (a) Jefferson, J. T. (b) Thompson, John

1st Attempt	2nd Attempt	3rd Attempt	
_____	_____	_____	Gather materials (equipment and supplies) listed under *Conditions*.
____/3	____/3	____/3	1. _____ (a) Henrietta S. Lamar (b) Greta Lee Mason (c) Mary Lou LaMotte
____/3	____/3	____/3	2. _____ (a) Raymond Lorenzana (b) R. Lorenzo (c) Tony Lorenzen
____/3	____/3	____/3	3. _____ (a) Roger N. Stephens (b) Garland N. St. John (c) Robert Sprague
____/3	____/3	____/3	4. _____ (a) Walter E. Johnston (b) Willard L. Johnson (c) Geo. W. Johnstone
____/3	____/3	____/3	5. _____ (a) Hugh M. MacAdoo (b) Bruce T. McCall (c) Robert A. Macall
____/3	____/3	____/3	6. _____ (a) Lt. Margaret Kim (b) Margaret LaForgeaus (c) Mrs. M. LeMaster (Loretta)
____/3	____/3	____/3	7. _____ (a) H. King IV (b) H. M. King Jr. (c) Mrs. H. M. King (Alice)
____/3	____/3	____/3	8. _____ (a) Mrs. Tina Simmons (Leonard) (b) Richard K. Simmons (c) R. K. Simons-Steele
____/3	____/3	____/3	9. _____ (a) J. W. Winn, MD, 1404 Rosealea Rd., Cleveland, Ohio (b) James W. Winn, 1203 Venetta Drive, Cleveland, Ohio (c) J. W. Winn, 18 Maple St., Cleveland, Ohio

JOB SKILL 8-2 (*continued*)

_____/3 _____/3 _____/3 10. _____ (a) Mary Sue Shelton (b) Martha Lee Shelton-Alston
(c) Sheila-Lynn Alston (Mrs. Shelton A.)

_____/3 _____/3 _____/3 11. _____ (a) Willard Champs, 1072 Main St. (b) Willard Champs, 290 Main St.
(c) Wilfred Champs, 10234 Main St.

_____/3 _____/3 _____/3 12. _____ (a) Jas. E. McBean (b) J. L. MacBeen (c) Jason McBean

_____/3 _____/3 _____/3 13. _____ (a) W. L. Arthur-Davis (b) Carolyn Archer (Mrs. David)
(c) Sister Arletta-Marie

_____/3 _____/3 _____/3 14. _____ (a) Grace Ayers (b) A. Joseph Almonzaz (c) Mrs. Anthony Ayers
(Gloria)

_____/3 _____/3 _____/3 15. _____ (a) Norman Gilliam (b) N. Gilliam (c) Mrs. N. R. Gilliam (Norma)

_____/3 _____/3 _____/3 16. _____ (a) Matthew Kuboushek (b) Toshi Kubota (c) I. M. Kuchenberg

_____/3 _____/3 _____/3 17. _____ (a) Dr. Vincent DeLucca (b) Victoria Deems (c) Dr. Carl Deams Jr.

_____/3 _____/3 _____/3 18. _____ (a) Mrs. Loretta Maggio (b) Bokker T. Magallon Sr. (c) B. L. Magill,
Rev.

_____ _____ _____ Complete within specified time.

_____/56 _____/56 _____/56 **Total points earned** (To obtain a percentage score, divide the total points
earned by the number of points possible.)

Comments:

National Curriculum Competency: CAAHEP: Cognitive: VI.C.7; Psychomotor: VI.P.5   ABHES: 7.a

JOB SKILL 8-3
File Patient and Business Names Alphabetically

Name _____ Date _____ Score _____

Performance Objective

Task: Sort patient names and business names in alphabetical order according to standardized alphabetical filing rules. Note: This is an advanced exercise.

Conditions: Need:

- Groups of names found in the following exercise
- Pen or pencil

  Refer to:

- *Textbook* "Alphabetical Filing Rules" used for indexing
- *Textbook* Procedure 8-4 for step-by-step directions

Standards: Complete all steps listed in this skill in _____ minutes with a minimum score of _____.
(Time element and accuracy criteria may be given by instructor.)

Time: **Start:** _____ **Completed:** _____ **Total:** _____ minutes

Scoring: One point for each step performed satisfactorily unless otherwise listed or weighted by instructor.

Directions with Performance Evaluation Checklist

After each group of four names, indicate by letter the order in which the names would be arranged in a file.

1st Attempt	2nd Attempt	3rd Attempt		
_____	_____	_____		Gather materials (equipment and supplies) listed under *Conditions*.
____/4	____/4	____/4	1. _____	a. Mrs. Allene Baker
				b. A. Baker
				c. A. Barker, MD
				d. Dr. Barker
____/4	____/4	____/4	2. _____	a. The Apple Advertising Co.
				b. Apple-Cornwall, Inc.
				c. Appling Health Care
				d. Allan Applesey Corp.
____/4	____/4	____/4	3. _____	a. Brother Brian Advertising
				b. The Bonita Rehab Facility
				c. B and B Clinic
				d. Bonita Rd. Care
____/4	____/4	____/4	4. _____	a. Larue-McGuire Canyon Hospital
				b. Los Angeles Community Care
				c. Laruem Medical Clinic
				d. Las Robles Medical Center
____/4	____/4	____/4	5. _____	a. Fortieth St. Convalescent Center
				b. The Forrest Hospital
				c. The Frew-Forrest Medical Group
				d. Forrest Medical Facility

JOB SKILL 8-3 (*continued*)

____/4 ____/4 ____/4 6. _____ a. Professor Sam A. Zimmer
                                                            b. Zimmer-Kliev Agency
                                                            c. Prof. A. Zimmer
                                                            d. Z and Z Druggists

____/4 ____/4 ____/4 7. _____ a. Robin Persy-Doerr
                                                            b. Philip Persico Retirement Care
                                                            c. Poinsettia Residential Care
                                                            d. Persicona-Philips Mortuary

____/4 ____/4 ____/4 8. _____ a. Mcdonald, Calvin
                                                            b. MacDonald, Carl, MD
                                                            c. Macdonald, C. A.
                                                            d. Dr. McDermott

____/4 ____/4 ____/4 9. _____ a. Tyler-Hill Medical Assn
                                                            b. Mark Tyler-Hill Mortuary
                                                            c. The Pleasant Hills Pharmacy
                                                            d. Phyllis G. Hills

____/4 ____/4 ____/4 10. _____ a. Kevin St. Mann Jr.
                                                            b. Chauncey A. Southern
                                                            c. Kevin St. Mann
                                                            d. Southwest St. Pharmaceuticals

_____ _____ _____ Complete within specified time.

____/42 ____/42 ____/42 **Total points earned** (To obtain a percentage score, divide the total points earned by the number of points possible.)

Comments:

Evaluator's Signature: _____ **Need to Repeat:** _____

National Curriculum Competency: CAAHEP: Cognitive: VI.C.7; Psychomotor: VI.P.5   ABHES: 7.a

JOB SKILL 8-4

Index Names on File Folder Labels and Arrange File Cards in Alphabetical Order

Name _____ Date _____ Score _____

Performance Objective

Task: Key names on file labels uniformly in correct indexing order. Affix labels to file cards or type names on file cards and alphabetize.

Conditions: Need:

- Computer with Internet connection
- Online Form 18, 19, and 20 (file labels) located at www.cengagebrain.com with student resources
- Sixty file folder labels (optional)
- Sixty 3" by 5" index cards (or slips of paper)

Refer to:

- *Textbook* "Alphabetical Filing Rules" used for indexing
- *Textbook* Procedure 8-4 for step-by-step directions

Standards: Complete all steps listed in this skill in _____ minutes with a minimum score of _____. (Time element and accuracy criteria may be given by instructor.)

Time: **Start:** _____ **Completed:** _____ **Total:** _____ minutes

Scoring: One point for each step performed satisfactorily unless otherwise listed or weighted by instructor.

Directions with Performance Evaluation Checklist

Dr. Practon has asked you to key or type patient names on file folder labels, as if they were to be attached to folder tabs, in proper indexing order. These can be printed neatly by hand using the forms provided, typed using a typewriter, or keyed and printed from a computer on actual file folder labels. Affix labels to or type names at the top right of index cards and arrange in alphabetical order. These may be spread out on your desk, or a small recipe box may be used for sorting. Note: *There are several options for completing this job skill. Please read through all the steps prior to starting and determine if you will be using the worksheet (forms) provided for file labels or actual file folder labels and index cards.*

1st Attempt	2nd Attempt	3rd Attempt	
_____	_____	_____	Gather materials (equipment and supplies) listed under *Conditions*.
____/30	____/30	____/30	1. Use the labels on Forms 18, 19, and 20 as a worksheet and write (in pencil) each patient's name in the correct indexing order. Check with the instructor if you have problems determining units and indexing sequence. If you are not using actual file folder labels for this job skill, you may use a blank sheet of paper for the worksheet and these labels for printing or typing patient names. They will then be cut up into slips of paper.
_____	_____	_____	2. Use blank labels marked "X" at the end of Form 20 for any names that need to be cross-referenced; these may vary per student.
____/30	____/30	____/30	3. Key or type names uniformly on file folder labels in indexing order starting at the left margin. At the right margin, key or type the reference number that appears by the patient's name as if it were an account number.

JOB SKILL 8-4 (*continued*)

EXAMPLE—FILE LABEL

> 1. Walter Louis McDougall
>   McDougall, Walter Louis   Acct. #1

____/30 ____/30 ____/30   4. Affix labels to index cards (top right), or key/type each name and number at the top of a card.

____/30 ____/30 ____/30   5. Alphabetize all cards or slips.

____/10 ____/10 ____/10   6. Complete an answer sheet by either listing the account numbers in the order they were filed or keying each name in the sequence you have determined.

EXAMPLE—ANSWER SHEET

> 34. Albert, Frank
> 17. *Benjamin, Thomas
> 57. Bennett, C. Richard

_____   _____   _____   Complete within specified time.

____/133 ____/133 ____/133   **Total points earned** (To obtain a percentage score, divide the total points earned by the number of points possible.)

Comments:

Evaluator's Signature: _____ **Need to Repeat:** _____

National Curriculum Competency: CAAHEP: Cognitive: VI.C.7; Psychomotor: VI.P.5, 6   ABHES: 7.a

JOB SKILL 8-5
Color-Code File Cards

Name _____ Date _____ Score _____

Performance Objective

Task: Color-code 60 file cards.

Conditions: Need:
- File index cards from Job Skill 8-4
- Highlight pens (orange, red, green, blue, and violet)

Refer to:
- *Textbook* section on colored labels
- *Textbook* Figures 8-3 and 8-10 to view color-coded labels

Standards: Complete all steps listed in this skill in _____ minutes with a minimum score of _____.
(Time element and accuracy criteria may be given by instructor.)

Time: Start: _____ Completed: _____ Total: _____ minutes

Scoring: One point for each step performed satisfactorily unless otherwise listed or weighted by instructor.

Directions with Performance Evaluation Checklist

Dr. Practon may ask you to add color coding to the medical office filing system to enhance the speed of filing and retrieval. When a file is placed in a cabinet or drawer, or a card in a box, alphabetical dividers will indicate the first letter of the first filing unit. Then, the names are filed according to the color code of the *second* letter of the last name.

1st Attempt	2nd Attempt	3rd Attempt	
_____	_____	_____	Gather materials (equipment and supplies) listed under *Conditions*.
___/60	___/60	___/60	1. Highlight the top edge of each 3" by 5" index card by color coding the *second* letter in the first unit of each name. Use the color guide in the following box. To help you remember the five divisions of the alphabetical system, notice that the first letter of each of the five groups is a vowel except for the last group, which begins with the letter "r."

If the second letter of the patient's surname is:	The tab guide color is:
a, b, c, or d	orange
e, f, g, or h	red
i, j, k, l, m, or n	green
o, p, or q	blue
r, s, t, u, v, w, x, y, or z	violet

1st	2nd	3rd	
_____	_____	_____	Complete within specified time.
___/62	___/62	___/62	**Total points earned** (To obtain a percentage score, divide the total points earned by the number of points possible.)

JOB SKILL 8-5 (*continued*)

Comments:

Evaluator's Signature: _____ **Need to Repeat:** _____

National Curriculum Competency: CAAHEP: Cognitive: VI.C.7; Psychomotor: VI.P.5, 6   ABHES: 7.a

Medical Records

STOP AND THINK CASE SCENARIOS

Refer to the end of Chapter 9 in the *textbook* for the following scenarios:

- Physician Roles and Titles
- Chart Documentation

EXAM-STYLE REVIEW QUESTIONS

Refer to the end of Chapter 9 in the *textbook*.

Abbreviation and Spelling Review

Read the patient's chart note and write the meanings for the abbreviations following the note. To decode any abbreviations you do not understand or that appear unfamiliar to you, refer to the list of abbreviations in Appendix B of this *Workbook*. Step-by-step directions for this exercise are in Procedure 1-1 of Chapter 1 in the *textbook*. Medical terms in the chart note are italicized; study them for spelling. Use your medical dictionary to look up their definitions. Your instructor may give a spelling and definition test that includes these words and abbreviations.

Elizabeth A. Warner

November 16, 20XX CC: *constipation*, *rectal* bleeding & pain after BM. CPX reveals int & ext *hemorrhoids*. BP 150/95. *Sigmoidoscopy* to 15 cm. Rx: adv outpatient surgery for removal of hemorrhoids and fistula repair. Dg: bleeding hemorrhoids, int & ext; anal *fistula*; HBP. Will call pt when surgery is scheduled.

Gerald Practon, MD
Gerald Practon, MD

CC _____   Cm _____

BM _____   Rx _____

CPX _____   Adv _____

int _____   Dg _____

ext _____   HBP _____

BP _____   Pt _____

Review Questions

Review the objectives, glossary, and chapter information before completing the following review questions.

1. List five reasons for keeping medical records.

   a. _____

   b. _____

   c. _____

   d. _____

   e. _____

2. Name two laws that were established to permit patient access to medical records.

   a. _____

   b. _____

3. List five disadvantages of a paper-based medical record system.

   a. _____

   b. _____

   c. _____

   d. _____

   e. _____

4. Define "meaningful use." _____

   _____

5. What equipment is necessary to digitize medical records when converting from a paper-based system to

   an electronic-based system? _____

6. Why are flow sheets, charts, and graphs used in the medical record? _____

   _____

   _____

   _____

7. State the differences between an electronic medical record (EMR) and an electronic health record (EHR) practice management system. _____

_____

_____

_____

_____

8. What were the most common features used in an EHR system according to doctors?

    a. _____

    b. _____

    c. _____

    d. _____

    e. _____

    f. _____

9. Name several ways a health care provider can document clinical findings in an EMR.

    a. _____

    b. _____

    c. _____

    d. _____

10. Name five advantages of using a medical record organizational system such as the problem-oriented medical record (POMR).

    a. _____

    b. _____

    c. _____

    d. _____

    e. _____

11. Name the most common paper-based management system. _____

_____

12. Besides keying information directly into the computer, a medical assistant acting as a "scribe" can enter data from a _____ or _____, use a _____, or _____ or _____ can be completed as the physician narrates findings and recommendations.

13. True or False. All medical assistants can perform computerized provider order entry (CPOE) into an EHR system. _____

14. Match the physician titles in the left column with the definitions in the right column and insert the correct letter in the blank space.

_____ attending physician   a. provider who sends the patient for testing

_____ consulting physician   b. provider whose opinion is requested

_____ ordering physician   c. medical staff member who is legally responsible for care of patient

_____ referring physician   d. provider who renders service to patient

_____ treating or performing physician   e. provider directing selection, preparation, or administration of tests, medication, or treatment

15. Since all documenters must sign their name to the portions of the medical record that they documented, when can initials legally be used? _____

_____

_____

16. Which is more secure, an electronic signature or a digital signature? _____

_____

17. True or False. EMRs follow the same documentation requirements as a paper-based system. _____

18. Using the "Documentation Guidelines," state briefly what is said about the following.

a. Patient encounters: _____

b. The assessment: _____

c. Risk factors: _____

d. Diagnostic and ancillary services: _____

e. Abbreviations: _____

f. Procedure and diagnostic codes: _____

g. Staff members assisting physician: _____

h. Patient education and instructions: _____

19. List items that should be documented in the medical record for skin lacerations and lesions.

a. _____

b. _____

c. _____

d. _____

e. _____

20. List the four basic elements of a patient history and their abbreviations.

a. _____

b. _____

c. _____

d. _____

21. If a patient is seen in the office, a history and physical is dictated, and then the patient is admitted to the hospital, can the dictated history and physical be used for the hospital documentation? _____

_____

_____

22. Name ways in which the physician collects objective data during a physical examination.

    a. _____

    b. _____

    c. _____

    d. _____

23. Name the three technical elements needed in a progress note.

    a. _____

    b. _____

    c. _____

24. List what the abbreviations stand for in the following documentation format and briefly describe each term.

    a. S: _____

    b. O: _____

    c. A: _____

    d. P: _____

25. Name three common medical reports that appear in patient records.

    a. _____

    b. _____

    c. _____

26. Name two main types of audits and briefly describe their differences.

    a. _____

    b. _____

Critical Thinking Exercises

1. The following phrases appeared on a history and physical. Place an *S* after those that are *subjective* and an *O* after those considered *objective*.

    a. Patient complains of feeling faint   _____

    b. BP 120/80   _____

    c. Headache   _____

    d. Skin shows no rashes   _____

    e. Patient denies chest pain   _____

    f. Mother L&W   _____

    g. No inguinal hernia   _____

    h. Heart tones normal   _____

    i. No masses palpable   _____

    j. Patient had an episode of nausea   _____

    k. Patient feels lethargic   _____

    l. Temperature 101.1°F   _____

   m. Blood in stool   _____

    n. Stomachache   _____

    o. Leg cramping   _____

    p. Blurred vision   _____

    q. Vision 20/40 R. eye   _____

    r. Hematocrit (HCT) 40%   _____

    s. Pap smear class II   _____

    t. Heel pain   _____

    u. Lump in left breast   _____

    v. Joint stiffness   _____

   w. X-ray showed fracture R. ulna   _____

    x. Urinalysis negative   _____

    y. Acne   _____

    z. Patient feels tired all the time   _____

2. Pair with another student and role-play the following scenario to practice documentation skills. Use the date, Friday, July 30, 20XX, and correct abbreviations.

   Participants—two students: Patient and receptionist

   An established patient presents at the reception desk of Practon Medical Group Inc. with no appointment. He or she just walked in and wants to be seen as soon as possible. The schedule is busy, so the receptionist asks the office manager what to do. The office manager advises the receptionist to take the chief complaint and vital signs.

   Patient: Make up a reason for being there and communicate it to the receptionist.

   Your blood pressure is 180/92 and your weight is 185 pounds.

   Receptionist: Record the chief complaint and vital signs.

   _____

   _____

   _____

3. Dr. Practon has had a busy morning and is ready to go to a lunch meeting. He has just finished dictating and approaches the medical assistant with all the morning charts. He asks the assistant to schedule the following tests for the patients who have been seen. Schedule all tests and procedures (making up the dates and times), and then document them in the patients' medical records. Use critical thinking skills to instruct the patient according to each test or procedure protocol.

   Patient A: Magnetic resonance imaging of the brain at College Hospital for headaches and visual changes—sometime next week.

   _____

   _____

   _____

Patient B: Pulmonary function test at College Hospital for asthma—sometime next week.

_____

_____

_____

Patient C: Mammogram at the Women's Clinic for breast screening—no hurry.

_____

_____

_____

Patient D: Blood culture at College Hospital for unresolved fever of unknown origin, lethargy, and malaise—immediately.

_____

_____

_____

Patient E: Chest x-ray at College Hospital for chest congestion, rule out pneumonia—as soon as possible.

_____

_____

_____

Patient F: Five-hour glucose tolerance test at College Hospital for elevated fasting blood sugar and frequency of urination—sometime next week.

_____

_____

_____

JOB SKILL 9-1
Prepare a Patient Record and Insert Progress Notes

Name _____ Date _____ Score _____

Performance Objective

Task: Complete a patient record form with demographic information and progress notes; type a file card and file folder label.

Conditions: Need:

- Computer with Internet connection
- Online Form 21 (patient record) located at www.cengagebrain.com with student resources
- One file folder
- One file folder label
- One 3" by 5" file card

Standards: Complete all steps listed in this skill in _____ minutes with a minimum score of _____. (Time element and accuracy criteria may be given by instructor.)

Time: **Start:** _____ **Completed:** _____ **Total:** _____ minutes

Scoring: One point for each step performed satisfactorily unless otherwise listed or weighted by instructor.

Directions with Performance Evaluation Checklist

Today is October 24, 20XX, and new patient Wayne G. Weather has come in as an emergency case; he was hurt on the job and has an injury to his lower back. He completed the patient information form (see Figure 7-1 in *Workbook* Job Skill 7-5).

Complete the demographic information on the patient record form (21), file folder label, and file card. His wife, Nancy Weather, is a receptionist. His patient record number is 1180, which is keyed in the right corner of the record, file card, and file label. Use the detailed information listed in the directions to Job Skill 7-5 pertaining to Mr. Weather's condition, and enter the progress notes for today and the day of his hospital admit.

1st Attempt	2nd Attempt	3rd Attempt	
_____	_____	_____	Gather materials (equipment and supplies) listed under *Conditions*.
____/2	____/2	____/2	1. Complete the file folder label with patient name and medical record number; affix to the file folder.
____/2	____/2	____/2	2. Complete the file card with patient name and medical record number.
____/25	____/25	____/25	3. Key the patient record number and demographic information on the top portion of the patient record.
____/15	____/15	____/15	4. Key the progress note for 10/24/20XX noting emergency office visit, on-the-job injury, diagnosis, surgical scheduling information, and preadmission testing.
____/5	____/5	____/5	5. Key the note for 10/28/20XX regarding his hospital admit.
____/4	____/4	____/4	6. Proofread the form, checking capitalization, punctuation, spelling, and spacing.
____/2	____/2	____/2	7. Finalize the record for the correct physician's signature.

JOB SKILL 9-1 (*continued*)

_____ _____ _____   Complete within specified time.

___/57 ___/57 ___/57   **Total points earned** (To obtain a percentage score, divide the total points earned by the number of points possible.)

Comments:

Evaluator's Signature: _____   **Need to Repeat:** _____

National Curriculum Competency: CAAHEP: Cognitive: VI.C.3; Psychomotor: V.P.3; 11; X.P.3   ABHES: 4.a, b.2; 7.a

JOB SKILL 9-2
Prepare a Patient Record and Format Chart Notes

Name _____ Date _____ Score _____

Performance Objective

Task: Format and complete a patient record, label a file folder, and type a file card.

Conditions: Need:

- Computer with Internet connection
- Online Form 22 (patient record) located at www.cengagebrain.com with student resources
- One file folder
- One file label
- One 3" by 5" file card

Refer to:

- *Textbook* Figure 9-7 for chart note example

Standards: Complete all steps listed in this skill in _____ minutes with a minimum score of _____.
(Time element and accuracy criteria may be given by instructor.)

Time: **Start:** _____ **Completed:** _____ **Total:** _____ minutes

Scoring: One point for each step performed satisfactorily unless otherwise listed or weighted by
instructor.

Directions with Performance Evaluation Checklist

You will be preparing a patient record, filling in the top portion with demographic information and the bottom portion with progress notes. Refer to Figure 9-7 in the *textbook* for an example of the charting format using the chief complaint (CC), physical examination (PE), diagnosis (DX), and treatment plan (Plan) as headings for the appropriate lines.

1st Attempt	2nd Attempt	3rd Attempt	
_____	_____	_____	Gather materials (equipment and supplies) listed under *Conditions*.
____/2	____/2	____/2	1. Use the name Krista Lee Carlisle and medical record number 1181. Complete a file folder label; affix to file folder.
____/2	____/2	____/2	2. Type a 3" by 5" file card with patient name and medical record number at top right.
____/25	____/25	____/25	3. Complete the top portion of the medical record (Form 22) for Krista Carlisle using your own personal information, or interview a person in class or someone at home to obtain this information (address, telephone number, insurance name, and so forth).
____/5	____/5	____/5	4. Complete the bottom portion of the medical record using the data found in *Workbook* Figure 9-1. Use a format similar to that found in *textbook* Figure 9-7 and abbreviate medical terms when appropriate.
____/10	____/10	____/10	5. Make a separate entry for Dr. Fran Practon's examination on October 25, 20XX.
____/10	____/10	____/10	6. Make a separate entry for the follow-up visit on October 28, 20XX.
____/10	____/10	____/10	7. Make a separate entry for the follow-up visit on November 15, 20XX.
____/4	____/4	____/4	8. Make a separate entry for the canceled appointment.

JOB SKILL 9-2 (*continued*)

_____   _____   _____   Complete within specified time.

___/70   ___/70   ___/70   **Total points earned** (To obtain a percentage score, divide the total points earned by the number of points possible.)

10/25/XX   Height: 5'10". Weight: 222 pounds. Blood pressure 140/60. Chief complaint: Patient complained of several weeks' history of fatigue, lack of appetite, and headache; has lost approximately 8 pounds since October 1, 20XX, denies smoking. Averages three beers a day. On examination liver appears somewhat enlarged, tender on palpitation. All other systems appear normal. No apparent jaundice. Urinalysis findings: dark amber urine, bilirubinemia and proteinuria 2+. Patient sent to laboratory for blood workup; complete blood count, chemistry panel, liver panel, hepatitis panel. Diagnosis: hepatomegaly, rule out hepatitis. Patient instructed to adhere to strict bed rest, low-fat, high-carbohydrate diet. Disability for 2 weeks; instructions given. Return to the office in three days. Call sooner if symptoms increase, Tylenol tablets every 4 to 6 hours for headache.

Fran Practon, MD
Fran Practon, MD

10/28/XX   Weight: 220 pounds. Blood pressure 128/64.Chief complaint: Follow-up visit for laboratory results. Definitive diagnosis: hepatitis A. All other laboratory results normal. Patient to increase disability to 8 weeks, mild activity as tolerated. Instructions to use no alcohol, continue same diet, fluids as tolerated. Tylenol as needed. Call office immediately if unable to tolerate fluids or diet. Return to office in 1 week.

Fran Practon, MD
Fran Practon, MD

1/15/XX   Weight: 224 pounds. Blood pressure 130/66. Chief complaint: Follow-up visit. Patient states "Is feeling much better," tolerating diet and fluids, good weight gain. On examination, no tenderness on palpitation of abdomen. Urinalysis: Clear yellow urine, protein-trace. Patient to follow up in 2 weeks. Continue modified activity as tolerated. Call if symptoms increase.

Fran Practon, MD
Fran Practon, MD

12/03/XX   Pt called to cancel appointment (3:00 p.m.); did not reschedule.

Margaret Dun, MA
Marqaret Dun, MA

FIGURE 9-1

Comments:

Evaluator's Signature: _____   **Need to Repeat:** _____

National Curriculum Competency: CAAHEP: Cognitive: VI.C.3; Psychomotor: V.P.11; X.P.3   ABHES 4.a, b.2; 7.a

JOB SKILL 9-3
Correct a Medical Record

Name _____ Date _____ Score _____

Performance Objective

Task: Make a correction on a medical record.

Conditions: Need:

          • Patient medical record for Krista Lee Carlisle (No. 1181 from Job Skill 9-2)

          Refer to:

          • *Textbook* Procedure 9-3 for step-by-step directions

          • *Textbook* Figure 9-5 for an illustration

Standards: Complete all steps listed in this skill in _____ minutes with a minimum score of _____.
          (Time element and accuracy criteria may be given by instructor.)

Time: **Start:** _____ **Completed:** _____ **Total:** _____ minutes

Scoring: One point for each step performed satisfactorily unless otherwise listed or weighted by
          instructor.

Directions with Performance Evaluation Checklist

On October 28, 20XX, Dr. Fran Practon indicated the patient would be disabled for eight weeks. On November 15, she realized she should have indicated the disability for six weeks. Correct the medical record.

1st Attempt	2nd Attempt	3rd Attempt	
_____	_____	_____	Gather materials (equipment and supplies) listed under *Conditions*.
___/2	___/2	___/2	1. Make the necessary change on the patient record by crossing out the incorrect entry ("~~X 8 weeks~~").
___/2	___/2	___/2	2. Handwrite, in ink, the correct entry above the words "~~X 8 weeks~~."
___/4	___/4	___/4	3. In the margin, write the word "correction," your initials, and the date you are making the correction.
_____	_____	_____	Complete within specified time.
___/10	___/10	___/10	**Total points earned** (To obtain a percentage score, divide the total points earned by the number of points possible.)

Comments:

Evaluator's Signature: _____ **Need to Repeat:** _____

National Curriculum Competency: CAAHEP: Psychomotor: V.P.3, 11; X.P.3   ABHES: 4.a; b.2; 7.a

JOB SKILL 9-4
Abstract from a Medical Record

Name _____ Date _____ Score _____

Performance Objective

Task: Abstract information from a patient record to answer questions and fill in a medical record abstract form.

Conditions: Need:

  • Patient medical record no. 1181 for Krista Lee Carlisle from Job Skill 9-2

  • Computer with Internet connection

  • Online Form 23 (medical record abstract) located at www.cengagebrain.com with student resources

  • Pen or pencil

  Refer to:

  • *Textbook* Procedure 9-4 for step-by-step directions

Standards: Complete all steps listed in this skill in _____ minutes with a minimum score of _____. (Time element and accuracy criteria may be given by instructor.)

Time: **Start:** _____ **Completed:** _____ **Total:** _____ minutes

Scoring: One point for each step performed satisfactorily unless otherwise listed or weighted by instructor.

Directions with Performance Evaluation Checklist

1st Attempt	2nd Attempt	3rd Attempt	
_____	_____	_____	Gather materials (equipment and supplies) listed under *Conditions*.
___/25	___/25	___/25	1. Abstract information from the medical record (No. 1181) and answer each question on the abstract form; complete the form.
_____	_____	_____	Complete within specified time.
___/27	___/27	___/27	**Total points earned** (To obtain a percentage score, divide the total points earned by the number of points possible.)

Comments:

Evaluator's Signature: _____   **Need to Repeat:** _____

National Curriculum Competency: CAAHEP: Psychomotor: V.P.3   ABHES: 4.a, b.2; 7.a

JOB SKILL 9-5

Prepare a History and Physical (H&P) Report

Name _____ Date _____ Score _____

Performance Objective

Task: Complete a patient record with demographic information, key a H&P report, prepare a file folder with file label, type a 3" by 5" file card, and print two copies or make a photocopy of the H&P report.

Conditions: Need:

- Computer with Internet connection
- Online Form 24 (patient record) located at www.cengagebrain.com with student resources
- Printer or photocopy machine
- *Workbook* Figure 9-2 (patient information form for Sun Low Chung)
- *Workbook* Figure 9-3 (history and physical data)
- One file folder
- One file folder label
- One file card (3" by 5")
- Two sheets of 8½" by 11" white paper

Refer to:

- *Textbook* Figures 9-6A and 9-6B for H&P format examples

Standards: Complete all steps listed in this skill in _____ minutes with a minimum score of _____. (Time element and accuracy criteria may be given by instructor.)

Time: Start: _____ Completed: _____ Total: _____ minutes

Scoring: One point for each step performed satisfactorily unless otherwise listed or weighted by instructor.

Directions with Performance Evaluation Checklist

You will be completing the demographic information on a patient record for Sun Low Chung and keying the history and physical examination in report form on separate paper.

1st Attempt	2nd Attempt	3rd Attempt	
_____	_____	_____	Gather materials (equipment and supplies) listed under *Conditions*.
_____	_____	_____	1. Prepare a file folder label for Sun Low Chung with medical record no. 1182; affix to the file folder.
_____	_____	_____	2. Prepare a 3" by 5" file card for Sun Low Chung.
____/20	____/20	____/20	3. Use Sun Low Chung's patient information form (*Workbook* Figure 9-2) to key his patient record number and demographic information on the top portion of the patient record (Form 24).
_____	_____	_____	4. Read the H&P in *Workbook* Figure 9-3.
____/3	____/3	____/3	5. Highlight the proper headings and subheadings that will be used when keying the data in a history and physical examination format (see *textbook* Figures 9-6A and 9-6B for examples).
_____	_____	_____	6. Insert patient name and medical record number, and then date the report using current dates as dictated and transcribed dates.
_____	_____	_____	7. Key in full block style.

JOB SKILL 9-5 (*continued*)

_____	_____	_____	8. Set margins so they are even, equal, and of correct size.
___/20	___/20	___/20	9. Key data in using proper history and physical format. Note: You will not be using the bottom portion of the patient record (Form 24) for this patient because a complete H&P report is being prepared for the medical record; reference it in the area of the progress notes.
___/15	___/15	___/15	10. Insert main topic headings and correct paragraphing.
___/7	___/7	___/7	11. Insert subtopic headings.
___/4	___/4	___/4	12. Insert capitalization, punctuation, tab stops, and correct spacing.
___/4	___/4	___/4	13. Insert page 2 heading.
___/3	___/3	___/3	14. Place a signature line at the end of H&P; Dr. Gerald Practon is the physician.
_____	_____	_____	15. Insert the typist's identifying signoff data for the H&P.
___/2	___/2	___/2	16. Proofread the H&P report for spelling and typographical errors.
___/2	___/2	___/2	17. Finalize the document for the physician to review and sign.
_____	_____	_____	18. Print two copies or make a photocopy of the completed H&P report.
_____	_____	_____	Complete within specified time.
___/90	___/90	___/90	**Total points earned** (To obtain a percentage score, divide the total points earned by the number of points possible.)

Comments:

JOB SKILL 9-5 *(continued)*

Insurance cards copied ☐
Date: __10/25/XX__

Patient Registration
Information
Please PRINT AND complete ALL sections below!

Account # : _____
Insurance # : _____
Co-Payment: $ _____

Is your condition a result of a work injury? YES (NO)   An auto accident? YES (NO)   Date of injury: _____

PATIENT'S PERSONAL INFORMATION Marital Status: ☐ Single ☑ Married ☐ Divorced ☐ Widowed Sex: ☑ Male ☐ Female

Name: _____Chung_____ _____Sun_____ _____Low_____
_{last name} _{first name} _{initial}

Street address: ___2375 Laney Street___ (Apt #____) City: _Woodland Hills_ State: _XY_ Zip: _12345_

Home phone: (555) 278-6135   Work phone: (555) 271-4811   Social Security # _XXX_ - _XX_ - _6712_

Date of Birth: _5_ / _20_ / _45_ Driver's License: (State & Numebr) _6-0065-178_
_{month} _{day} _{year}

Employer / Name of School _Civil Service Maintenance_   ☐ Full Time ☐ Part Time

Spouse's Name: ___Chung___ ___Song___ ___Su___ Spouse's Work phone: (555) 279 4827
_{last name} _{first name} _{initial}

How do you wish to be addressed? _____ Social Security # _____ - _____ - _____

PATIENT'S / RESPONSIBLE PARTY INFORMATION

Responsible party: _____ Date of Birth: _____

Relationship to Patient: ☐ Self ☐ Spouse ☐ Other _____ Social Security # _____ - _____ - _____

Responsible party's home phone: (____) _____ Work phone: (____) _____

    Address: _____ (Apt # ____) City: _____ State: _____ Zip: _____

Employer's name: _____ Phone number: (____) _____

    Address: _____ City: _____ State: _____ Zip: _____

    Your occupation: _____

Spouse's Employer's name: _____ Spouse's Work phone: (____) _____

    Address: _____ City: _____ State: _____ Zip: _____

PATIENT'S INSURANCE INFORMATION Please present insurance cards to receptionist.

PRIMARY insurance company's name: ____Blue Shield____

Insurance address: ___2751 Courntney St.___ City: _Woodland Hills_ State: _XY_ Zip: _12345_

Name of insured: _____ Date of Birth: _____ Relationship to insured: ☐ Self ☐ Spouse ☐ Other ☐ Child

Insurance ID number: ___27894B___ Group number: _____

SECONDARY insurance company's name: _____

Insurance address: _____ City: _____ State: _____ Zip: _____

Name of insured: _____ Date of Birth: _____ Relationship to insured: ☐ Self ☐ Spouse ☐ Other ☐ Child

Insurance ID number: _____ Group number: _____

Check if appropriate: ☐ Medigap policy ☐ Retiree coverage

PATIENT'S REFERRAL INFORMATION   (please circle one)

Referred by: _____ If referred by a friend, may we thank her or him? YES NO

Name(s) of other physician(s) who care for you: _____
_____

EMERGENCY CONTACT

Name of person not living with you: _Pat Chung_ Relationship: _brother_

Address: ___2851 Laney St___ City: _Woodland Hills_ State: _XY_ Zip: _12345_

Phone number (home): (555) 278-7812   Phone number (work): (____) _____

Assignment of Benefits • Financial Agreement   _Gerald Practon_

I hereby give lifetime authorization for payment of insurance benefits to be made directly to _____ , and any assisting physicians for services rendered. I understand that I am financially responsible for all charges whether or not they are covered by insurance. In the event of default, I agree to pay all costs of collection, and reasonable attorney's fees. I hereby authorize this healthcare provider to release all information necessary to secure the payment of benefits.

I further agree that a photocopy of this agreement shall be as valid as the original.

Sun Low Chung

Date: _____ Your Signature: _____

Method of Payment: ☐ Cash ☐ Check ☐ Credit Card

FORM # 58-8424 • BIBBERO SYSTEMS, INC. • PETALUMA, CA. • TO ORDER CALL TOLL FREE : 800-BIBBERO (800-242-2376) • FAX (800) 242-9330 © 7/94

PATIENT REGISTRATION

FIGURE 9-2

JOB SKILL 9-5 (*continued*)

Sun Low Chung

History. Chief complaint. Palpitations for 1 week. Present illness. This patient has had known hypertension for 4 years. He has been taking Serpasil 0.25 mg daily. About 1 month ago, the medication was changed to Dyazide 250 mg, one tablet per day. Since that time, the patient has felt more nervous and anxious, with occasional chest tightness. One week ago the patient noted some skipped heartbeats occurring in the evening. There were no other associated symptoms and no history of paroxysmal nocturnal dyspnea, orthopnea, or ankle edema. Palpitation subsided spontaneously but recurred the following night, with a fast throbbing sensation in his right ear. He was seen by Dr. Chan 2 weeks later and had a chest x-ray and cardiac enzymes done. These were normal values. An electrocardiogram showed normal sinus rhythm, with nonspecific ST abnormalities. He experiences palpitations in the evening. The patient has been asked to avoid any strenuous exercise and to stay at home until he is seen by the undersigned physician. Past, family, and social history. The patient was born in Hankow, China, but has lived in the United States since 1952. He has worked in the Air Force and airplane industry but lately is working for civil service at Port Davis. He has been subjected to some work pressure recently. There was no history of coronary artery disease, heart murmurs, rheumatic fever, or joint problems in childhood. Malaria in his youth in China. Hypothyroidism diagnosed about 10 years ago, and he has been on thyroid 1 grain q.d. Operations none. Allergies none. Medication as stated above, and Valium 5 milligrams one b.i.d. to t.i.d. p.r.n., Thyroid 1 grain q.d. Social history. The patient smoked one pack of cigarettes per day for 10 years but has discontinued for about 15 years. He does not drink. He consumes about two cups of coffee per day and very little tea. The family history. Most of the family members were separated during the war, and their health conditions are not known. Mother died from an unknown illness at the age of 35. The patient has two children, 36 and 27, both in good health. No known diabetes, hypertension, or heart problems in the family. The review of systems. General. No recent weight gain or weight loss. No unusual fatigue. No recent fevers. The patient has myopia in both eyes. Glasses have not been checked for the past 5 years, and distant vision is not good. EENT. Negative. CV/R. As in PI. No history of hemoptysis or chronic cough. GI. Negative. GU. Nocturia once a night for many years. CNS. No history of headache, syncope, or light-headedness. No history of paralysis. MS. No history of joint problems. Physical examination. General. This patient is an elderly Asian male in no acute distress. Blood pressure in right arm 148 over 80 and left arm 138 over 88. Pulse 80 and regular. Respirations 18. Height 5 feet, 7 inches. Weight 176 1/4 pounds. The patient is afebrile. HEENT. Not pale or cyanotic. Tympanic membranes intact. Fundus normal in the left; right cannot be visualized because of question of early cataract or marked refractive error. Neck. Supple. No jugular venous pulse, thyromegaly, or lymphadenopathy. Carotid upstrokes normal. Chest. Point of maximum, impulse in the fifth intercostal space in the mid-clavicular line. S1, S2 normal. A soft S4 was heard. No S3. No murmurs. Lungs clear. Abdomen. Soft, nontender. No hepatosplenomegaly. No masses felt. No abdominal bruits. Neurological. No gross abnormalities. Musculoskeletal. Bilateral hallux valgus. No edema or clubbing. All peripheral pulses normal and equal. Diagnosis. 1. Palpitations, probably premature ventricular contractions. Rule out coronary artery disease. Rule out malignant arrhythmias. 2. History of hypertension. 3. History of hypothyroidism. Therapeutic Plan. 1. Review old records. 2. Tumor skin test. 3. EKG with 12-hour Hotter monitor. 4. Measure blood pressure once a week x 3 weeks. Decide whether long-term hypertensive medication is necessary. 5. Ophthalmology consult.

FIGURE 9-3

Evaluator's Signature: _____   **Need to Repeat:** _____

National Curriculum Competency: CAAHEP: Cognitive: VI.C.3, 4; Psychomotor: V.P.3, 8, 11; X.P.3   ABHES: 4.a, 8.a

JOB SKILL 9-6
Record Test Results on a Flow Sheet

Name _____ Date _____ Score _____

Performance Objective

Task: Record laboratory test results for triglycerides, cholesterol, and glucose on a patient flow sheet.

Conditions: Need:

- Computer with Internet connection
- Online Form 25 (flow sheet) located at www.cengagebrain.com with student resources
- *Workbook* Figure 9-4 (test results)
- Pen

Refer to:

- *Textbook* Example 9-3 for a completed flow sheet

Standards: Complete all steps listed in this job skill in _____ minutes with a minimum score of _____. (Time element and accuracy criteria may be given by instructor.)

Time: Start: _____ Completed: _____ Total: _____ minutes

Scoring: One point for each step performed satisfactorily unless otherwise listed or weighted by instructor.

Directions with Performance Evaluation Checklist

Record test results for patient Richard Freeman on a flow sheet.

1st Attempt	2nd Attempt	3rd Attempt	
_____	_____	_____	Gather materials (equipment and supplies) listed under *Conditions*.
_____/2	_____/2	_____/2	1. Record the date of the laboratory report on Richard Freeman's flow sheet.
_____/2	_____/2	_____/2	2. Record his triglycerides on the flow sheet.
_____/2	_____/2	_____/2	3. Record his total cholesterol on the flow sheet.
_____/2	_____/2	_____/2	4. Record his high-density lipoprotein (HDL) cholesterol on the flow sheet.
_____/2	_____/2	_____/2	5. Record his low-density lipoprotein (LDL) cholesterol on the flow sheet.
_____/2	_____/2	_____/2	6. Record his cholesterol/high-density lipoprotein cardiac risk ratio on the flow sheet.
_____/2	_____/2	_____/2	7. Record his fasting glucose on the flow sheet.
_____/2	_____/2	_____/2	8. Distinguish between normal and abnormal test results and list any that were out of range, indicating if they were high or low. _____
_____	_____	_____	Complete within specified time.
____/18	____/18	___/18	**Total points earned** (To obtain a percentage score, divide the total points earned by the number of points possible.)

Comments:

JOB SKILL 9-6 *(continued)*

```
PRACTON MEDICAL GROUP, INC.                          LABORATORY REPORT
4567 BROAD AVENUE
WOODLAND HILLS, XY 12345-4700
```

PATIENT NAME		PATIENT ID		ROOM NO	AGE	SEX	PHYSICIAN
FREEMAN, RICHARD E		08051944RF			64	M	Practon, Gerald M

PAGE	REQUISITION NO.	ACCESSION NO.	LAB REF. #	COLLECTION DATE & TIME	LOG-IN DATE	REPORT DATE	& TIME
1	0013188	EN77346IN		072120XX 1044	07212009		4:25PM

REMARKS
FASTING   **PACIFIC
                                                                                TIME**

REPORT STATUS	FINAL	TEST	RESULT IN RANGE	RESULT OUT OF RANGE	UNITS	REFERENCE RANGE	SITE CODE
	rth: 08/05						
Patient Phone: (555)487-7892							
GLUCOSE				171 H	mg/dL	65-99	EN
						FASTING REFERENCE INTERVAL	
LIPID PANEL							
TRIGLYCERIDES			127		mg/dL	⟨150	EN
CHOLESTEROL, TOTAL			156		mg/dL	125-200	EN
HDL CHOLESTEROL			40		mg/dL	⟩ OR = 40	EN
LDL CHOLESTEROL			91		mg/dL ⟨CALC⟩	⟨130	EN
DESIRABLE RANGE ⟨100 MG/DL FOR PATIENTS WITH CHD OR DIABETES AND ⟨70 MG/DL FOR DIABETIC PATIENTS WITH KNOWN HEART DISEASE.							
CHOL/HDLC RATIO			3.9		⟨CALC⟩	⟨ OR = 5.0	EN

FIGURE 9-4

Evaluator's Signature: _____   **Need to Repeat:** _____

National Curriculum Competency: CAAHEP: Cognitive: II.C.6; Psychomotor: II.P.3	ABHES: 4.a, b.2; 7.a

Drug and Prescription Records

STOP AND THINK CASE SCENARIOS

Refer to the end of Chapter 10 in the *textbook* for the following scenarios:

• Determine Correct Medication   • Determine Food and Drug Allergies

EXAM-STYLE REVIEW QUESTIONS

Refer to the end of Chapter 10 in the *textbook*.

Abbreviation and Spelling Review

Read the patient's chart note and write the meanings for the abbreviations following the note. To decode any abbreviations you do not understand or that appear unfamiliar to you, refer to the list of abbreviations in Appendix B of this *Workbook*. Step-by-step directions for this exercise are found in Procedure 1-1 of Chapter 1 in the *textbook*. Medical terms in the chart note are italicized; study them for spelling. Use your medical dictionary to look up their definitions. Your instructor may give a spelling and definition test that includes these words and abbreviations.

Lillian M. Chan

February 17, 20XX, OB case. LMP 12-14-20XX. Pt had D & C in 20XX following *spontaneous abortion*. First child delivered by C-section. Ordered CBC, UA, and WR. Pt to ret in 1 mo.

Fran Practon, MD
Fran Practon, MD

OB   _____   CBC   _____

LMP   _____   UA   _____

Pt   _____   WR   _____

D & C   _____   ret   _____

C-section _____   mo   _____

Review Questions

Review the objectives, glossary, and chapter information before completing the following review questions.

1. Fill in the following blanks:

   a. Most Americans have taken at least _____ prescription medication in the last decade.

   b. In the years 2007–2008, _____% of adults 60 years of age or older used two or more prescription drugs.

   c. In the years 2007–2008, _____% of adults 60 years of age or older used five or more prescription drugs.

2. Match the law or agency in the right column with the description in the left column by writing the correct letters in the blanks.

   _____ Law requiring transfer tax for those who sold marijuana.

   _____ Federal law that requires the pharmaceutical industry to maintain physical security and strict recordkeeping for scheduled drugs.

   _____ First law to control the prescription, sale, and possession of narcotic drugs.

   _____ Organization that regulates the manufacturing and dispensing of dangerous and potentially abused drugs.

   _____ Law that prohibited the manufacture, transportation, and sale of beverages containing more than 0.5% alcohol.

   _____ Agency that determines the safety of drugs before it permits them to be marketed.

   _____ First law that required the labeling of drugs with directions for safe use

   a. Harrison Narcotic Act

   b. Volstead Act

   c. Marijuana Tax Act

   d. Food, Drug, and Cosmetic Act

   e. Controlled Substances Act

   f. Food and Drug Administration

   g. Drug Enforcement Administration

3. True or False. Recreational marijuana is now legal in several states. _____

4. Where must the physician register for a narcotic license and when must the license be renewed?

   _____

5. Refer to *textbook* Table 10-1, Five Schedules of Controlled Substances, and answer the following questions:

   a. On which schedule(s) may prescriptions be written by the health care worker?

   _____

   b. On which schedule(s) will the medical assistant most likely be handling triplicate forms for the doctor?

   _____

   c. On which schedule(s) do drugs have the most potential for abuse?

   _____

6. If a medical practice dispenses controlled substances, how long must an inventory be kept for Schedule I and II drugs? _____

_____

7. Name and define the three types of drug names.

    a. _____

    b. _____

    c. _____

8. Define *generic drug*. _____

_____

9. In the *Physician's Desk Reference*, which section is used most frequently by the medical assistant?

_____

10. Name and define the four components of a prescription.

    a. _____

    b. _____

    c. _____

    d. _____

11. Match the drug route in the right column with the correct definition in the left column by writing the correct letters in the blanks.

    _____ medication administered into a joint   a. ophthalmic

    _____ medication administered through the ear   b. otic

    _____ medication absorbed through the skin using a patch c. endotracheal

    _____ medication placed between the cheek and gum   d. intra-articular

    _____ medication administered to the eye   e. buccal

    _____ medication placed under the tongue   f. sublingual

    _____ medication administered through the trachea   g. transdermal

12. Write the abbreviation or symbol for the following pharmaceutical terms.

    a. after meals _____

    b. drops _____

    c. every morning _____

    d. every two hours _____

    e. intramuscular _____

    f. when necessary _____

13. True or False. All medical assistants can enter medication orders into a computerized system for CMS prescription incentive programs. _____

14. When charting medication refills, list the items needed to record:

    a. _____

    b. _____

    c. _____

    d. _____

    e. _____

    f. _____

15. Name several ways the medical assistant can instruct the patient about drug dosages to be sure the patient understands the directions.

    a. _____

    b. _____

    c. _____

    d. _____

    e. _____

16. Name three important items to include when instructions are given to patients taking antibiotics.

    a. _____

    b. _____

    c. _____

17. Name three ways a medical assistant can track a patient's drug use habits.

    a. _____

    b. _____

    c. _____

18. Name five ways to protect prescription pads from being misused.

    a. _____

    b. _____

    c. _____

    d. _____

    e. _____

19. Name some common side effects associated with medications.

    a. _____   g. _____

    b. _____   h. _____

    c. _____   i. _____

    d. _____   j. _____

    e. _____   k. _____

    f. _____   l. _____

20. If the patient does not have any known allergies, what is the abbreviation listed on the "alert tag" on the front of the patient's chart? _____

Critical Thinking Exercises

1. If a pharmacist calls the office and the physician approves a refill on Mr. Hamilton's prescription, what administrative task should the medical assistant then perform (list details)?

   _____

   _____

   _____

   _____

2. Mrs. Schwartz telephones and says that the doctor prescribed Hytrin, but she cannot remember why. With the physician's permission, you would tell her that the medication is being prescribed for her:

   a. Headaches

   b. Hypertension

   c. Nerves

   d. Hypotension

   (Find the answer in the *PDR* or other drug reference book.)

3. Rewrite the following statements as they would appear on a prescription, using Latin abbreviations.

   a. Proventil (albuterol) inhaler, one hundred milligrams per five milliliters, one or two inhalations every four hours whenever necessary.

   _____

   b. Cardizem CD (diltiazem HCl) capsules, 180 milligrams, number one hundred, once a day before meals, and one before bedtime.

   _____

   c. Lanoxin (digoxin) tablets, zero point one hundred and twenty-five milligrams, number sixty, one every day.

   _____

   d. Vantin (cefpodoxime proxetil) tablets, two hundred milligrams, number twenty-eight, one by mouth, every twelve hours for fourteen days.

   _____

JOB SKILL 10-1
Spell Drug Names

Name _____ Date _____ Score _____

Performance Objective

Task: Correctly spell brand or generic drug names.

Conditions: Need:

- Pen or pencil
- Drug reference books such as the *Physicians' Desk Reference, Delmar Healthcare Drug Handbook, Instant Drug Index, Hospital Formulary,* or *Pharmaceutical Terminology*

Refer to:

- Ten drug names listed next to each step
- *Textbook* Procedure 10-1 for step-by-step directions

Standards: Complete all steps listed in this skill in _____ minutes with a minimum score of _____. (Time element and accuracy criteria may be given by instructor.)

Time: **Start:** _____ **Completed:** _____ **Total:** _____ minutes

Scoring: One point for each step performed satisfactorily unless otherwise listed or weighted by instructor.

Directions with Performance Evaluation Checklist

Dr. Practon has dictated 10 drug names for several patients, and you have written them phonetically. Find and record the correct spelling for each drug. Be sure to begin all brand names with a capital letter and all generic names with a lowercase letter.

1st Attempt	2nd Attempt	3rd Attempt	
_____	_____	_____	Gather materials (equipment and supplies) listed under *Conditions*.
____/3	____/3	____/3	1. Spell **CAR-de-zem** _____
____/3	____/3	____/3	2. Spell **di-ah-BEN-eze** _____
____/3	____/3	____/3	3. Spell **FEE-a-sol** _____
____/3	____/3	____/3	4. Spell **NAP-ro-sin** _____
____/3	____/3	____/3	5. Spell **LIP-a-tour** _____
____/3	____/3	____/3	6. Spell **LAY-six** _____
____/3	____/3	____/3	7. Spell **eye-bu-PRO-fen** _____
____/3	____/3	____/3	8. Spell **die-AS-a-pam** _____
____/3	____/3	____/3	9. Spell **TEN-or-min** _____
____/3	____/3	____/3	10. Spell **aug-MEN-tin** _____
_____	_____	_____	Complete within specified time.
____/32	____/32	____/32	**Total points earned** (To obtain a percentage score, divide the total points earned by the number of points possible.)

JOB SKILL 10-1 (*continued*)

Comments:

JOB SKILL 10-2
Determine the Correct Spelling of Drug Names

Name _____ Date _____ Score _____

Performance Objective

Task: Determine the correct spellings for brand, generic, or over-the-counter drug names.

Conditions: Need:

- Drug reference books such as the *PDR*, *Delmar Healthcare Drug Handbook*, *Instant Drug Index*, *Hospital Formulary*, or *Pharmaceutical Terminology*
- Pen or pencil

Refer to:

- *Textbook* Procedure 10-1 for step-by-step directions
- Common knowledge, an over-the-counter drug book, or visit a local drug store to locate the medication on the shelf

Standards: Complete all steps listed in this skill in _____ minutes with a minimum score of _____. (Time element and accuracy criteria may be given by instructor.)

Time: Start: _____ Completed: _____ Total: _____ minutes

Scoring: One point for each step performed satisfactorily unless otherwise listed or weighted by instructor.

Directions with Performance Evaluation Checklist

Use the 10 sentences in the following steps, each has two spellings of a medication, and then circle the correct spelling from each pair of generic or brand-name medications. These sentences contain some frequently misspelled drug names.

1st Attempt	2nd Attempt	3rd Attempt	
_____	_____	_____	Gather materials (equipment and supplies) listed under *Conditions*.
____/3	____/3	____/3	1. Dr. Practon's last chart note on Mr. Hoy Cho states, "advised the patient to take (a) Aspirin, (b) aspirin, 1 tab b.i.d."
____/3	____/3	____/3	2. After Ray Nunez suffered a mild heart attack, the physician prescribed a (a) nitroglycerin, (b) nitroglycerine patch daily.
____/3	____/3	____/3	3. Maria Sanchez telephones stating she has a cold and wants to know if it is all right to take (a) Contac, (b) Contact, an over-the-counter drug.
____/3	____/3	____/3	4. Mrs. Hatakeyama's allergy is easily treated with (a) Actafed, (b) Actifed.
____/3	____/3	____/3	5. Rosaria LaMaccia suffered a mild respiratory infection and Dr. Practon gave her a prescription for (a) Ceclor, (b) Seklor.
____/3	____/3	____/3	6. The patient is complaining of muscle spasms in the lumbar region, so a prescription for (a) Flexeril, (b) Flexoril is given.
____/3	____/3	____/3	7. Fayetta Brown's diagnosis is duodenal ulcer, so she is given a prescription for (a) Bentil, (b) Bentyl.
____/3	____/3	____/3	8. A year ago Mae James had a urinary tract infection and was prescribed (a) Ceptra, (b) Septra.

JOB SKILL 10-2 (*continued*)

____/3   ____/3   ____/3   9. Ventricular arrhythmias are diagnosed in Cameron Lesser's case, so (a) Quiniglute, (b) Quinaglute is given.

____/3   ____/3   ____/3   10. After the death of her spouse, Danielle La Fleur became depressed and Dr. Practon prescribed (a) amatriptyline, (b) amitriptyline.

_____   _____   _____   Complete within specified time.

____/32   ____/32   ____/32   **Total points earned** (To obtain a percentage score, divide the total points earned by the number of points possible.)

Comments:

Evaluator's Signature: _____   **Need to Repeat:** _____

National Curriculum Competency: ABHES: 6.c, d

JOB SKILL 10-3
Use a Drug Reference Book to Locate Information

Name _____ Date _____ Score _____

Performance Objective

Task: Locate medication in a drug reference book; read and make determinations regarding its use.

Conditions: Need:

- Drug reference books such as the *PDR, Delmar Healthcare Drug Handbook, Instant Drug Index, Hospital Formulary,* or *Pharmaceutical Terminology*
- Pen or pencil

Refer to:

- *Textbook* Figure 10-3 for a visual example
- *Textbook* Procedure 10-1 for step-by-step directions

Standards: Complete all steps listed in this skill in _____ minutes with a minimum score of _____. (Time element and accuracy criteria may be given by instructor.)

Time: **Start:** _____ **Completed:** _____ **Total:** _____ minutes

Scoring: One point for each step performed satisfactorily unless otherwise listed or weighted by instructor.

Directions with Performance Evaluation Checklist

Dr. Practon has just received a prothrombin time report on Mrs. Darcuiel. He asks you to call the patient and verify her present dosage of Coumadin before he makes an adjustment. When you call the patient, she states she put all the pills in a medication container and no longer remembers her dosage. She says it is the only medication she is taking and it is *blue*. Answer the following questions regarding the Coumadin medication.

1st Attempt	2nd Attempt	3rd Attempt	
_____	_____	_____	Gather materials (equipment and supplies) listed under *Conditions*.
____/3	____/3	____/3	1. Refer to the *PDR*, a pill identification section online or in a drug reference book, or *textbook* Figure 10-3 to determine how many milligrams Mrs. Darcuiel is taking. What is the dosage she is taking? _____
____/3	____/3	____/3	2. Where did you find the information? _____
__(optional)	__(optional)	__(optional)	3. If using a *PDR*, in what section did you find the information? _____
____/3	____/3	____/3	4. Locate the medication in a drug reference book. What is the generic name for Coumadin? _____
____/3	____/3	____/3	5. What type of medication is Coumadin? _____
____/6	____/6	____/6	6. Name the most common gastrointestinal side effects. _____
_____	_____	_____	Complete within specified time.
____/20	____/20	____/20	**Total points earned** (To obtain a percentage score, divide the total points earned by the number of points possible.)

JOB SKILL 10-3 (*continued*)

Comments:

Evaluator's Signature: _____ **Need to Repeat:** _____

National Curriculum Competency: ABHES: 6.a, c, d

JOB SKILL 10-4
Translate Prescriptions

Name _____ Date _____ Score _____

Performance Objective

Task: Translate prescriptions from Latin into common English.

Conditions: Need:

- One sheet of plain paper
- Pen or pencil

Refer to:

- *Workbook* Figure 10-1 for nine written prescriptions
- *Textbook* Table 10-4 or *Workbook* Appendix B, Table B-7, Common Prescription Abbreviations and Symbols
- *Textbook* Procedure 10-2 step-by-step directions

Standards: Complete all steps listed in this skill in _____ minutes with a minimum score of _____. (Time element and accuracy criteria may be given by instructor.)

Time: Start: _____ Completed: _____ Total: _____ minutes

Scoring: One point for each step performed satisfactorily unless otherwise listed or weighted by instructor.

Directions with Performance Evaluation Checklist

Translate and write out the prescriptions in *Workbook* Figure 10-1 into common English by referring to *textbook* Table 10-4.

EXAMPLE:

```
Valium 10 mg
#21
Sig.: c̄ p.o. t.i.d.
```

Translation: Valium, ten milligrams, number
twenty-one, one by mouth three times a day.

1st Attempt	2nd Attempt	3rd Attempt	
_____	_____	_____	Gather materials (equipment and supplies) listed under *Conditions*.
____/5	____/5	____/5	1. Translate prescription for Tagamet.
____/5	____/5	____/5	2. Translate prescription for Darvocet.
____/5	____/5	____/5	3. Translate prescription for Diovan.
____/5	____/5	____/5	4. Translate prescription for Tenormin.
____/5	____/5	____/5	5. Translate prescription for Robitussin.
____/5	____/5	____/5	6. Translate prescription for Isordil.
____/5	____/5	____/5	7. Translate prescription for Compazine.

JOB SKILL 10-4 (*continued*)

____/5 ____/5 ____/5   8. Translate prescription for Vanceril.

____/5 ____/5 ____/5   9. Translate prescription for Timoptic Solution.

_____ _____ _____   Complete within specified time.

____/47 ____/47 ____/47   **Total points earned** (To obtain a percentage score, divide the total points earned by the number of points possible.)

Comments:

1
Tagamet 400 mg
#30
Sig.: ṫ p.o. h.s.

2
Darvocet N-100
#60 Tabs
Sig.: ṫṫ every 4h.
p.r.n. pain

3
Diovan HCT
160mg/12.5mg
#100
sig.: ṫ p.o. every day

4
Tenormin 50 mg
#100
ṫ every day

5
Robitussin DAC
4 oz. bottle
2 tsp every 4h. p.r.n.
cough

6
Isordil
(isosorbide dinitrate)
20 mg
#30
ṫ p.o every 12°

7
Compazine
25 mg suppositories
#14
ṫ rectally b.i.d.
p.r.n. vomiting

8
Vanceril Inhalation Aerosol
42 mcg
#1 bottle
2 inhalations q.i.d
p.r.n. asthma

9
Timoptic Solution
0.25%
1 bottle
ṫ gt. each eye b.i.d.

FIGURE 10-1

Evaluator's Signature: _____   **Need to Repeat:** _____

National Curriculum Competency: CAAHEP: Cognitive: II.C.5   ABHES: 3.b; 6.c.1, 2, 3

JOB SKILL 10-5
Record Prescription Refills in Medical Records

Name _____ Date _____ Score _____

Performance Objective

Task: Record four prescription refills in patient medical records.

Conditions: Need:

- Computer with Internet connection
- Online Form 26 (four large file folder labels) located at www.cengagebrain.com with student resources
- Medical record for Wayne G. Weather completed in Job Skill 7-5 and Job Skill 9-1
- Medical record for Krista Lee Carlisle completed in Job Skill 9-2
- Medical record for Sun Low Chung completed in Job Skill 9-5
- Pen or pencil

Refer to:

- *Textbook* Procedure 10-3 for step-by-step directions
- *Textbook* Table 10-4 or *Workbook* Appendix B, Table B-7, Common Prescription Abbreviations and Symbols

Standards: Complete all steps listed in this skill in _____ minutes with a minimum score of _____. (Time element and accuracy criteria may be given by instructor.)

Time: Start: _____ Completed: _____ Total: _____ minutes

Scoring: One point for each step performed satisfactorily unless otherwise listed or weighted by instructor.

Directions with Performance Evaluation Checklist

Read the following scenarios and abstract the prescription information. Record each transaction on a label, use the current date, initial it, and then secure the label in the patient's medical record.

1st Attempt	2nd Attempt	3rd Attempt	
_____	_____	_____	Gather materials (equipment and supplies) listed under *Conditions*.
___/10	___/10	___/10	1. Record: The ABC Pharmacy calls about a prescription for Wayne G. Weather. Dr. Practon approves a refill for Darvocet N-100, number twenty, one tablet every four hours whenever necessary for pain.
___/10	___/10	___/10	2. Record: The Dalton Pharmacy calls about Krista Lee Carlisle. The pharmacist asks if a refill on Sonata, ten-milligram capsules, number ten, one by mouth at bedtime, can be approved. Dr. Practon approves.
___/10	___/10	___/10	3. Record: The Georgetown Pharmacy calls regarding Sun Low Chung. He has a urinary tract infection again and would like a refill on his Bactrim, double strength, number twenty-eight, one by mouth two times a day for fourteen days. Dr. Practon approves.
___/10	___/10	___/10	4. Record: Two days later, Sun Low Chung calls Dr. Practon reporting an adverse reaction to the Bactrim. Dr. Practon calls the Main Street Pharmacy to order Macrodantin, one-hundred milligram capsules, number forty, one by mouth four times a day with milk or meals for ten days.
___/4	___/4	___/4	5. Secure prescription documentation (on labels) in correct medical records.

JOB SKILL 10-5 (*continued*)

_____ _____ _____   Complete within specified time.

___/46 ___/46 ___/46   **Total points earned** (To obtain a percentage score, divide the total points earned by the number of points possible.)

Comments:

National Curriculum Competency: CAAHEP: Cognitive II.C.5; Psychomotor: X.P.3   ABHES: 3.d; 6.c.1, 2, 3

JOB SKILL 10-6
Write a Prescription

Name _____ Date _____ Score _____

Performance Objective

Task: Write a prescription.

Conditions: Need:

- Computer with Internet connection
- Online Form 27 (one prescription) located at www.cengagebrain.com with student resources

Refer to:

- *Textbook* Figure 10-5 for a visual example
- *Textbook* Table 10-4 or *Workbook* Appendix B, Table B-7, Common Prescription Abbreviations and Symbols

Standards: Complete all steps listed in this skill in _____ minutes with a minimum score of _____.
(Time element and accuracy criteria may be given by instructor.)

Time: Start: _____ Completed: _____ Total: _____ minutes

Scoring: One point for each step performed satisfactorily unless otherwise listed or weighted by instructor.

Directions with Performance Evaluation Checklist

In some regions, medical assistants may be allowed to write prescriptions for patients; the physician must approve and sign all originals. This exercise is designed to help understand the different components of a prescription and the abbreviations used. Read the following scenario and write a prescription using today's date.

Scenario: Felisha Weiss, 456 Los Angeles Avenue, Woodland Hills, XY 12345, needs prophylactic treatment for migraine headache syndrome. She will be given verapamil, one hundred eighty milligrams, sustained release, number one hundred and twenty tablets. Directions are to take one by mouth every morning; she may have two refills.

1st Attempt	2nd Attempt	3rd Attempt	
_____	_____	_____	Gather materials (equipment and supplies) listed under *Conditions*.
____/5	____/5	____/5	1. Complete patient demographic information and enter today's date.
____/4	____/4	____/4	2. Complete inscription.
____/2	____/2	____/2	3. Complete subscription.
____/4	____/4	____/4	4. Complete signature.
_____	_____	_____	5. Indicate number of refills.
_____	_____	_____	6. Proofread form prior to physician's signature.
_____	_____	_____	Complete within specified time.
____/19	____/19	____/19	**Total points earned** (To obtain a percentage score, divide the total points earned by the number of points possible.)

JOB SKILL 10-6 (*continued*)

Comments:

Evaluator's Signature: _____   **Need to Repeat:** _____

National Curriculum Competency: CAAHEP: Psychomotor: X.P.3	ABHES: 3.d; 6.1, 2, 3

JOB SKILL 10-7
Interpret a Medication Log

Name _____ Date _____ Score _____

Performance Objective

Task: Determine the drug use habits of a patient.

Conditions: Need:
  • Pen or pencil
  Refer to:
  • *Workbook* Figure 10-2 (medication log)

Standards: Complete all steps listed in this skill in _____ minutes with a minimum score of _____.
(Time element and accuracy criteria may be given by instructor.)

Time: **Start:** _____ **Completed:** _____ **Total:** _____ minutes

Scoring: One point for each step performed satisfactorily unless otherwise listed or weighted by instructor.

Directions with Performance Evaluation Checklist

It is November 17, current year, and Mary Beth Foley calls to request a refill on her Glucotrol. Study the medication log and answer the following questions.

1st Attempt	2nd Attempt	3rd Attempt	
_____	_____	_____	Gather materials (equipment and supplies) listed under *Conditions*.
____/2	____/2	____/2	1. Has Mary Beth Foley been prescribed the medication? YES/NO
____/2	____/2	____/2	2. How many days has it been since she got her last refill? _____ days
____/2	____/2	____/2	3. Is it time to refill the medication? YES/NO
____/2	____/2	____/2	4. When may she call for the next refill? _____
_____	_____	_____	Complete within specified time.
___/10	___/10	___/10	**Total points earned** (To obtain a percentage score, divide the total points earned by the number of points possible.)

Comments:

JOB SKILL 10-7 (*continued*)

<table>
<tr><td colspan="11" align="center">MEDICATION LOG</td></tr>
<tr><td colspan="6">PATIENT NAME: FOLEY, Mary Beth</td><td colspan="5">DATE OF BIRTH: 9-30-52</td></tr>
<tr><td colspan="11">ALLERGIES: NKA</td></tr>
<tr>
<th>DATE</th>
<th>MEDICATIONS</th>
<th>DOSE</th>
<th>#</th>
<th>INSTRUCTIONS (SIG)</th>
<th>PRN REG</th>
<th>TEL WRIT</th>
<th>PHARMACY</th>
<th>DR. SIG.</th>
</tr>
<tr><td>8/5/XX</td><td>Amitriptyline</td><td>100 mg</td><td>90</td><td>i p.o. h.s.</td><td>R</td><td>T</td><td>ABC Pharm</td><td>GMP</td></tr>
<tr><td>9/23/XX</td><td>Glucotrol</td><td>10 mg</td><td>30</td><td>i p.o. a.c./a.m.</td><td>R</td><td>T</td><td>ABC Pharm</td><td>GMP</td></tr>
<tr><td>9/23/XX</td><td>Verapamil SR</td><td>240 mg</td><td>30</td><td>i p.o. q.a.m.</td><td>R</td><td>T</td><td>ABC Pharm</td><td>GMP</td></tr>
<tr><td>10/7/XX</td><td>Glucotrol</td><td>10 mg</td><td>90</td><td>i p.o. a.c./a.m.</td><td>R</td><td>W</td><td>mail order pharmacy</td><td>GMP</td></tr>
<tr><td>10/7/XX</td><td>Tetracycline</td><td>250 mg</td><td>30</td><td>i p.o. T.I.D. p.r.n. yellow sputum</td><td>P</td><td>T</td><td>ABC Pharm</td><td>GMP</td></tr>
<tr><td>10/16/XX</td><td>Verapamil SR</td><td>240 mg</td><td>90</td><td>i p.o. q.a.m.</td><td>R</td><td>W</td><td>mail order pharmacy</td><td>GMP</td></tr>
<tr><td>10/28/XX</td><td>Amitriptyline</td><td>100 mg</td><td>90</td><td>i p.o. h.s.</td><td>R</td><td>T</td><td>ABC Pharm</td><td>GMP</td></tr>
<tr><td></td><td></td><td></td><td></td><td></td><td></td><td></td><td></td><td></td></tr>
<tr><td></td><td></td><td></td><td></td><td></td><td></td><td></td><td></td><td></td></tr>
<tr><td></td><td></td><td></td><td></td><td></td><td></td><td></td><td></td><td></td></tr>
<tr><td></td><td></td><td></td><td></td><td></td><td></td><td></td><td></td><td></td></tr>
</table>

FIGURE 10-2

Evaluator's Signature: _____   **Need to Repeat:** _____

National Curriculum Competency: CAAHEP: Psychomotor: X.P.3	ABHES: 3.d; 6.c2, 3

JOB SKILL 10-8
Record on a Medication Schedule

Name _____ Date _____ Score _____

Performance Objective

Task: Record medication name, dosage, and instructions on a medication schedule.

Conditions: Need:
- Computer with Internet connection
- Online Form 28 (medication schedule) located at www.cengagebrain.com with student resources
- Pen or pencil

Refer to:
- *Textbook* Figure 10-6 for a visual example

Standards: Complete all steps listed in this skill in _____ minutes with a minimum score of _____. (Time element and accuracy criteria may be given by instructor.)

Time: Start: _____ Completed: _____ Total: _____ minutes

Scoring: One point for each step performed satisfactorily unless otherwise listed or weighted by instructor.

Directions with Performance Evaluation Checklist

Mr. Delbert Silva has just seen Dr. Fran Practon. She has prescribed Paxil for his depression. The dosage is 20 milligrams every morning. He is very confused, and Dr. Practon would like you to record all of his prescription information on a medication schedule. There is information in his chart indicating he is also taking Sinemet 20/250 milligrams for his Parkinson's disease. He takes two tablets four times a day. He is also on Lopressor, 100 milligrams twice a day, for his hypertension. You have verified that Mr. Silva is still on these medications. Please set up and fill out the medication schedule for Mr. Silva.

1st Attempt	2nd Attempt	3rd Attempt	
_____	_____	_____	Gather materials (equipment and supplies) listed under *Conditions*.
___/2	___/2	___/2	1. Fill in patient name and physician name.
___/4	___/4	___/4	2. Set up schedule for "a.m.," "NOON," "p.m.," and "BED."
___/4	___/4	___/4	3. Record information for Paxil medication.
___/8	___/8	___/8	4. Record information for Sinemet medication.
___/5	___/5	___/5	5. Record information for Lopressor medication.
_____	_____	_____	6. Proofread schedule prior to giving it to the patient.
_____	_____	_____	Complete within specified time.
___/26	___/26	___/26	**Total points earned** (To obtain a percentage score, divide the total points earned by the number of points possible.)

Comments:

Evaluator's Signature: _____ **Need to Repeat:** _____

National Curriculum Competency: CAAHEP: Cognitive: II.C.5 Psychomotor: X.P.3 | ABHES: 3.d; 6.c.2

C H A P T E R **11**

Written Correspondence

STOP AND THINK CASE SCENARIOS

Refer to the end of Chapter 11 in the *textbook* for the following scenarios:

- Edit a Thank-You Letter for Final Copy
- Edit a Transcribed Medial Report
- Select the Correct Homonyms in a Medical Report

EXAM-STYLE REVIEW QUESTIONS

Refer to the end of Chapter 11 in the *textbook*.

Abbreviation and Spelling Review

Read the patient's chart note and write the meanings for the abbreviations following the note. To decode any abbreviations you do not understand or that appear unfamiliar to you, refer to the list of abbreviations in Appendix B of this *Workbook*. Step-by-step directions for this exercise are in Procedure 1-1 of Chapter 1 in the *textbook*. Medical terms in the chart note are italicized; study them for spelling. Use your medical dictionary to look up their definitions. Your instructor may give a spelling and definition test that includes these words and abbreviations.

DATE	PROGRESS
1/3/20XX	Maria K Morgan CC: Pt complains of back pain, *nausea, dysuria,* & *oliguria* of 1 wk. PH: *Congenital stricture* rt. *ureter* at *ureterovesical junction.* UA: Occ WBC, occ epith., pH 7, alb 1, sugar O. Dr. Woodman's summary rev. Dilat to K35 c̄ Brev sodium, ordered IVP. *Unilateral nephrectomy* may be indicated. Dx: possible *urinary calculi.* RTO 1 wk. for UA & possible Dilat.
	Gerald Practon, MD
	Gerald Practon, MD

CC	_____	alb	_____
pt	_____	rev	_____
wk	_____	dilat	_____
PH	_____	K35	_____
rt	_____	$\bar{c}$	_____
UA	_____	Brev	_____
occ	_____	IVP	_____
WBC	_____	Dx	_____
epith.	_____	RTO	_____
pH	_____		

Review Questions

Review the objectives, glossary, and chapter information before completing the following review questions.

1. How should a letter of an official or legal nature be sent when there is a need to expedite it? _____

   _____

2. When keying a letter on a computer, what type of software would you use? _____

3. List three flaws that would make a letter unmailable.

   a. _____

   b. _____

   c. _____

4. Which style is the least personal of the various letter formats? _____

5. Which two punctuation styles are most commonly used? Briefly describe each.

   a. _____

   b. _____

6. What are the typical default settings for right and left margins? _____

7. Name three devices you could use to arouse the reader's interest in the first paragraph of a letter you are writing for the physician.

   a. _____

   b. _____

   c. _____

8. Explain the following text-editing features of electronic word processors.

   a. Directional keys _____

   b. Function keys _____

   c. Memory functions _____

   d. Tool features _____

   _____

   e. Edit features _____

   _____

   f. Printing feature _____

   _____

   g. Format functions _____

   _____

   _____

9. When checking for layout or format prior to printing, what software program option would you use to view an entire page of a document? _____

   _____

10. Transcription needs in the physician's office will be based on the following factors:

    a. _____

    b. _____

    c. _____

    d. _____

11. What procedure should be followed when the transcriptionist researches but still cannot understand a word or phrase of a physician's dictation? _____

    _____

12. The following are three methods the physician may use to create letters. Briefly describe the physician's and medical transcriber's roles when using these methods.

    a. Dictation equipment: _____

    _____

    _____

    b. Voice-activated software: _____

    _____

    _____

    c. Remote device (e.g., PDA): _____

    _____

    _____

13. List five ways to increase the productivity of photocopy machines.

a. _____

b. _____

c. _____

d. _____

e. _____

Critical Thinking Exercises

1. The following examples are parts of a letter. Read each example, and then identify and name the part of the letter.

   a. Attn: Philip Kellogg, MD

   _____

   b. Re: *Administrative Medical Assisting*, 8th edition

   _____

   c. P.S. Please call me if you need directions.

   _____

   d. Sincerely,

   _____

   e. Arthur Miller, MD
      2300 Broad Avenue
      Woodland Hills, XY 12345-4700

   _____

   f. Dear Dr. Rogers:

   _____

   g. CC: Bernice Brantley, MD

   _____

   h. Enc. (3)

   _____

JOB SKILL 11-1
Spell Medical Words

Name _____ Date _____ Score _____

Performance Objective

Task: Identify correctly spelled medical terms.

Conditions: Need:
                  • Pen or pencil

Standards: Complete all steps listed in this skill in _____ minutes with a minimum score of _____.
                  (Time element and accuracy criteria may be given by instructor.)

Time: Start: _____ Completed: _____ Total: _____ minutes

Scoring: One point for each step performed satisfactorily unless otherwise listed or weighted by
                  instructor.

Directions with Performance Evaluation Checklist

Select and circle the correctly spelled medical word from the choices given.

1st Attempt	2nd Attempt	3rd Attempt				
_____	_____	_____	Gather materials (equipment and supplies) listed under *Conditions*.			
_____	_____	_____	1. conchiousness	consciousness	consceousness	
_____	_____	_____	2. exhaustion	exsaustion	exhausion	
_____	_____	_____	3. theraputic	therapuetic	therapeutic	
_____	_____	_____	4. antidiarrheal	antidiarrhial	antidiarheal	
_____	_____	_____	5. neurolysis	nuerolysis	neurolosis	
_____	_____	_____	6. medisinal	medicinal	medicenal	
_____	_____	_____	7. roentegenogram	rentegenogram	roentgenogram	
_____	_____	_____	8. kinesiology	kenesiology	kenisiology	
_____	_____	_____	9. pharmasuetical	pharmaceutical	pharmaceutical	
_____	_____	_____	10. humeris	humerus	humerous	
_____	_____	_____	11. esophaglagia	esophagalgia	esopagalgia	
_____	_____	_____	12. critereon	criterion	creiterion	
_____	_____	_____	13. cauterisation	caterization	cauterization	
_____	_____	_____	14. methastasize	metastasize	metasthasize	
_____	_____	_____	15. spontaneous	spontenous	spontaneous	
_____	_____	_____	16. capitation	captation	capitasion	
_____	_____	_____	17. pancretectomy	pancraetectomy	pancreatectomy	
_____	_____	_____	18. indemity	endemnity	indemnity	
_____	_____	_____	19. negoteable	negotiable	negotable	
_____	_____	_____	20. intemperance	intemperance	intemparance	

JOB SKILL 11-1 (*continued*)

_____	_____	_____	21. ajudicate	adjudicate	adgudicate
_____	_____	_____	22. cursor	curser	courser
_____	_____	_____	23. stethoscope	steathescope	stethescrope
_____	_____	_____	24. purelent	purulent	peurulent
_____	_____	_____	25. ausculation	auscultation	auscultasion
_____	_____	_____	Complete within specified time.		
___/27	___/27	___/27	**Total points earned** (To obtain a percentage score, divide the total points earned by the number of points possible.)		

Comments:

Evaluator's Signature: _____ **Need to Repeat:** _____

National Curriculum Competency: CAAHEP: Cognitive: V.C.7 Psychomotor: V.P.3

JOB SKILL 11-2
Key a Letter of Withdrawal

Name _____ Date _____ Score _____

Performance Objective

Task: Key a letter of withdrawal for the physician's signature.

Conditions: Need:

* Computer with Internet connection
* Online Form 29 (letterhead for Practon Medical Group, Inc.) located at www.cengagebrain.com with student resources, or formatted in a word processing program on one sheet of letterhead

Refer to:

* *Textbook* Figure 11-3 and Figure 11-4 for format
* *Textbook* Figure 3-11 (Chapter 3) for an example
* *Textbook* Procedure 11-1 for step-by-step directions

Standards: Complete all steps listed in this skill in _____ minutes with a minimum score of _____. (Time element and accuracy criteria may be given by instructor.)

Time: **Start:** _____ **Completed:** _____ **Total:** _____ minutes

Scoring: One point for each step performed satisfactorily unless otherwise listed or weighted by instructor.

Directions with Performance Evaluation Checklist

Mrs. Stanfield refused to follow the treatment prescribed by Dr. Gerald Practon, and he has asked you to prepare a letter of withdrawal on his letterhead. Follow the steps below to complete this job skill.

1st Attempt	2nd Attempt	3rd Attempt	
_____	_____	_____	Gather materials (equipment and supplies) listed under *Conditions*.
_____	_____	_____	1. Format letterhead or use Form 29.
_____	_____	_____	2. Use the current date.
_____	_____	_____	3. Address the letter to Constance M. Stanfield, 2090 Hope Street, Woodland Hills, XY 12345.
_____	_____	_____	4. Use the correct salutation.
_____	_____	_____	5. Key in full block style.
_____	_____	_____	6. Use open punctuation.
_____	_____	_____	7. Use even and equal left and right margins.
_____	_____	_____	8. Place the letter on stationery with correct spacing.
___/10	___/10	___/10	9. Compose an appropriate letter with wording that is legally correct.
___/2	___/2	___/2	10. Use clear wording and correct grammar.
_____	_____	_____	11. Check paragraphing and punctuation.
___/2	___/2	___/2	12. Place the complimentary close and signature line in the appropriate place.
_____	_____	_____	13. Key reference initials.
_____	_____	_____	14. Key an enclosure notation.
_____	_____	_____	15. Proofread for spelling and typographical errors while on-screen.

JOB SKILL 11-2 (*continued*)

_____ _____ _____   16. Correct, print, and proofread again.

_____ _____ _____   17. Correct all errors and ready for the physician's signature.

_____ _____ _____   Complete within specified time.

____/30 ____/30 ____/30   **Total points earned** (To obtain a percentage score, divide the total points earned by the number of points possible.)

Comments:

Evaluator's Signature: _____ **Need to Repeat:** _____

National Curriculum Competency: CAAHEP: Cognitive: V.C.7; Psychomotor: V.P.3, 8, 11   ABHES: 7.b, g, h

JOB SKILL 11-3
Edit Written Communication

Name _____ Date _____ Score _____

Performance Objective

Task: Edit sentences for improvement.

Conditions: Need:

• Pen or pencil

Standards: Complete all steps listed in this skill in _____ minutes with a minimum score of _____. (Time element and accuracy criteria may be given by instructor.)

Time: Start: _____ Completed: _____ Total: _____ minutes

Scoring: One point for each step performed satisfactorily unless otherwise listed or weighted by instructor.

Directions with Performance Evaluation Checklist

Read each of the following sentences and edit to eliminate words, change the sequence of words, and eliminate redundant phrases.

1st Attempt	2nd Attempt	3rd Attempt	
_____	_____	_____	Gather materials (equipment and supplies) listed under *Conditions*.
_____	_____	_____	1. Mrs. Benson just recovered from an attack of pneumonia.
_____	_____	_____	2. The letter arrived at a time when we were busy.
_____	_____	_____	3. During the year of 20XX the unpaid accounts were numerous.
_____	_____	_____	4. If the population, as in the general case, increases, we'll plan on expanding our practice.
_____	_____	_____	5. The water is for drinking purposes only.
_____	_____	_____	6. The close proximity of the police department scared the thief.
_____	_____	_____	7. It costs the sum of 20 dollars.
_____	_____	_____	8. The young secretary has a beautiful future before her.
_____	_____	_____	9. The wreck occurred at the corner of Fourth and Rampart Streets.
_____	_____	_____	10. The color of the prize rose was dark red.
_____	_____	_____	11. We are now engaged in building a new medical office.
_____	_____	_____	12. Somebody or other must assume the responsibility.
_____	_____	_____	13. The file is made out of steel.
_____	_____	_____	14. There is much construction in the city of Ventura.
_____	_____	_____	15. It happened at the hour of midnight.
_____	_____	_____	16. The package should be there in three weeks' time.
_____	_____	_____	17. We will ship the office supplies at a later date.
_____	_____	_____	18. The character of the road was smooth.

JOB SKILL 11-3 (*continued*)

_____ _____ _____ 19. The physician spoke at a meeting held in Miami Beach.

_____ _____ _____ 20. The patient appeared for her appointment at the hour of 2:30 p.m.

_____ _____ _____ Complete within specified time.

___/22 ___/22 ___/22 **Total points earned** (To obtain a percentage score, divide the total points earned by the number of points possible.)

Comments:

National Curriculum Competency: CAAHEP: Cognitive: V.C.7; Psychomotor: V.P.3, 8, 11   ABHES: 7.b, g, h

JOB SKILL 11-4
Compose and Key a Letter for a Failed Appointment

Name _____ Date _____ Score _____

Performance Objective

Task: Compose and key an original letter dealing with a failed appointment.

Conditions: Need:

- Computer with Internet connection
- Online Form 30 (letterhead for Practon Medical Group, Inc.) located at www.cengagebrain.com with student resources, or formatted in a word processing program on one sheet of letterhead
- Dictionary

Refer to:

- *Textbook* Figure 11-3 and Figure 11-4 for format
- *Textbook* Procedure 11-1 for step-by-step directions

Standards: Complete all steps listed in this skill in _____ minutes with a minimum score of _____. (Time element and accuracy criteria may be given by instructor.)

Time: **Start:** _____ **Completed:** _____ **Total:** _____ minutes

Scoring: One point for each step performed satisfactorily unless otherwise listed or weighted by instructor.

Directions with Performance Evaluation Checklist

Margaret B. Hanson of 2319 Warren Street, Woodland Hills, XY 12345 calls on September 20 to make a 4 p.m. appointment for her 18-year-old son, James P. Hanson, on September 25. The patient does not show (DNS) for the appointment. Write a letter to Mrs. Hanson with a reference line notifying her about her son's failure to keep his appointment. Remember that this is a legal document that must be prepared for Dr. Fran Practon's signature. Key this letter in full block style with mixed punctuation; assume a file copy will be made.

1st Attempt	2nd Attempt	3rd Attempt	
_____	_____	_____	Gather materials (equipment and supplies) listed under *Conditions*.
_____	_____	_____	1. Design letterhead or use Form 30.
_____	_____	_____	2. Date the letter using the current date.
_____	_____	_____	3. Key the inside address.
_____	_____	_____	4. Key an appropriate salutation.
_____	_____	_____	5. Key the reference or subject line.
_____	_____	_____	6. Use full block style.
_____	_____	_____	7. Use mixed punctuation.
_____	_____	_____	8. Center the letter with even margins.
____/5	____/5	____/5	9. Mention the failed appointment with date and time in the body of the letter in a clear, concise manner.
_____	_____	_____	10. Insert proper paragraphing.
____/2	____/2	____/2	11. Key an appropriate complimentary close and signature line.

JOB SKILL 11-4 (*continued*)

_____	_____	_____	12. Insert proper reference initials.
____/5	____/5	____/5	13. Proofread while the document is on-screen for correct grammar and spelling, punctuation, capitalization, and typing errors.
_____	_____	_____	14. Correct, print, and proofread again.
_____	_____	_____	15. Make corrections and ready for the physician's signature.
_____	_____	_____	Complete within specified time.
____/26	____/26	____/26	**Total points earned** (To obtain a percentage score, divide the total points earned by the number of points possible.)

Comments:

Evaluator's Signature: _____   **Need to Repeat:** _____

National Curriculum Competency: CAAHEP: Cognitive: V.C.7; Psychomotor: V.P.3, 8, 11   ABHES: 7.b, g, h

JOB SKILL 11-5
Compose and Key a Letter for an Initial Visit

Name _____ Date _____ Score _____

Performance Objective

Task: Compose and key an original letter to a new patient explaining procedures for the initial visit and requesting insurance information.

Conditions: Need:

- Computer with Internet connection
- Form 31 (letterhead for Practon Medical Group, Inc.) located at www.cengagebrain.com with student resources, or formatted in a word processing program on one sheet of letterhead
- Dictionary

Refer to:

- *Textbook* Figure 11-3 and Figure 11-4 for format
- *Textbook* Procedure 11-1 for step-by-step directions

Standards: Complete all steps listed in this skill in _____ minutes with a minimum score of _____. (Time element and accuracy criteria may be given by instructor.)

Time: **Start:** _____ **Completed:** _____ **Total:** _____ minutes

Scoring: One point for each step performed satisfactorily unless otherwise listed or weighted by instructor.

Directions with Performance Evaluation Checklist

You are an administrative medical assistant. Write a letter over your own signature to Raymond E. Stokes Jr., 4053 Magnolia Boulevard, Woodland Hills, XY 12345. Remind him of his appointment with Dr. Fran Practon at 2:30 p.m. on Thursday, October 2, (current year). Inform him that the fee for an initial office visit is approximately $70.92. Suggest that he bring all insurance information if he has insurance coverage. Use full block style with mixed punctuation.

1st Attempt	2nd Attempt	3rd Attempt	
_____	_____	_____	Gather materials (equipment and supplies) listed under *Conditions*.
_____	_____	_____	1. Design letterhead or use Form 31.
_____	_____	_____	2. Date the letter using the current date.
_____	_____	_____	3. Key the inside address.
_____	_____	_____	4. Key an appropriate salutation.
_____	_____	_____	5. Key a reference or subject line.
_____	_____	_____	6. Use full block style.
_____	_____	_____	7. Use mixed punctuation.
_____	_____	_____	8. Center the letter with even margins.
___/5	___/5	___/5	9. Mention the appointment time, date, fee, and insurance coverage information in the body of the letter using clear language.
_____	_____	_____	10. Insert proper paragraphing.
___/2	___/2	___/2	11. Key an appropriate complimentary close and signature line.
_____	_____	_____	12. Insert proper reference initials.

JOB SKILL 11-5 (*continued*)

____/5   ____/5   ____/5   13. Proofread while the document is on-screen for correct grammar and spelling, punctuation, capitalization, and typing errors.

_____   _____   _____   14. Correct, print, and proofread again.

_____   _____   _____   15. Make corrections and sign.

_____   _____   _____   Complete within specified time.

____/26   ____/26   ____/26   **Total points earned** (To obtain a percentage score, divide the total points earned by the number of points possible.)

Comments:

Evaluator's Signature: _____   **Need to Repeat:** _____

National Curriculum Competency: CAAHEP: Cognitive: V.C.7; Psychomotor: V.P.3, 8, 11	ABHES: 7.b, g, h

JOB SKILL 11-6
Compose and Key a Letter to Another Physician

Name _____ Date _____ Score _____

Performance Objective

Task: Compose and key an original letter referring a patient to another physician.

Conditions: Need:

- Computer with Internet connection
- Online Form 32 (letterhead for Practon Medical Group, Inc.) located at www.cengagebrain. com with student resources, or formatted in a word processing program on one sheet of letterhead
- Dictionary

Refer to:

- *Textbook* Figure 11-3 and Figure 11-4 for format
- *Textbook* Procedure 11-1 for step-by-step directions

Standards: Complete all steps listed in this skill in _____ minutes with a minimum score of _____. (Time element and accuracy criteria may be given by instructor.)

Time: **Start: _____ Completed: _____ Total: _____** minutes

Scoring: One point for each step performed satisfactorily unless otherwise listed or weighted by instructor.

Directions with Performance Evaluation Checklist

Write a letter to Dr. Manuel Madero-Gonzales, Av. Mexico 131, Parque San Andreas, Mexico 21, D.F., referring Dr. Fran Practon's patient, Mr. Hector Gutierrez, who may need medical attention while vacationing in Mexico from September 30 through October 21, 20XX. He has been treated for infectious hepatitis, and his recent laboratory studies and clinical evaluations were within normal limits; assume you are enclosing copies of the most recent laboratory report and clinical evaluation. Tell Dr. Madero-Gonzales that you have instructed Mr. Gutierrez to contact him if any medical problems develop during his three-week stay. Use modified block style and open punctuation; make a copy to mail to the patient.

1st Attempt	2nd Attempt	3rd Attempt	
_____	_____	_____	Gather materials (equipment and supplies) listed under *Conditions*.
_____	_____	_____	1. Design letterhead or use Form 32.
_____	_____	_____	2. Date the letter using the current date.
_____	_____	_____	3. Key the inside address.
_____	_____	_____	4. Key an appropriate salutation.
_____	_____	_____	5. Key the reference or subject line.
_____	_____	_____	6. Use modified block style.
_____	_____	_____	7. Use open punctuation.
_____	_____	_____	8. Center the letter with even margins.
____/5	____/5	____/5	9. Mention the enclosed clinical evaluation in the body of the letter.
_____	_____	_____	10. Use clear language and insert proper paragraphing.
____/2	____/2	____/2	11. Key the appropriate complimentary close and signature line.

JOB SKILL 11-6 (*continued*)

_____	_____	_____	12. Insert proper reference initials.
_____	_____	_____	13. Key the enclosure notation.
_____	_____	_____	14. Key the copy notation.
____/5	___/5	___/5	15. Proofread while the document is on-screen for correct grammar and spelling, punctuation, capitalization, and typing errors.
_____	_____	_____	16. Correct, print, and proofread again.
_____	_____	_____	17. Make corrections and prepare for the physician's signature.
_____	_____	_____	18. Make a copy to mail to the patient.
_____	_____	_____	Complete within specified time.
___/29	___/29	___/29	**Total points earned** (To obtain a percentage score, divide the total points earned by the number of points possible.)

Comments:

Evaluator's Signature: _____   **Need to Repeat:** _____

National Curriculum Competency: CAAHEP: Cognitive: V.C.7; Psychomotor: V.P.3, 8, 11   ABHES: 7.b, g, h

JOB SKILL 11-7
Compose and Key a Letter Requesting Payment

Name _____ Date _____ Score _____

Performance Objective

Task: Compose and key a letter requesting payment on an overdue bill.

Conditions: Need:

• Computer with Internet connection

• Online Form 33 (letterhead for Practon Medical Group, Inc.) located at www.cengagebrain.com with student resources, or formatted in a word processing program on one sheet of letterhead

• Dictionary

Refer to:

• *Textbook* Figure 11-3 and Figure 11-4 for format

• *Textbook* Procedure 11-1 for step-by-step directions

Standards: Complete all steps listed in this skill in _____ minutes with a minimum score of _____. (Time element and accuracy criteria may be given by instructor.)

Time: Start: _____ Completed: _____ Total: _____ minutes

Scoring: One point for each step performed satisfactorily unless otherwise listed or weighted by instructor.

Directions with Performance Evaluation Checklist

When checking the financial records, you find that Christine LaMairre, 247 South Lincoln Boulevard, Apartment 5, Topanga, XY 12345, has not paid her bill for three months. She was seen for a consultation and complete physical examination; the fee was $70.92. She has no insurance coverage. Write a firm letter requesting payment by a specific date so it is not necessary to turn her account over to a collection agency. Enclose a copy of the current statement. Compose and key an original letter over Dr. Gerald Practon's signature in modified block style with open punctuation; assume a file copy of the letter will be made.

1st Attempt	2nd Attempt	3rd Attempt	
_____	_____	_____	Gather materials (equipment and supplies) listed under *Conditions*.
_____	_____	_____	1. Design letterhead or use Form 33.
_____	_____	_____	2. Date the letter using the current date.
_____	_____	_____	3. Key the inside address.
_____	_____	_____	4. Key an appropriate salutation.
_____	_____	_____	5. Key the reference or subject line.
_____	_____	_____	6. Use modified block style.
_____	_____	_____	7. Use open punctuation.
_____	_____	_____	8. Center the letter with even margins.
____/5	____/5	____/5	9. Request payment, stating the amount owed in the body of the letter using firm language.
_____	_____	_____	10. Insert proper paragraphing.
____/2	____/2	____/2	11. Key an appropriate complimentary close and signature line.
_____	_____	_____	12. Insert proper reference initials.

JOB SKILL 11-7 (*continued*)

_____	_____	_____	13. Key the enclosure notation.
____/5	____/5	____/5	14. Proofread while the document is on-screen for correct grammar and spelling, punctuation, capitalization, and typing errors.
_____	_____	_____	15. Correct, print, and proofread again.
_____	_____	_____	16. Make corrections and prepare for the physician's signature.
_____	_____	_____	17. Make a file copy.
_____	_____	_____	Complete within specified time.
___/28	___/28	___/28	**Total points earned** (To obtain a percentage score, divide the total points earned by the number of points possible.)

Comments:

Evaluator's Signature: _____   **Need to Repeat:** _____

National Curriculum Competency: CAAHEP: Cognitive: V.C.7; Psychomotor: V.P.3, 8, 11   ABHES: 7.b, g, h

JOB SKILL 11-8
Key Two Interoffice Memorandums

Name _____ Date _____ Score _____

Performance Objective

Task: Key two interoffice memorandums from handwritten notes.

Conditions: Need:

* Computer with Internet connection
* Online Form 34 and 35 (two interoffice memos) located at www.cengagebrain.com with student resources

Refer to:

* Handwritten notes *(Workbook* Figure 11-1 and Figure 11-2)
* *Textbook* Figure 11-6 for an example

Standards: Complete all steps listed in this skill in _____ minutes with a minimum score of _____.
(Time element and accuracy criteria may be given by instructor.)

Time: **Start:** _____ **Completed:** _____ **Total:** _____ minutes

Scoring: One point for each step performed satisfactorily unless otherwise listed or weighted by instructor.

Directions with Performance Evaluation Checklist

Scenario A: Dr. Gerald Practon has written a note *(Workbook* Figure 11-1) and asked you to key a memorandum to Dr. Yong Hall. Abstract information from his handwritten note and key the message accurately on an interoffice memo. Use guide words such as those found on Form 34.

Scenario B: Dr. Fran Practon has written you a note *(Workbook* Figure 11-2) asking you to key a memorandum to the physical therapist Cathy Crowe, RPT. Dr. Practon will take it to the hospital and place it in Cathy's box. Key the appropriate memo using guidewords such as those found on Form 35.

1st Attempt	2nd Attempt	3rd Attempt	
_____	_____	_____	Gather materials (equipment and supplies) listed under *Conditions*.
____/2	____/2	____/2	1. Read each note before beginning to compose the memos.
____/2	____/2	____/2	2. Prepare a rough draft of each memo.
____/2	____/2	____/2	3. Align and key memo headings (or use those on Forms 34 and 35).
____/2	____/2	____/2	4. Fill in spaces after each guide word with appropriate data.
____/2	____/2	____/2	5. Choose appropriate information for the subject heading.
____/10	____/10	____/10	6. Write a concise message using clear language and appropriate sentence structure.
____/2	____/2	____/2	7. Include all relevant information.
____/5	____/5	____/5	8. Proofread the memos while the documents are on-screen for correct grammar and spelling, punctuation, capitalization, and typing errors.
____/2	____/2	____/2	9. Print hard copies.
_____	_____	_____	Complete within specified time.
____/31	____/31	____/31	**Total points earned** (To obtain a percentage score, divide the total points earned by the number of points possible.)

JOB SKILL 11-8 (*continued*)

Comments:

Evaluator's Signature: _____ **Need to Repeat:** _____

National Curriculum Competency: CAAHEP: Cognitive: V.C.7; Psychomotor: V.P.3, 8, 11   ABHES: 7.b, g, h

JOB SKILL 11-8 (*continued*)

From the Desk of... G. P.

3-22

Jean:
Ask Dr. Hall if he saw article "Evaluation of Biofeedback Training + Its Effects upon pt's with Tension Headaches" - Jan, 20XX. AMA Journal by Dr. Hugh James, pgs 21-25 - relevant to his research: very informative!

G. P.

P.S. Does he need a reprint?

FIGURE 11-1

From the Desk of... Fran

3-22

J:-
Please type a memo so I can take it to the hospital today to Cathy Crowe, RPT. Tell her we haven't rec'd copy of muscle strength Evaluation form for pt. Eric Willard. I desperately need it by 24th before I see Eric.

Thanks!
F.P.

FIGURE 11-2

JOB SKILL 11-9
Abstract Information from a Medical Record; Compose and Key a Letter

Name _____ Date _____ Score _____

Performance Objective

Task: Abstract patient information from a chart note, and then key a letter to a referring physician.

Conditions: Need:

- Computer with Internet connection
- Online Form 36 (letterhead for Practon Medical Group, Inc.) located at www.cengagebrain.com with student resources, or formatted in a word processing program on one sheet of letterhead
- *Workbook* Figure 11-3 for chart note
- Dictionary

Refer to:

- *Textbook* Figure 11-3 and Figure 11-4 for format
- *Textbook* Procedure 11-1 for step-by-step directions

Standards: Complete all steps listed in _____ this skill in minutes with a minimum score of _____.
                   (Time element and accuracy criteria may be given by instructor.)

Time: **Start:** _____ **Completed:** _____ **Total:** _____ minutes

Scoring: One point for each step performed satisfactorily unless otherwise listed or weighted by instructor.

Directions with Performance Evaluation Checklist

Dr. Fran Practon has asked you to review the chart notes of Ben Olman *(Workbook* Figure 11-3) and send a letter, dated March 22, 20XX, to the referring physician outlining the treatment since the last letter. Use full block style with mixed punctuation and key the letter for the physician's signature.

1st Attempt	2nd Attempt	3rd Attempt	
_____	_____	_____	Gather materials (equipment and supplies) listed under *Conditions*.
_____	_____	_____	1. Design letterhead or use Form 36.
_____	_____	_____	2. Date the letter.
_____	_____	_____	3. Key the inside address.
_____	_____	_____	4. Key an appropriate salutation.
_____	_____	_____	5. Key the reference or subject line.
_____	_____	_____	6. Use full block style.
_____	_____	_____	7. Use mixed punctuation.
_____	_____	_____	8. Center the letter with even margins.
___/3	___/3	___/3	9. Include the patient's name and the purpose of the letter at the beginning of the letter.
___/10	___/10	___/10	10. Include all dates and medical information since the previous letter.
_____	_____	_____	11. Use clear language and insert proper paragraphing.
___/2	___/2	___/2	12. Key an appropriate closing sentence.
___/2	___/2	___/2	13. Key an appropriate complimentary close and signature line.

JOB SKILL 11-9 (*continued*)

_____	_____	_____	14.	Insert proper reference initials.
____/5	____/5	____/5	15.	Proofread while the document is on-screen for correct grammar and spelling, punctuation, capitalization, and typing errors.
_____	_____	_____	16.	Correct, print, and proofread again.
_____	_____	_____	17.	Make corrections and prepare for the physician's signature.
_____	_____	_____		Complete within specified time.
____/36	____/36	____/36		**Total points earned** (To obtain a percentage score, divide the total points earned by the number of points possible.)

DATE	PROGRESS	Olman, Ben A.
2/3/XX	Pt moved recently to area and was referred to me by Dr. Ann Coleman, 4021 Indiana Ave, Ste 2, Pacific Palisades, CA 90272. States he has a long HX of tonsillitis. Pt seen in ofc complaining of chills, sore throat since January 26. Temp. 102.6° F. CPX shows tonsils that appear enlarged & red. Throat culture taken. llf	*Fran Practon, MD*
2/5/XX	Pt improved. Tonsils appear less swollen. Throat culture neg. for strep. Continue penicillin Rx for 10 days p.o. t.i.d. Call if not improved. llf	*Fran Practon, MD*
2/20/XX	Pt comes in again with severe sore throat. Began 3 days after penicillin was dc. Malaise. Temp 101.4° F. Tonsil culture taken and await results before prescribing antibiotic. Ret 3 days. llf	*Fran Practon, MD*
2/23/XX	Pt presents with acute sore throat, red & inflamed. Temp 102.4° F. Adv tonsillectomy after acute phase subsides. Rx antibiotic, Suprax, 20 mg q. 12 h. llf	*Fran Practon, MD*
2/23/XX	Letter mailed to Dr. Coleman.	
3/2/XX	Pt RTO. Throat improved. Scheduled T & A at College Hospital for 3/15/XX. llf	*Fran Practon, MD*
3/15/XX	Pt adm to outpatient surgery at College Hospital. T & A with disc. same day. llf	
3/21/XX	PO; no complaints. Temp 98.4° F. To retn p.r.n.	*Fran Practon, MD*

FIGURE 11-3

Comments:

Evaluator's Signature: _____ **Need to Repeat:** _____

National Curriculum Competency: CAAHEP: Cognitive: V.C.7; Psychomotor: V.P.3, 8, 11	ABHES: 7.b, g, h

JOB SKILL 11-10
Key a Two-Page Letter

Name _____ Date _____ Score _____

Performance Objective

Task: Key a two-page letter using an appropriate second-page heading.

Conditions: Need:

- Computer with Internet connection
- Online Form 37 (letterhead for Practon Medical Group, Inc.) located at www.cengagebrain.com with student resources, or formatted in a word processing program on one sheet of letterhead
- One piece of plain white paper for second page
- *Workbook* Figure 11-4 for text of letter
- Dictionary

Refer to:

- *Textbook* Figure 11-3 and Figure 11-4 for format
- *Textbook* Example 11-21 for a second-page heading
- *Textbook* Procedure 11-1 for step-by-step directions

Standards: Complete all steps listed in this skill in _____ minutes with a minimum score of _____. (Time element and accuracy criteria may be given by instructor.)

Time: **Start:** _____ **Completed:** _____ **Total:** _____ minutes

Scoring: One point for each step performed satisfactorily unless otherwise listed or weighted by instructor.

Directions with Performance Evaluation Checklist

Using the current date, format and key a two-page letter to the attention of the education chair of your local county medical society; use their address. The subject for the letter is "Work Experience for the Medical Office Student," and the text is a summary written by Dr. Gerald Practon, and found in *Workbook* Figure 11-4. Set 1½-inch margins, use full block style with open punctuation, determine paragraphing, and make capitalization corrections as required.

1st Attempt	2nd Attempt	3rd Attempt	
_____	_____	_____	Gather materials (equipment and supplies) listed under *Conditions*.
_____	_____	_____	1. Design letterhead or use Form 37 and one sheet of plain paper for the second page.
_____	_____	_____	2. Date the letter using the current date.
_____	_____	_____	3. Key the inside address.
_____	_____	_____	4. Include the attention line.
_____	_____	_____	5. Key an appropriate salutation.
_____	_____	_____	6. Key the reference or subject line.
_____	_____	_____	7. Use full block style.
_____	_____	_____	8. Use open punctuation.
_____	_____	_____	9. Center the letter using 1½-inch margins.
_____/6	_____/6	_____/6	10. Determine and insert proper paragraphing.

JOB SKILL 11-10 (*continued*)

_____	_____	_____	11. Make necessary capitalization corrections.
_____	_____	_____	12. Choose the appropriate line to end page 1.
___/3	___/3	___/3	13. Insert a second-page heading.
___/5	___/5	___/5	14. Key all information accurately.
_____	_____	_____	15. Key an appropriate concluding sentence.
___/2	___/2	___/2	16. Key an appropriate complimentary close and signature line.
_____	_____	_____	17. Insert proper reference initials.
___/5	___/5	___/5	18. Proofread while the document is on-screen for correct grammar and spelling, punctuation, capitalization, and typing errors.
_____	_____	_____	19. Correct, print, and proofread again.
_____	_____	_____	20. Make corrections and prepare for the physician's signature.
_____	_____	_____	Complete within specified time.
___/38	___/38	___/38	**Total points earned** (To obtain a percentage score, divide the total points earned by the number of points possible.)

In reply to your request for information on work experience, I am enclosing a summary of the material I have found for your group, and I hope it answers some of your questions. Physicians, administrators, educational and medical associations, and officials of school districts have expressed increased interest in the value of on-the-job training and career-related work-study programs for their medical office students. Some colleges have instituted major curriculum changes to provide for internships and hospital work-study assignments. As a result of this interest, employers, including medical agencies, as well as federal agencies, are being asked to support the objectives of this new educational concept by providing new training opportunities for medical office students. Many agencies have inquired as to the role that they may play in making medical facilities available and in providing training to support these work-study medical programs. These inquiries have requested clarification in three general program areas: (1) programs established through legislation; (2) part-time, intermittent, or temporary employment; and (3) the selective exposure of students, in a nonpaid status, to learning projects related to educational objectives. Agencies are now providing and are encouraged to expand work-study opportunities for students and enrollees in programs authorized by legislation. Such legislation includes the Higher Education, Vocational Education Training, Economic Opportunity, and Social Security acts. Under these programs, students receive stipends from financial grants provided by statute. Similar support is urged for part-time, intermittent, and cyclic employment programs for students. Hospital programs such as cooperative work-study, summer and vacation employment, and part-time employment during the school year offer agencies an excellent opportunity to make significant contributions through medical-related assignments. These programs are also in keeping with federal long-range recruitment objectives. I hope this summarizes for your group the information you requested. If I can be of any further assistance in setting up the program in your area, please feel free to contact me.

FIGURE 11-4

JOB SKILL 11-10 *(continued)*

Comments:

Processing Mail and Electronic Correspondence

STOP AND THINK CASE SCENARIOS

Refer to the end of Chapter 12 in the *textbook* for the following scenarios:

- Practice Mail Security
- Classify Outgoing Mail
- Select the Best Communication Method

EXAM-STYLE REVIEW QUESTIONS

Refer to the end of Chapter 12 in the *textbook*.

Abbreviation and Spelling Review

Read the patients' chart notes and write the meanings for the abbreviations following the notes. To decode any abbreviations you do not understand or that appear unfamiliar to you, refer to the list of abbreviations in Appendix B of this *Workbook*. Step-by-step directions for this exercise are found in Procedure 1-1 of Chapter 1 in the *textbook*. Medical terms in the chart note are italicized; study them for spelling. Use your medical dictionary to look up their definitions. Your instructor may give a spelling and definition test that includes these words and abbreviations.

Stephen L. Boasberg

January 17, 20XX OC: Biopsy report pos. for CA of *prostate*. TURP & *bilateral orchiectomy, scrotal*. Adm to hosp in 2 days. Est. TD: 6 wks. Adv dc pain medication in 3 days.

Fran Practon, MD
Fran Practon, MD

OC	_____	est. _____
pos.	_____	TD _____
CA	_____	wks _____
TURP	_____	adv _____
adm	_____	dc _____
hosp	_____	

Terence O. Williams

January 17, 20XX Sunday, 4 a.m. pt seen in ER complaining of pain, R ear, abt 3 days, PX revealed fluid & pus. Temp. 100°F.

Fran Practon, MD
Fran Practon, MD

---

a.m.	_____	abt _____
pt	_____	PX _____
ER	_____	temp. _____
R	_____	F _____

Review Questions

Review the objectives, glossary, and chapter information before completing the following review questions.

1. According to the U.S. Postal Service, the *domestic mail* zone includes _____

    _____

2. OCR stands for _____

3. List three advantages of using a postage meter.

    a. _____

    b. _____

    c. _____

4. Name three ways in which postage stamps can be obtained in addition to purchasing them at the post office.

    a. _____

    b. _____

    c. _____

5. List the items that should be available when opening mail.

    a. _____

    b. _____

    c. _____

    d. _____

    e. _____

    f. _____

6. Why should all incoming correspondence be dated? _____

_____

7. Generally, a letter marked _____ or _____
   is not opened by the medical assistant.

8. *Standard post* is also known as _____ or _____
   mail.

9. The most expedient and economic way to send a letter that weighs under 13 ounces is

   _____, and the most expedient way to send a letter that weighs over

   13 ounces is _____.

10. The fastest and most reliable delivery service offered by the U.S. Postal Service, which guarantees a

    delivery date and time (next day, second day), is called _____

11. OCR envelope guidelines require keying the attention line _____

    _____

12. Name four service endorsements that can be placed on envelopes to notify the U.S. Postal Service of
    action to take when a piece of mail is undeliverable as addressed.

    a. _____

    b. _____

    c. _____

    d. _____

13. A type of mail service that electronically sends, receives, stores, and forwards messages in digital form

    over telecommunication lines is known as _____

14. An email business communication should follow the format of a _____

15. Answer "True" or "False" to the following statements.

    a. _____ Informal salutations may be used with email.

    b. _____ Informal complementary closings may be used with email.

    c. _____ Pronouns are recommended in the composition of all emails.

    d. _____ It is all right to forward chain letters via office email as long as it is done quickly.

    e. _____ Email attachments should never be sent with office email.

    f. _____ Even though HIPAA does not directly address email in its standards, both the privacy and
       security rules apply.

    g. _____ A secure messaging service allows email to be encrypted.

    h. _____ It is recommended that you check your email box at work every hour.

16. Describe three situations in which the physician might use facsimile (fax) transmission from the office.

    a. _____

    b. _____

    c. _____

17. What method of mailing should be used to send a patient chart to a lawyer for use in a malpractice

    court hearing? _____

18. Name two reasons a fax cover sheet is mandatory.

    a. _____

    b. _____

19. Complete the following statement: "*Fax health information only when* _____

    _____

    _____."

20. What is it important to remember when faxing a document to be signed?

    _____

    _____.

◤ Critical Thinking Exercises

1. Select the best statement regarding composing email messages and comment on your answers.

    a. There is no need to worry about typographical or spelling errors.

    b. It is *important* to proofread for spelling and accuracy.

    c. It is permissible to use abbreviations because the recipient will understand what you mean.

    _____

    _____

    _____

2. Select the best statement regarding answering email messages and comment on your answers.

    a. Respond as soon as possible, but after you finish the task you are doing.

    b. Answer immediately.

    c. Print the message, put it in your inbox with other fax and telephone requests, and answer when convenient.

    d. Always acknowledge that the message has been received.

    _____

    _____

3. Respond to the following statements regarding the insertion of your telephone number on email messages.

    a. It is not necessary because you reply directly to the sender of the message.

    b. Always include it.

    c. It depends on the preference of the employer or individual sending the message.

    _____

    _____

    _____

4. Select the best statement regarding printing email messages and comment on your answers.

    a. If the message is important or if a hardcopy record is needed, then print the message.

    b. Always print the message.

    c. Never print the message.

    _____

    _____

    _____

5. Read the following scenario, then search each Internet site for the shipping companies listed and compare what it would cost to send a package by (1) United States Postal Service, (2) United Parcel Service, and (3) Federal Express.

    Scenario: You are working for Practon Medical Group, Inc., and have been asked to mail a package that is 18 inches long by 4 inches high by 10 inches wide; it weighs 2 pounds, and needs to arrive in 2 days (anytime). You are mailing it from Clifton Park, New York 12065, to Ventura, California 93003. Search each carrier via the Internet to "calculate shipping" prices.

    List the cost of each company and determine which is the most reasonable:

    a. USPS:

    _____

    _____

    b. UPS:

    _____

    _____

    c. FedEx:

    _____

    _____

JOB SKILL 12-1
Process Incoming Mail

Name _____ Date _____ Score _____

Performance Objective

Task:　　　　Sort and process incoming mail; determine the disbursement and action for each communication.

Conditions:　Need:
- Pen or pencil

Refer to:
- *Workbook* Figure 12-1 for a list of incoming mail categories

Standards:　Complete all steps listed in this skill in _____ minutes with a minimum score of _____. (Time element and accuracy criteria may be given by instructor.)

Time:　　　　Start: _____ Completed: _____ Total: _____ minutes

Scoring:　　One point for each step performed satisfactorily unless otherwise listed or weighted by instructor.

Directions with Performance Evaluation Checklist

You will be opening today's mail and determining what action needs to take place for each piece. Some of the mail will be placed on the physician's desk; please designate its importance by indicating "top," "middle," or "bottom" of the mail stack. You may need to read and annotate some mail, route mail to other office workers, pull a patient's chart and possibly place the chart on the physician's desk (if the office does not use electronic medical records [EMRs]), record items on the physician or medical assistant's calendar, or set up a file folder. All money received needs to be posted or recorded on the patient's ledger or account, the daysheet or journal, and the bank deposit (you can simply check "record payment") and then put in a safe place (locked drawer or safe). You will need to verify the address on all checks received against the office records to make sure each address is current. You have the ability to write checks if an invoice needs to be paid and you may simply file or discard an item.

Study the following list of mail items and use critical thinking skills to determine what action needs to be taken. Refer to the headings in *Workbook* Figure 12-1 and indicate with a checkmark (✓) how each piece of mail is to be handled (check all that apply).

1st Attempt	2nd Attempt	3rd Attempt	
_____	_____	_____	Gather materials (equipment and supplies) listed under *Conditions*.
_____	_____	_____	1. Letter and check from a patient.
_____	_____	_____	2. Announcement of a medical society meeting.
_____	_____	_____	3. Advertisement for an x-ray machine.
_____	_____	_____	4. Mail-order gardening catalog.
_____	_____	_____	5. Letter from patient, Charles J. Conway.
_____	_____	_____	6. Check from patient Mr. Bill Owen.
_____	_____	_____	7. Advertisement about a new tranquilizer drug.
_____	_____	_____	8. *Journal of the American Medical Association* (current issue).
_____	_____	_____	9. A request for a reprint of an article written by Dr. Practon.
_____	_____	_____	10. Letter marked "Personal" to Dr. Fran Practon.

JOB SKILL 12-1 (*continued*)

_____ _____ _____ 11. A drug sample.

_____ _____ _____ 12. Letter referring a patient to Dr. Gerald Practon.

_____ _____ _____ 13. A piece of pornographic literature.

_____ _____ _____ 14. Letter announcing an evening professional meeting in 2 months.

_____ _____ _____ 15. License tax-due notice.

_____ _____ _____ 16. Charity solicitation letter.

_____ _____ _____ 17. Insurance query about patient Mrs. Dorothy Ranger.

_____ _____ _____ 18. Medicare payment for patient Beth Cook.

_____ _____ _____ 19. Lab test results on patient Mary Murdock.

_____ _____ _____ 20. Consultant report on patient Bill McKean.

_____ _____ _____ 21. Check from Aetna Insurance Company for service rendered to Samantha Boatman.

_____ _____ _____ 22. Prudential insurance questionnaire on patient Tom Patten.

_____ _____ _____ 23. Invoice from V. Mueller Supply Company.

_____ _____ _____ 24. Letter from patient Clarice Stark without date or return address (these do appear on the envelope).

_____ _____ _____ 25. Letter from Dr. Lees concerning a research project.

_____ _____ _____ 26. Letter about cancellation of appointment by a patient who is on vacation.

_____ _____ _____ 27. *Time* magazine.

_____ _____ _____ 28. Mutual funds investment letter.

_____ _____ _____ 29. Local medical society agenda for monthly meeting.

_____ _____ _____ 30. Ad for new filing equipment.

_____ _____ _____ 31. Mail-order medical instrument catalog.

_____ _____ _____ 32. Gift parcel from Mrs. Gaspar Whelan (patient).

_____ _____ _____ 33. Letter notifying Dr. Fran Practon of the death of a colleague.

_____ _____ _____ 34. Telegram from Dr. Perry Cardi congratulating Dr. Gerald Practon on his election as vice president of the local medical society.

_____ _____ _____ 35. Personal letter, opened by mistake.

_____ _____ _____ Complete within specified time.

___/37 ___/37 ___/37 **Total points earned** (To obtain a percentage score, divide the total points earned by the number of points possible.)

Comments:

Evaluator's Signature: _____ **Need to Repeat:** _____

National Curriculum Competency: ABHES: 7.a

No.	Place Mail on MD Desk			Read Mail	Annotate	Route Mail to:	Pull Patient Chart	Place Chart on MD Desk	Record on Calendar (MD/MA) or Appt Book	Setup File	Record Payment	Place Money in Secure Place	Verify Address on Check	Write Check	F=File D=Discard
	Top	Middle	Bottom												
1															
2															
3															
4															
5															
6															
7															
8															
9															
10															
11															
12															
13															
14															
15															
16															
17															
18															
19															

(continues)

FIGURE 12-1

No.	Place Mail on MD Desk			Read Mail	Annotate	Route Mail to:	Pull Patient Chart	Place Chart on MD Desk	Record on Calendar (MD/MA) or Appt Book	Setup File	Record Payment	Place Money in Secure Place	Verify Address on Check	Write Check	F=File D=Discard
	Top	Middle	Bottom												
20															
21															
22															
23															
24															
25															
26															
27															
28															
29															
30															
31															
32															
33															
34															
35															

FIGURE 12-1 *(continued)*

JOB SKILL 12-2
Annotate Mail

Name _____ Date _____ Score _____

Performance Objective

Task: Read a letter, annotate significant words or phrases, and make comments in the margin concerning the action to be taken.

Conditions: Need:

- Highlighter or colored pen

Refer to:

- *Workbook* Figure 12-2 (letter)
- *Textbook* Procedure 12-3 for step-by-step directions

Standards: Complete all steps listed in this skill in _____ minutes with a minimum score of _____. (Time element and accuracy criteria may be given by instructor.)

Time: Start: _____ Completed: _____ Total: _____ minutes

Scoring: One point for each step performed satisfactorily unless otherwise listed or weighted by instructor.

Directions with Performance Evaluation Checklist

Read the letter from Mr. Glen Marchall (*Workbook* Figure 12-2) that arrived today. Note significant words or phrases by highlighting them or by underlining with colored pen. Annotate any action requirements in the right margin using colored pen.

1st Attempt	2nd Attempt	3rd Attempt	
_____	_____	_____	Gather materials (equipment and supplies) listed under *Conditions*.
___/10	___/10	___/10	1. Underline important words or phrases.
___/5	___/5	___/5	2. Annotate action areas of letter.
_____	_____	_____	Complete within specified time.
___/17	___/17	___/17	**Total points earned** (To obtain a percentage score, divide the total points earned by the number of points possible.)

Comments:

JOB SKILL 12-2 *(continued)*

MARCHALL RENTS
23990 WEST VALLEY ROAD
SEPULVEDA, XY 93087

December 2, 20XX

Gerald Practon, MD
4567 Broad Avenue
Woodland Hills, XY 12345

Dear Dr. Practon:

We have recently opened a medical equipment rental-sales company in your area and are anxious for members of the medical profession to know of our specialized home-care equipment.

Our staff is highly trained to help you determine and meet the precise requirements for each patient's comfort and safety. We handle only the best equipment—from oxygen equipment to wheelchairs, hospital beds, and patient lifts—and we are on 24-hour call.

Our salesman will be in your area around January 13, so we are contacting you to see if we can set up an appointment for him to show and demonstrate pieces of equipment.

We will follow this communication with a personal telephone call to determine a date that is satisfactory. We hope that we can meet with you soon and work as a team to help satisfy your patients' needs.

Sincerely,

Glen Marchall

Mr. Glen Marchall
President

GM:jf

FIGURE 12-2

JOB SKILL 12-3
Classify Outgoing Mail

Name _____ Date _____ Score _____

Performance Objective

Task: Identify classes of mail.

Conditions: Need:

- Pen or pencil

Refer to:

- *Textbook* section: *Mail Classifications*
- *Textbook* Procedure 12-4 for step-by-step directions

Standards: Complete all steps listed in this skill in _____ minutes with a minimum score of _____.
(Time element and accuracy criteria may be given by instructor.)

Time: **Start:** _____ **Completed:** _____ **Total:** _____ minutes

Scoring: One point for each step performed satisfactorily unless otherwise listed or weighted by instructor.

Directions with Performance Evaluation Checklist

You will be mailing various pieces and types of mail for the physicians, and it will be helpful if you can determine classifications before going to the post office. After each piece of mail, indicate the appropriate classification or special services used.

1st Attempt	2nd Attempt	3rd Attempt	
_____	_____	_____	Gather materials (equipment and supplies) listed under *Conditions*.
_____	_____	_____	1. Income tax forms mailed on deadline date _____
_____	_____	_____	2. Proof that estimated income tax form was mailed by deadline _____
_____	_____	_____	3. Prescription _____
_____	_____	_____	4. Postal card _____
_____	_____	_____	5. Letter with photograph _____
_____	_____	_____	6. New patient letter with medical pamphlet _____
_____	_____	_____	7. Newspaper _____
_____	_____	_____	8. Bound 28-page manuscript _____
_____	_____	_____	9. Several CDs weighing 1 pound 2 ounces _____
_____	_____	_____	10. Green diamond border envelope to enclose an item weighing more than 2 pounds _____
_____	_____	_____	11. U.S. treasury bond _____
_____	_____	_____	12. X-rays with letter _____
_____	_____	_____	13. Cultured pearl necklace _____
_____	_____	_____	14. Sealed dental catalog _____
_____	_____	_____	15. Monthly statement _____
_____	_____	_____	16. Letter with check enclosed _____

JOB SKILL 12-3 *(continued)*

——— ——— ———   17. Laboratory report _____

——— ——— ———   18. Package weighing 36 pounds _____

——— ——— ———   19. Fastest delivery for a medical tape _____

——— ——— ———   20. Important item to be delivered within 24 hours; it is Saturday noon
_____

——— ——— ———   21. A final collection letter from medical office _____

——— ——— ———   22. Thirty-page book with advertising _____

——— ——— ———   23. Medical society journal _____

——— ——— ———   Complete within specified time.

___/25 ___/25 ___/25   **Total points earned** (To obtain a percentage score, divide the total points
earned by the number of points possible.)

Comments:

Evaluator's Signature: _____   **Need to Repeat:** _____

National Curriculum Competency:

JOB SKILL 12-4
Address Small Envelopes for OCR Scanning

Name _____ Date _____ Score _____

Performance Objective

Task: Address small envelopes for OCR scanning using acceptable abbreviations and correct ZIP codes.

Conditions: Need:

- Computer with Internet connection
- Online Forms 38 and 39 (small envelope templates) located at www.cengagebrain.com with student resources, or three small number 6 envelopes

Refer to:

- *Textbook* Figure 12-6 for envelope illustration
- *Textbook* Table 12-2 for recommended address formats
- *Textbook* Table 12-3 for address abbreviations
- *Textbook* Table 12-4 for two-letter state abbreviations
- *Workbook* Figure 12-3 for long address abbreviations and ZIP codes

Standards: Complete all steps listed in this skill in _____ minutes with a minimum score of _____. (Time element and accuracy criteria may be given by instructor.)

Time: Start: _____ Completed: _____ Total: _____ minutes

Scoring: One point for each step performed satisfactorily unless otherwise listed or weighted by instructor.

Directions with Performance Evaluation Checklist

Dr. Fran Practon has three letters that need to be mailed immediately. Key the addresses listed in this exercise on three number 6 envelopes using standard abbreviations and ZIP codes. If using real envelopes, key Dr. Practon's office address in the upper left corner of each envelope (see *Workbook* Appendix A).

1. Mr. and Mrs. Arthur L. Duncally
   Post Office Box 286
   West Boothbay Harbor, Maine

2. Coastal Community Hospital
   8900 West Elvingston Drive
   Brooklyn-Curtis Bay, Maryland
   Attn: Elizabeth Collingswood, MD

3. Mr. Randolph G. Greenworthy Jr.
   49021 67th Avenue North
   Apartment 8
   Washington Grove, Maryland

1st Attempt	2nd Attempt	3rd Attempt	
_____	_____	_____	Gather materials (equipment and supplies) listed under *Conditions*.
____/9	____/9	____/9	1. Key return address if not using Forms 37 and 38.
____/9	____/9	____/9	2. Key addresses for three envelopes.
____/9	____/9	____/9	3. Use OCR format.
____/9	____/9	____/9	4. Look up and use abbreviations.

JOB SKILL 12-4 (*continued*)

____/3   ____/3   ____/3   5. Look up and key correct ZIP codes.

_____   _____   _____   6. Place attention line in correct position.

_____   _____   _____   7. Proofread for typographical, spelling, and spacing errors.

_____   _____   _____   Complete within specified time.

____/43   ____/43   ____/43   **Total points earned** (To obtain a percentage score, divide the total points earned by the number of points possible.)

MAINE

ZIP code	City	Abbreviation
04006-0000	Biddeford Pool	BIDDEFRD POOL
04625-0000	Cranberry Isles	CRANBERRY IS
04021-0000	Cumberland Center	CUMBRLND CTR
04426-0000	Dover-Foxcroft	DOVR FOXCROFT
04940-0000	Farmington Falls	FARMINGTN FLS
04575-0000	West Boothbay Harbor	W BOOTHBY HBR

MARYLAND

ZIP code	City	Abbreviation
21005-0000	Aberdeen Proving Ground	ABRDN PRV GRD
20331-0000	Andrews Air Force Hospital	ANDRS AF HOSP
21225-0000	Brooklyn-Curtis Bay	BKLYN CTS BAY
20622-0000	Charlotte Hall	CHARLOTE HALL
20732-0000	Chesapeake Beach	CHESAPKE BCH
20904-0000	Ednor Cloverly	EDNR CLOVERLY
21713-0000	Fahrney Keedy Memorial Home	FHRN MEM HOME
20755-0000	Fort George G. Meade	FT MEADE
21240-0000	Friendship Airport	FRNDSHP ARPRT
21078-0000	Havre de Grace	HVRE DE GRACE
20014-0000	National Naval Medical Center	NAVAL MED CTR
20390-0000	Naval Air Facility	NAV AIR FACIL
20678-0000	Prince Frederick	PRNC FREDERCK
20788-0000	Prince Georges Plaza	PRNC GEO PLZ
21152-0000	Sparks Glencoe	SPRKS GLENCOE
21784-0000	Springfield State Hospital	SPRINFLD HOSP
20390-0000	U.S. Naval Communications Center	NAV COMMS CTR
20880-0000	Washington Grove	WASHINGTN GRV

FIGURE 12-3

Comments:

Evaluator's Signature: _____   **Need to Repeat:** _____

National Curriculum Competency: ABHES: 7.a, g

JOB SKILL 12-5
Complete a Mail-Order Form for Postal Supplies

Name _____ Date _____ Score _____

Performance Objective

Task: Complete a mail-order form for postal supplies and compute the total amount owed.

Conditions: Need:

- Computer with Internet connection
- Online Form 40 (Stamps by Mail Order Form) located at www.cengagebrain.com with student resources
- Calculator
- Pen

Standards: Complete all steps listed in this skill in _____ minutes with a minimum score of _____.
(Time element and accuracy criteria may be given by instructor.)

Time: **Start:** _____ **Completed:** _____ **Total:** _____ minutes

Scoring: One point for each step performed satisfactorily unless otherwise listed or weighted by instructor.

Directions with Performance Evaluation Checklist

Complete in ink the mail-order form for stamps. For each item ordered, list the quantity and multiply it by the price to obtain the cost, and then add all figures in the "cost" column to determine the total cost of the order. A check would ordinarily be made out to the U.S. Postmaster and enclosed with the order; however, since check writing is discussed in a future chapter, a check will not be written for this exercise.

1st Attempt	2nd Attempt	3rd Attempt	
_____	_____	_____	Gather materials (equipment and supplies) listed under *Conditions*.
_____/5	_____/5	_____/5	1. Print the medical practice's telephone number, name, and complete address.
_____/3	_____/3	_____/3	2. Order five roles of 49-cent stamps; 100 in each roll.
_____/3	_____/3	_____/3	3. Order one set of 1-cent stamps (20 stamps per set).
_____/2	_____/2	_____/2	4. Order one book of "Forever Stamps," which can be used for first-class mail regardless of future postal rate increases.
_____/3	_____/3	_____/3	5. Order forty 34-cent postcard stamps.
_____/3	_____/3	_____/3	6. Order two hundred 21-cent additional ounce stamps for first-class postage (20 stamps per set).
_____	_____	_____	7. Compute the total cost and insert.
_____	_____	_____	Complete within specified time.
_____/22	_____/22	_____/22	**Total points earned** (To obtain a percentage score, divide the total points earned by the number of points possible.)

JOB SKILL 12-5 (*continued*)

Comments:

Evaluator's Signature: _____ **Need to Repeat:** _____

National Curriculum Competency:

JOB SKILL 12-6
Compose a Letter and Prepare an Envelope for Certified Mail

Name _____ Date _____ Score _____

Performance Objective

Task: Compose and key a letter in a specified format; address and prepare a large envelope for OCR processing as Certified Mail.

Conditions: Need:

- Computer with Internet connection
- Online Form 41 (one letterhead) located at www.cengagebrain.com with student resources, or create a letterhead on a word-processing program
- Online Form 42 (large envelope) or one number 10 envelope
- Online Form 43 (Certified Mail Receipt and Domestic Return Receipt)
- Pen

Refer to:

- *Textbook* Figure 12-4 for a Certified Mail Receipt
- *Textbook* Figure 12-5 for a Domestic Return Receipt
- *Textbook* Figure 12-6 for an envelope illustration
- *Textbook* Procedures 12-5 and 12-6 for step-by-step directions
- *Textbook* Figure 3-13 (Chapter 3) for letter composition example

Standards: Complete all steps listed in this skill in _____ minutes with a minimum score of _____.
(Time element and accuracy criteria may be given by instructor.)

Time: **Start:** _____ **Completed:** _____ **Total:** _____ minutes

Scoring: One point for each step performed satisfactorily unless otherwise listed or weighted by instructor.

Directions with Performance Evaluation Checklist

Mrs. Jane K. Call of 199 Eisenhower Boulevard, Apartment 17-J, Canoga Park, XY 12345-0001, telephoned yesterday stating that she wanted no further treatment from Dr. Gerald Practon. Write a letter to confirm this discharge by the patient stating that Dr. Practon feels further treatment is necessary and recommends that she contact the Valley Medical Society at (555) 659-2234 to obtain the name of another physician. See *textbook* Figure 3-13 in Chapter 3 for help with letter composition. Read through and follow the format specifications listed for the letter, envelope, certification form, and Receipt for Certified Mail.

1st Attempt	2nd Attempt	3rd Attempt	
_____	_____	_____	Gather materials (equipment and supplies) listed under *Conditions*.

LETTER

_____	_____	_____	1. Use Practon letterhead.
_____	_____	_____	2. Use modified block style.
_____	_____	_____	3. Use mixed punctuation.
_____	_____	_____	4. Use current date.
_____	_____	_____	5. Center letter with even margins.
_____	_____	_____	6. Key inside address.

JOB SKILL 12-6 (*continued*)

_____ _____ _____ 7. Key appropriate salutation.

_____ _____ _____ 8. Mention patient name and purpose of letter at the beginning.

____/2 ____/2 ____/2 9. Compose appropriate letter with clear wording that is legally correct.

_____ _____ _____ 10. Insert proper paragraphing.

_____ _____ _____ 11. Key complementary closing line in correct position.

_____ _____ _____ 12. Key signature line.

_____ _____ _____ 13. Key reference initials.

_____ _____ _____ 14. Proofread letter while the document is on-screen for correct grammar and typographical, spelling, punctuation, and capitalization errors.

_____ _____ _____ 15. Correct errors.

_____ _____ _____ 16. Print letter and proofread again.

_____ _____ _____ 17. Present letter ready for the physician to read and sign.

ENVELOPE

____/8 ____/8 ____/8 18. Key large envelope in OCR format with no errors.

_____ _____ _____ 19. Determine the correct postage via the Internet or by calling your local post office, and write the amount where the stamp would be placed on the envelope.

CERTIFICATION FORM

____/5 ____/5 ____/5 20. Complete data on front of certification form.

____/5 ____/5 ____/5 21. Complete data on back of certification form.

DOMESTIC RETURN RECEIPT

____/5 ____/5 ____/5 22. Complete Domestic Return Receipt for Certified Mail.

_____ _____ _____ 23. Fold letter correctly and insert in envelope; do not seal.

_____ _____ _____ Complete within specified time.

____/45 ____/45 ____/45 **Total points earned** (To obtain a percentage score, divide the total points earned by the number of points possible.)

Comments:

Evaluator's Signature: _____ **Need to Repeat:** _____

National Curriculum Competency: CAAHEP: Cognitive: V.C.7; Psychomotor: V.P.8	ABHES: 7.a, g

JOB SKILL 12-7
Key and Fold an Original Letter; Address a Small Envelope for Certified Mail, Return Receipt Requested

Name _____ Date _____ Score _____

Performance Objective

Task: Key a letter using specified format, prepare a small envelope for OCR processing, fold and insert the letter into the envelope, and attach special mailing forms.

Conditions: Need:

- Computer with Internet connection
- Online Form 44 (one letterhead) located at www.cengagebrain.com with student resources, or create a letterhead on a word-processing program
- Online Form 45 (small envelope), or use a number 6 envelope
- Online Form 46 (Certified Mail form and Domestic Return Receipt form)
- Pen

Refer to:

- *Textbook* Figure 12-4 for Certified Mail form
- *Textbook* Figure 12-5 for Domestic Return Receipt
- *Textbook* Figure 12-6 envelope illustration
- *Textbook* Procedures 12-5 and 12-6 for step-by-step directions

Standards: Complete all steps listed in this skill in _____ minutes with a minimum score of _____. (Time element and accuracy criteria may be given by instructor.)

Time: **Start:** _____ **Completed:** _____ **Total:** _____ minutes

Scoring: One point for each step performed satisfactorily unless otherwise listed or weighted by instructor.

Directions with Performance Evaluation Checklist

Henry J. Stone, One April Circle, Pacoima, XY 91331-0000, has had surgery and is negligent about following Dr. Gerald Practon's advice; he is at risk of having complications. Compose an appropriate letter to Mr. Stone advising him of Dr. Practon's withdrawal from the case as of 30 days from the date of this letter. Refer to *textbook* Figure 3-11 in Chapter 3 for help with letter composition. Read and follow the format specifications listed for the letter, envelope, and special mailing forms.

1st Attempt	2nd Attempt	3rd Attempt	
_____	_____	_____	Gather materials (equipment and supplies) listed under *Conditions*.

LETTER

_____	_____	_____	1. Use Practon letterhead.
_____	_____	_____	2. Use full block style.
_____	_____	_____	3. Use mixed punctuation.
_____	_____	_____	4. Use current date.
_____	_____	_____	5. Center letter with even margins.
_____	_____	_____	6. Key inside address.
_____	_____	_____	7. Key appropriate salutation.

JOB SKILL 12-7 (*continued*)

____/3 ____/3 ____/3   8. Compose letter of withdrawal with clear wording that is legally correct.

_____ _____ _____   9. Insert proper paragraphing.

_____ _____ _____ 10. Key complementary closing line in correct position.

_____ _____ _____ 11. Key signature line.

_____ _____ _____ 12. Key reference initials.

_____ _____ _____ 13. Proofread letter while the document is on-screen for correct grammar and typographical, spelling, punctuation, and capitalization errors.

_____ _____ _____ 14. Correct errors.

_____ _____ _____ 15. Print letter and proofread again.

_____ _____ _____ 16. Present letter ready for the physician to read and sign.

ENVELOPE

____/8 ____/8 ____/8 17. Key small envelope in OCR format with no errors using correct address abbreviations.

_____ _____ _____ 18. Determine the correct postage via the Internet or by calling your local post office and write the amount where the stamp would be placed on the envelope.

CERTIFICATION FORM

____/5 ____/5 ____/5 19. Complete data on front of certification form.

____/5 ____/5 ____/5 20. Complete data on back of form.

DOMESTIC RETURN RECEIPT

____/5 ____/5 ____/5 21. Complete Domestic Return Receipt for Certified Mail.

_____ _____ _____ 22. Fold letter correctly and insert in envelope; do not seal.

_____ _____ _____   Complete within specified time.

____/45 ____/45 ____/45 **Total points earned** (To obtain a percentage score, divide the total points earned by the number of points possible.)

Comments:

Evaluator's Signature: _____ **Need to Repeat:** _____

National Curriculum Competency: CAAHEP: Cognitive: V.C.7; Psychomotor: V.P.8	ABHES: 7.a, g

JOB SKILL 12-8

Key and Fold an Original Letter; Address a Large Envelope for Certified Mail, Return Receipt Requested

Name _____ Date _____ Score _____

Performance Objective

Task: Key a letter, prepare a large envelope for OCR processing, fold and insert the letter into the envelope, and attach special mailing forms.

Conditions: Need:

- Computer with Internet connection
- Online Form 47 (one letterhead) located at www.cengagebrain.com with student resources, or create a letterhead on a word-processing program
- Online Form 48 (large envelope), or use one number 10 envelope
- Online Form 49 (Certified Mail form and Domestic Return Receipt)
- Pen

Refer to:

- *Textbook* Figure 12-4 for Certified Mail form
- *Textbook* Figure 12-5 for Domestic Return Receipt
- *Textbook* Figure 12-6 for envelope illustration
- *Textbook* Procedures 12-5 and 12-6 for step-by-step directions

Standards: Complete all steps listed in this skill in _____ minutes with a minimum score of _____. (Time element and accuracy criteria may be given by instructor.)

Time: **Start:** _____ **Completed:** _____ **Total:** _____ minutes

Scoring: One point for each step performed satisfactorily unless otherwise listed or weighted by instructor.

Directions with Performance Evaluation Checklist

Miss Henrietta M. Marskovskie of 4311 Eberly Street, Woodland Hills, XY 12345-4700, was referred to Practon Medical Group by Dr. Ambrose Kistler, 698 Madison Way, Gretna, NE 54321-0009, when she relocated to Woodland Hills. Dr. Gerald Practon went to medical school at the University of Omaha, Nebraska, with Dr. Kistler. Dr. Kistler and his wife, Julie, share the Practon's love for the game of golf; they have played many rounds together. Dr. Practon would like you to write a letter acknowledging this kind referral, and he will edit it prior to its finalization. He saw the patient yesterday and will be taking over her care. She is being treated for renal disease, which is now under control; the patient is doing well and looks very healthy. She is thrilled to be in her new home and close to her grandchildren. Write a friendly referral thank-you letter under Dr. Gerald Practon's signature.

1st Attempt	2nd Attempt	3rd Attempt	
_____	_____	_____	Gather materials (equipment and supplies) listed under *Conditions*.

LETTER

_____	_____	_____	1. Use Practon letterhead.
_____	_____	_____	2. Use modified block style.
_____	_____	_____	3. Use mixed punctuation.
_____	_____	_____	4. Use current date.
_____	_____	_____	5. Center letter with even margins.

JOB SKILL 12-8 (*continued*)

_____ _____ _____ 6. Key inside address.

_____ _____ _____ 7. Key appropriate salutation.

____/7 ____/7 ____/7 8. Compose a short, friendly letter thanking Dr. Kistler for the referral.

_____ _____ _____ 9. Insert proper paragraphing.

_____ _____ _____ 10. Key complementary closing line in correct position.

_____ _____ _____ 11. Key signature line.

_____ _____ _____ 12. Key reference initials.

_____ _____ _____ 13. Proofread letter while the document is on-screen for correct grammar and typographical, spelling, punctuation, and capitalization errors.

_____ _____ _____ 14. Correct errors.

_____ _____ _____ 15. Print letter and proofread again.

_____ _____ _____ 16. Present letter ready for the physician to read and edit.

_____ _____ _____ 17. Incorporate any changes into the letter, print, and present for signature.

ENVELOPE

____/8 ____/8 ____/8 18. Key large envelope in OCR format with no errors.

_____ _____ _____ 19. Determine the correct postage via the Internet or by calling your local post office, and write the amount where the stamp would be placed on the envelope.

CERTIFICATION FORM

____/5 ____/5 ____/5 20. Complete data on front of certification form.

____/5 ____/5 ____/5 21. Complete data on back of certification form.

DOMESTIC RETURN RECEIPT

____/5 ____/5 ____/5 22. Complete Domestic Return Receipt for Certified Mail.

_____ _____ _____ 23. Fold letter correctly and insert in envelope; do not seal.

_____ _____ _____ Complete within specified time.

____/50 ____/50 ____/50 **Total points earned** (To obtain a percentage score, divide the total points earned by the number of points possible.)

Comments:

Evaluator's Signature: _____ **Need to Repeat:** _____

National Curriculum Competency: CAAHEP: Cognitive: V.C.7; Psychomotor: V.P.8 | ABHES: 7.a, g

JOB SKILL 12-9
Prepare a Cover Sheet for Fax Transmission

Name _____ Date _____ Score _____

Performance Objective

Task: Prepare a transmission slip to accompany a message for fax communication.

Conditions: Need:

- Computer with Internet connection
- Online Form 50 (fax transmittal form) located at www.cengagebrain.com with student resources

Refer to:

- *Textbook* Figure 12-11 for a visual example of a cover sheet
- *Textbook* Procedure 12-9 for step-by-step directions

Standards: Complete all steps listed in this skill in _____ minutes with a minimum score of _____.
(Time element and accuracy criteria may be given by instructor.)

Time: Start: _____ Completed: _____ Total: _____ minutes

Scoring: One point for each step performed satisfactorily unless otherwise listed or weighted by instructor.

Directions with Performance Evaluation Checklist

Dr. Fran Practon is scheduled to speak at the Massachusetts American Women's Medical Association convention on November 20 in Boston. She asks you to prepare a fax cover sheet to accompany a two-page letter she will write for fax transmission. The fax will be directed to Dr. Elmo Reardon, 891 So. Revere Way, Boston, MA 02100; fax number: (555) 326-9923; phone number: (555) 326-9921. Abstract the necessary information and complete the fax cover sheet dated November 13, current year.

1st Attempt	2nd Attempt	3rd Attempt	
_____	_____	_____	Gather materials (equipment and supplies) listed under *Conditions*.
____/8	____/8	____/8	1. Complete the top portion of the fax cover sheet.
_____	_____	_____	2. Indicate number of pages sent.
____/3	____/3	____/3	3. Write in the "Remarks" section of the fax sheet requesting prompt confirmation of fax receipt by fax or telephone.
_____	_____	_____	4. List student name as contact.
_____	_____	_____	Complete within specified time.
____/15	____/15	____/15	**Total points earned** (To obtain a percentage score, divide the total points earned by the number of points possible.)

Comments:

Evaluator's Signature: _____ Need to Repeat: _____

National Curriculum Competency: ABHES: 7.a, g

C H A P T E R **13**

The Revenue Cycle: Fees, Credit, and Collection

STOP AND THINK CASE SCENARIOS

Refer to the end of Chapter 13 in the *textbook* for the following scenarios:

- Tackle Payment Obstacles
- Handle Collection Problems

EXAM-STYLE REVIEW QUESTIONS

Refer to the end of Chapter 13 in the *textbook*.

Abbreviation and Spelling Review

Read the patient's chart note and write the meanings for the abbreviations following the note. To decode any abbreviations you do not understand or that appear unfamiliar to you, refer to the list of abbreviations in Appendix B of this *Workbook*. Step-by-step directions for this exercise are found in Procedure 1-1 of Chapter 1 in the *textbook*. Medical terms in the chart note are italicized; study them for spelling. Use your medical dictionary to look up their definitions. Your instructor may give a spelling and definition test that includes these words and abbreviations.

> Robert M Feldman-Pt seen for *bronchial asthma*, ASHD, HBP & *sebaceous cyst*. ECG ordered stat. Lab & x-rays ordered. Comp PX to be done on Friday. PTR next wk for I & D of sebaceous cyst of ® *axilla*.
>
> *Fran Practon, MD*
> Fran Practon, MD

pt	_____	Comp	_____
ASHD	_____	PX	_____
HBP	_____	PTR	_____
ECG	_____	Wk	_____
stat.	_____	I & D	_____
lab	_____	®	_____

Review Questions

Review the objectives, glossary, and chapter information before completing the following review questions.

1. Match the terms in the right column with the definitions in the left column by writing the letters in the blanks.

   _____ analysis of accounts receivable showing 30, 60, 90, and 120 days' delinquency

   _____ a legal proceeding in which money (salary) and property are attached so they can be used to pay a debt

   _____ a list of the physician's procedures, services, and fees

   _____ a message to remind a patient about delinquent payment

   _____ record of business transactions on the books that represent an unsecured accounts receivable for which credit has been extended without a formal written contract

   _____ to trust in an individual's integrity to meet financial obligations

   _____ a debtor who moves and does not leave a forwarding address

   a. garnishment

   b. credit

   c. open accounts

   d. dun

   e. skip

   f. aging account

   g. fee schedule

2. Points of contact in the life of patient accounts from creation to payment is referred to as the

   _____

3. Name three reasons why a patient registration (information) form is valuable for the collection process.

   a. _____

   b. _____

   c. _____

4. How often should a patient information form be updated?_____

5. Name the following different types of fee schedules:

   a. Set schedule of fees: _____

   b. Based on individual physician charge profiles, considering similar groupings of physicians, geographic area, and experience: _____

   c. Fees determined by weighted value (unit value) of each procedure code: _____

   d. Method used by managed care plans, which pays a fixed, per capita amount every month for each patient enrolled: _____

   e. Medicare fee schedule: _____

6. Participating physicians receive _____%

   of the allowable fee paid by Medicare.

7. Circle correct answer. A [participating or nonparticipating] physician may not bill more than the Medicare limiting charge.

8. If a patient signs an assignment of benefits statement, where is the insurance payment sent? _____

   _____

9. Medicare fees based on diagnosis instead of time or services rendered are used in a _____

   and are called _____

   _____.

10. Historically, health care providers have been paid on a fee-for-service model that rewards the number of patients seen, testing performed, and hospital admissions; this is referred to as _____.

11. The new payment model emerging, which is centered around providing the minimum number of services necessary to improve a patient's condition is called _____ _____.

12. Physician outpatient fees may be discounted if they are:

    a. _____

    b. _____

    c. _____

13. The job of discussing and collecting fees is usually relegated to the _____.

14. When is the best time to collect for an office visit and why? _____ _____ _____.

15. Every patient coming to the medical office should have heard about the practice's financial policy at least _____ times.

16. When is a managed care co-payment usually collected? _____

17. Name several things to look for in a deadbeat patient.

    a. _____

    b. _____

    c. _____

    d. _____

    e. _____

    f. _____

    g. _____

    h. _____

18. What are some names used for the form that serves as a combination bill, insurance form, and routing document?

    a. _____

    b. _____

    c. _____

    d. _____

    e. _____

    f. _____

    g. _____

    h. _____

    i. _____

19. Explain cycle billing. _____

_____

_____

20. Name four advantages of using a billing service.

    a. _____

    b. _____

    c. _____

    d. _____

21. A document from the insurance company that arrives with a check for payment of an insurance claim is

    called a/an _____. In the

    Medicare program, this document is called a/an _____,

    and the one sent to patients is called a/an _____.

22. If a patient is called about a delinquent bill at 10 p.m., what federal law is being violated? _____

    _____

23. If credit is refused to a patient, what federal legislation must be complied with? _____

    _____

24. If, in an obstetrical case, a patient is asked for monthly payments before delivery of the baby, what form

    must be completed, signed, and given to the patient? _____ If

    there are fewer than _____ payment installments, this form is not necessary.

25. If interest is charged on a monthly billing statement, what law requires the disclosure of these costs

    before the time of service? _____

    _____

26. Which law states the requirements and limitations for the patient and the medical practice when a

    complaint is registered about a billing statement error? _____

    _____

27. Name the time limit for collection on an open account in your state. _____

28. Explain aging an account and state why it is necessary. _____

    _____

    _____

29. An itemized billing statement is usually sent every _____ days, and when an account

    becomes delinquent a _____ message is sent to prompt payment.

30. What is the average time frame for turning an account over to a collection agency? _____

    _____

31. If a physician asks you to file a claim in small-claims court, where would you go to get the form and

    detailed information about the process? _____

    _____

    _____

32. Define wage garnishment. _____

_____

33. Name two types of bankruptcy that are typically applicable to patients' debts in a medical practice.

a. _____

b. _____

Critical Thinking Exercises

1. Mr. Hernandez starts an argument with you about the physician's fee. What would be your response?

_____

_____

_____

_____

2. Dr. Practon expects you to ask patients to pay at the time of their office visits. Mr. Owen passes your desk without stopping after seeing the doctor. What would you say?

_____

_____

_____

_____

3. What are the most important precautions to take in case a patient becomes a *skip* and you have to conduct a *trace?* _____

_____

_____

_____

_____

JOB SKILL 13-1
Use a Physician's Fee Schedule to Determine Correct Fees

Name _____ Date _____ Score _____

Performance Objective

Task: Determine appropriate fees using a mock fee schedule.

Conditions: Need:
  • Pen or pencil
  Refer to:
  • *Workbook*, Appendix A (Fee Schedule)

Standards: Complete all steps listed in this job skill in _____ minutes with a minimum score of _____.
(Time element and accuracy criteria may be given by instructor.)

Time: Start: _____ Completed: _____ Total: _____ minutes

Scoring: One point for each step performed satisfactorily unless otherwise listed or weighted by instructor.

Directions with Performance Evaluation Checklist

Refer to Appendix A at the end of the *Workbook*, Appendix for Practon Medical Group, Inc., and study the "Fee Schedule" to familiarize yourself with how it is set up. There are main headings (in capital letters) and subheadings to help you find various types of services. The columns under the headings include (1) procedure codes, (2) levels of service or description of procedures, (3) mock fees (used by private payers or private insurance companies), (4) Medicare participating provider fees, (5) Medicare nonparticipating provider fees, and (6) Medicare limiting charges. After familiarizing yourself with the schedule, determine correct fees for the following services and procedures.

1st Attempt	2nd Attempt	3rd Attempt	
_____	_____	_____	Gather materials (equipment and supplies) listed under *Conditions*.
____/2	____/2	____/2	1. Evaluation and Management (E/M) services for a new private pay patient (99204). $ _____
____/2	____/2	____/2	2. Medicare participating physician E/M services for an established patient, level III. $ _____
____/2	____/2	____/2	3. Medicare participating physician E/M services for an initial hospital admit (99223). $ _____
____/2	____/2	____/2	4. Medicare nonparticipating fee for an emergency department visit; established patient (99281). $ _____
____/2	____/2	____/2	5. Rest home visit for an established patient who has private insurance (99335). $ _____
____/2	____/2	____/2	6. Preventive medicine office visit for a 35-year-old new patient. $ _____
____/2	____/2	____/2	7. Initial neonatal intensive care services for a 25-day-old newborn; the baby is covered on the family's private insurance plan. $ _____
____/2	____/2	____/2	8. Medicare participating physician performs destruction of a benign skin lesion (Integumentary System) on a 66-year-old established patient. $ _____

JOB SKILL 13-1 (*continued*)

____/2 ____/2 ____/2 9. Nasal fracture repair (complicated open treatment) on a 16-year-old high school football player with school insurance. $ _____

____/2 ____/2 ____/2 10. Routine venipuncture (36415) performed by the medical assistant on a private pay patient. $ _____

____/2 ____/2 ____/2 11. Cystourethroscopy performed by a Medicare nonparticipating physician. $ _____

____/2 ____/2 ____/2 12. Routine vaginal delivery with total OB care on a 29-year-old patient with private insurance. $ _____

____/2 ____/2 ____/2 13. Chest x-ray, 1 view on a 77-year-old Medicare patient performed by a participating radiologist. $ _____

____/2 ____/2 ____/2 14. Hemoglobin (85018) performed on a private insurance patient. $ _____

____/2 ____/2 ____/2 15. Supplies provided during an office surgical procedure on a patient with Blue Cross. $ _____

_____ _____ Complete within specified time.

____/32 ____/32 ____/32 **Total points earned** (To obtain a percentage score, divide the total points earned by the number of points possible.)

Comments:

Evaluator's Signature: _____   **Need to Repeat:** _____

National Curriculum Competency: CAAHEP: Cognitive: II.C.1; VII.C.1	ABHES: 7.c

JOB SKILL 13-2
Complete Cash Receipts

Name _____ Date _____ Score _____

Performance Objective

Task: Locate fees, calculate charges, subtract payments, and complete four cash receipt forms.

Conditions: Need:
- Computer with Internet connection
- Online Form 51 (cash receipts) located at www.cengagebrain.com with student resources
- Calculator
- Photocopy machine
- Pen

Refer to:
- *Workbook*, Appendix A (Fee Schedule)
- *Workbook*, Appendix B, Table B-2 (Appointment and Patient Care Abbreviations), also found in Chapter 7, Table 7-1)

Standards: Complete all steps listed in this skill in _____ minutes with a minimum score of _____. (Time element and accuracy criteria may be given by instructor.)

Time: Start: _____ Completed: _____ Total: _____ minutes

Scoring: One point for each step performed satisfactorily unless otherwise listed or weighted by instructor.

Directions with Performance Evaluation Checklist

The following private-pay patients have paid in full for professional services, and their entries have been posted to their accounts. Locate the correct fees in the fee schedule, calculate charges, subtract payments, and fill out cash receipts. Make a copy of each receipt for Dr. Practon's file (which you can keep for your records). Give the original receipts to the instructor for grading; these originals in a real situation would be given to the patient for his or her records.

1st Attempt	2nd Attempt	3rd Attempt	
_____	_____	_____	Gather materials (equipment and supplies) listed under *Conditions*.
_____	_____	_____	1. Use February 16 of the current year as the date of service on all cash receipts.
_____	_____	_____	2. The first patient is Beth T. Hobson; record the last name first.
_____	_____	_____	3. Refer to the number in the bottom right corner of the receipt, and insert it in the "reference" column.
___/3	___/3	___/3	4. Beth Hobson is an established patient and had a Level I office visit. Locate the fee in the "fee schedule" and insert the amount above "Charges." Use correct abbreviations to list the description.
___/2	___/2	___/2	5. She has no previous balance and pays in full by cash. Add the charge and subtract the payment to determine the current balance.
_____	_____	_____	6. Indicate in "Other" area if the payment is by cash, or write "check" and check number.

JOB SKILL 13-2 (*continued*)

____/10 ____/10 ____/10 7. Follow steps 2 through 6 to locate fees, calculate charges, subtract payments, and produce a cash receipt for new patient Henry P. Morgan. He has a Level IV examination and pays in cash.

____/12 ____/12 ____/12 8. Follow steps 2 through 6 to locate fees, calculate charges, subtract payments, and produce a cash receipt for a Level II office consultation for Harriet F. Garber. She also had an electrocardiogram (see Medicine Section). Indicate both services above the "Description" column and add both fees to calculate total charge. She pays in cash.

____/15 ____/15 ____/15 9. Follow steps 2 through 6 to locate fees, calculate charges, subtract payments, and produce a cash receipt for established patient Carole V. Putnam. She has a Level III office visit and a two-view x-ray of her right wrist. Previous balance $50; she pays the account in full with check No. 4706. Add the previous balance to the total charges to determine the amount of the check.

_____ _____ _____ Complete within specified time.

____/48 ____/48 ____/48 **Total points earned** (To obtain a percentage score, divide the total points earned by the number of points possible.)

Comments:

Evaluator's Signature: _____ **Need to Repeat:** _____

National Curriculum Competency: CAAHEP: Cognitive: II.C.1	ABHES: 7.c

JOB SKILL 13-3
Interpret an Explanation of Benefits Form

Name _____ Date _____ Score _____

Performance Objective

Task: Interpret payment details and verify figures on an EOB form.

Conditions: Need:

- Calculator
- Pen or pencil

Refer to:

- *Workbook* Figure 13-1 (Explanation of Benefits)
- *Workbook*, Appendix A (Fee Schedule)

Standards: Complete all steps listed in this skill in _____ minutes with a minimum score of _____. (Time element and accuracy criteria may be given by instructor.)

Time: Start: _____ Completed: _____ Total: _____ minutes

Scoring: One point for each step performed satisfactorily unless otherwise listed or weighted by instructor.

Directions with Performance Evaluation Checklist

Study the EOB form in *Workbook* Figure 13-1, then calculate various figures and answer the following questions.

1st Attempt	2nd Attempt	3rd Attempt		
_____	_____	_____		Gather materials (equipment and supplies) listed under *Conditions*.
____/2	____/2	____/2	1.	How many patients' payment information is included on this EOB? _____
____/4	____/4	____/4	2.	For patient **Bradley Capell**: What are the two dates procedures were performed? _____ and _____
____/2	____/2	____/2	3.	What was the total charge for both procedures? $ _____
____/4	____/4	____/4	4.	Subtract the total amount allowed for both procedures from the total amount charged and indicate the "write-off" amount. $ _____
____/2	____/2	____/2	5.	What is the total amount applied to the deductible for both procedures? $ _____
____/2	____/2	____/2	6.	What was the total co-payment collected? $ _____
____/4	____/4	____/4	7.	Subtract the total amount of the co-payment collected from the total amount allowed, then compare this amount with the total amount paid on Bradley Capell's claim; write this amount. $ _____
____/3	____/3	____/3	8.	For patient **Margaret Champion**: What service is being billed for on this claim? _____
____/4	____/4	____/4	9.	What is the amount that will be written off the books? $ _____

JOB SKILL 13-3 (*continued*)

____/4 ____/4 ____/4   10. What is the total amount paid on Margaret Champion's claim? Indicate the math to verify this amount. _____

____/2 ____/2 ____/2   11. What is the total amount paid for both patients on this claim? $ _____

_____ _____ _____   Complete within specified time.

____/35 ____/35 ____/35   **Total points earned** (To obtain a percentage score, divide the total points earned by the number of points possible.)

EXPLANATION OF BENEFITS

ABC Insurance Company
PO Box 27894
Chicago, IL 95927-0004

Practon Medical Group, Inc.
4567 Broadway Avenue
Woodland Hills, XY 12345-4700

Issue Date: 10-31-XX
Page: 1
Check No: 021820377

Physician: Gerald M. Practon, MD
Member: Yes
Provider Number: 46278897XX

PATIENT NAME ID NUMBER GROUP NUMBER	PATIENT ACCOUNT NUMBER CLAIM NUMBER	DATES OF SERVICE	PROCEDURE NUMBER	UNITS OF SERVICE	BILLED AMOUNT	ALLOWED AMOUNT	NOTES	DEDUCTIBLE	CO-PAY AMOUNT	AMOUNT PAID
CAPELL BRADLEY	CAP107	0716XX	52281	1	1000.00	243.75	2	0.00	73.13	170.62
		0917XX	52281	1	1000.00	243.75	2	0.00	73.13	170.62
					2000.00	487.50		0.00	146.26	341.24

NOTES: 1
BECAUSE THE PHYSICIAN OR OTHER HEALTH CARE PROVIDER IS A MEMBER OF ABC INSURANCE, THE ALLOWED AMOUNT IS ACCEPTED AS PAYMENT IN FULL. THE SUBSCRIBER IS RESPONSIBLE ONLY FOR DEDUCTIBLES, CO-PAYMENT AMOUNTS AND NONCOVERED ITEMS.
THE PATIENT'S CO-PAYMENT PORTION IS $146.26.
FOR QUESTIONS REGARDING THE ABOVE CLAIM PLEASE CALL (800) 123-4567.

PATIENT NAME ID NUMBER GROUP NUMBER	PATIENT ACCOUNT NUMBER CLAIM NUMBER	DATES OF SERVICE	PROCEDURE NUMBER	UNITS OF SERVICE	BILLED AMOUNT	ALLOWED AMOUNT	NOTES	DEDUCTIBLE	CO-PAY AMOUNT	AMOUNT PAID
CHAMPION MARGARET	CAP140	1007XX	99213	2	96.97	51.29	1	0.00	45.00	6.29
					96.97	51.29		0.00	45.00	6.29

NOTES: 2
BECAUSE THE PHYSICIAN OR OTHER HEALTH CARE PROVIDER IS A MEMBER OF ABC INSURANCE, THE ALLOWED AMOUNT IS ACCEPTED AS PAYMENT IN FULL. THE SUBSCRIBER IS RESPONSIBLE ONLY FOR DEDUCTIBLES, CO-PAYMENT AMOUNTS AND NONCOVERED ITEMS.
THE PATIENT'S CO-PAYMENT PORTION IS $45.00.

					BILLED	ALLOWED		DEDUCTIBLE	CO-PAY	AMOUNT PAID
TOTAL:					2090.00	538.79		0.00	191.26	347.53

NOTES: 3
BECAUSE THE PHYSICIAN OR OTHER HEALTH CARE PROVIDER IS A MEMBER OF ABC INSURANCE, THE ALLOWED AMOUNT IS ACCEPTED AS PAYMENT IN FULL. THE SUBSCRIBER IS RESPONSIBLE ONLY FOR DEDUCTIBLES, CO-PAYMENT AMOUNTS AND NONCOVERED ITEMS.
THE PATIENT'S CO-PAYMENT PORTION IS $146.26.
FOR QUESTIONS REGARDING THE ABOVE CLAIM PLEASE CALL (800) 123-4567.

FIGURE 13-1

JOB SKILL 13-3 *(continued)*

Comments:

National Curriculum Competency: CAAHEP: Cognitive: II.C.1; VII.C.1	ABHES: 7.c

JOB SKILL 13-4
Role-Play Collection Scenarios

Name _____ Date _____ Score _____

Performance Objective

Task: State how you would handle fee collection in 20 scenarios illustrated in this exercise.

Conditions: Need:
- Two sheets of plain bond paper
- Computer
- Pen or pencil

Refer to:
- *Workbook*, Appendix A (Practon Medical Group, Inc., office policy*)*
- *Workbook*, Appendix A (Fee Schedule)
- *Textbook* Procedure 13-4 and 13-6 for debt collection

Standards: Complete all steps listed in this skill in _____ minutes with a minimum score of _____. (Time element and accuracy criteria may be given by instructor.)

Time: **Start:** _____ **Completed:** _____ **Total:** _____ minutes

Scoring: One point for each step performed satisfactorily unless otherwise listed or weighted by instructor.

Directions with Performance Evaluation Checklist

Refer to Appendix A at the end of the *Workbook*, Appendix for Practon Medical Group, Inc., and read about "Office Policies" and "Payment Policies and Health Insurance Protocol." After reading this section, use critical thinking skills to determine how you would handle each of the following collection situations.

1st Attempt	2nd Attempt	3rd Attempt	
_____	_____	_____	Gather materials (equipment and supplies) listed under *Conditions*.
_____/5	_____/5	_____/5	1. A new private pay patient, Anne Rule, calls for an appointment for Monday morning. It is your office policy to collect the physician's fee at the time of the first visit. Convey this information during your conversation.
_____/5	_____/5	_____/5	2. An established patient, Sylvia Cone, came in on Wednesday for a Level IV examination. She calls today and says she is not going to pay the bill because she is not satisfied with the treatment. She says, "Go ahead and send my account to a collection agency. I'll call my attorney. I can make trouble for you and Dr. Practon." Prepare your response.
_____/5	_____/5	_____/5	3. Mrs. Katrina Frenzel calls to ask you about the bill she just received for her son, Paul, who recently made his first visit to the office. She thinks the bill for $132.28 is "very high" and wonders if there is a mistake because the fee seems out of line. She says she has recently moved into this area. Prepare your response and state what action you would take.
_____/5	_____/5	_____/5	4. Today you call Miss Wendy Snow about her account, which is overdue. You have sent her two statements, telephoned her, and finally sent a letter asking her to call the office about the $80 she owes. She has not responded. According to your records, she was seen on November 2, she lives at home with her parents, and she has health insurance but has not paid the deductible. Prepare questions you would ask her.

JOB SKILL 13-4 (*continued*)

_____/5 _____/5 _____/5 5. Recently, Dr. Gerald Practon performed a two-hour operation and billed the patient his standard fee, which is what physicians generally charge in your region. However, the patient's husband considers the fee exorbitant and has paid only part of it. What action would you take, and how would you collect the outstanding amount?

_____/5 _____/5 _____/5 6. Last week, Dr. Fran Practon made a lengthy long-distance telephone call to check on a postoperative patient who had a complicated major surgery. Should you bill the patient for the telephone charges? Explain your answer.

_____/5 _____/5 _____/5 7. Recently, a patient whose account you have turned over to a collection agency saw you in the supermarket and mentioned that she would be telephoning for an appointment soon. Before making the appointment, you notify Dr. Practon of this circumstance. He insists she pay what she owes, and requires any future bills be paid in cash. Is this ethical? Explain your answer.

_____/5 _____/5 _____/5 8. You routinely bill Dr. Practon's patients the amount that appears on the established fee schedule. In reviewing an account, Dr. Practon finds that a certain patient has been charged more than was intended. The patient makes no complaint and pays the bill in full. What action would you take?

_____/5 _____/5 _____/5 9. Sister Mary Benedict Ramer, a new patient, is seen in consultation. She gives you her insurance card and asks whether she will be given a discount because she is a member of the clergy. How would you respond?

_____/5 _____/5 _____/5 10. Dr. Practon's fee for an appendectomy is $568.36 (*CPT* code 44950). Mr. Jefferson's hospital stay for his appendectomy was unusually troublesome. His first symptoms appeared after midnight, and he was admitted to the hospital as an emergency patient. A decision to operate immediately was postponed by Dr. Practon when the patient began to improve; however, he had several abnormal laboratory results. During the following night, the patient's condition worsened, and the appendectomy was performed, thereby interrupting Dr. Practon's sleep for a second night. After the operation, the patient had a bad case of postanesthesia nausea and was quite demanding while in the hospital. Would Dr. Practon be justified in charging him extra because he was "a lot of trouble"? Explain.

_____/5 _____/5 _____/5 11. You send a bill for $1500 to Mrs. Jamison for a major surgery. She tells you that the physician told her in a presurgery conversation that the charge would be "about $1300." Dr. Practon says he does not remember quoting the figure to her. If the usual charge is $1500 for this procedure, what should you do about the bill? Explain.

_____/5 _____/5 _____/5 12. Mr. French calls in complaining about an overdue refund. He, as well as the insurance company, paid for a procedure, and he is owed a return of his payment. You have been swamped with billing and reply that the statements come first and when you can "get to it" you will mail the refund. What is the proper procedure in this instance? Describe.

_____/5 _____/5 _____/5 13. Patient Joanie Franklin comes in to see Dr. Practon for an initial visit. When asked about insurance coverage, she states, "According to our divorce settlement, my husband's insurance should be billed first." How would you respond?

_____/5 _____/5 _____/5 14. An established patient telephones and says, "The letter I received from the insurance company said you charged too much." How would you respond?

JOB SKILL 13-4 *(continued)*

___/5 ___/5 ___/5 15. New patient Bill Songer comes in to see Dr. Gerald Practon. He says, "My wife handles all the bills, so you will have to call her." How would you reply?

___/5 ___/5 ___/5 16. An established patient was seen by Dr. Fran Practon and returned the following week to have a treadmill test. His insurance was billed; however, the EOB was sent to the patient denying payment for the test. The patient came in and stated, "My insurance should have covered that service." What questions would you ask and what action would you take?

___/5 ___/5 ___/5 17. You call patient Mary Edwards regarding an overdue account and reach an answering machine—the patient is not home. What will you do?

___/5 ___/5 ___/5 18. A patient who has not seen Dr. Practon in a long time comes in for an office visit. Upon leaving, the patient states, "My attorney told me not to pay the bill." What would you say and what question(s) would you ask?

___/5 ___/5 ___/5 19. A long-standing patient owes over $500, which is now past due. She calls stating, "I have just declared bankruptcy." How would you respond?

___/5 ___/5 ___/5 20. You are calling Jana Lynn Rose about an overdue account. Her spouse answers the phone and states that the patient is deceased. How would you respond?

_____ _____ _____ Complete within specified time.

___/102 ___/102 ___/102 **Total points earned** (To obtain a percentage score, divide the total points earned by the number of points possible.)

Comments:

Evaluator's Signature: _____ **Need to Repeat:** _____

National Curriculum Competency: CAAHEP: Cognitive: VII.C.3, 6; Psychomotor: VII.P.3, 4; Affective: VII.A.1; VIII.A.3	ABHES: 7.c

JOB SKILL 13-5
Compose a Collection Letter and Prepare an Envelope

Name _____ Date _____ Score _____

Performance Objective

Task: Compose a collection letter and address a business envelope. Make a photocopy of the completed letter and envelope.

Conditions: Need:

- Computer with Internet connection
- Online Form 52 (one letterhead) located at www.cengagebrain.com with student resources
- Online Form 53 (one number 10 envelope)
- Photocopy machine

Refer to:

- *Textbook* Procedure 11-1 (Chapter 11; written correspondence)
- *Textbook* Procedure 12-6 (Chapter 12; addressing a business envelope)
- *Textbook* Figure 12-6 (Chapter 12; envelope illustration)
- *Workbook* Appendix A (Fee Schedule)

Standards: Complete all steps listed in this skill in _____ minutes with a minimum score of _____. (Time element and accuracy criteria may be given by instructor.)

Time: **Start:** _____ **Completed:** _____ **Total:** _____ minutes

Scoring: One point for each step performed satisfactorily unless otherwise listed or weighted by instructor.

Directions with Performance Evaluation Checklist

Mrs. Mae Van Alystine is a patient of Dr. Gerald Practon. Her home address is 2381 Maple Street, Woodland Hills, XY 12345. Her home telephone number is (555) 421-8700. She is insured with Mutual Insurance Company, policy number J148, and employed by TBC Import Company, work telephone number (555) 421-0707. Her date of birth is 4/12/56.

On July 10, current year, she is a new patient and has a 30-minute office visit (Level III) and an intrauterine device inserted (58300). The insurance company is billed on the same day services are rendered.

On July 25, the insurance company denies payment because the visit was for a contraceptive device. The patient is billed for all services rendered. The patient is billed a second time on August 25. The patient is billed a third time on September 25. No payment has been received.

1st Attempt	2nd Attempt	3rd Attempt	
_____	_____	_____	Gather materials (equipment and supplies) listed under *Conditions*.

LETTER

____/4	____/4	____/4	1. Compose a rough draft of a collection letter to be sent with a copy of the statement.
____/8	____/8	____/8	2. Use letterhead to produce the collection letter, centered on the page with full block style, even and equal margins, consistent punctuation, and appropriate paragraphing, capitalization, and abbreviations.
_____	_____	_____	3. Date the letter October 25 of the current year.
____/3	____/3	____/3	4. Use proper address format for the inside address.

JOB SKILL 13-5 (*continued*)

_____ _____ _____ 5. Place a salutation identifying the person to whom the letter is being written.

____/3 ____/3 ____/3 6. Locate the charges in the fee schedule and include a reference line indicating the date of service and charges.

____/6 ____/6 ____/6 7. In the body of the letter, state the reason for the letter and indicate the expected response.

____/2 ____/2 ____/2 8. Place a complimentary close and signature line.

_____ _____ _____ 9. Insert the proper enclosure notation.

_____ _____ _____ 10. Proofread for correct grammar, spelling and typographical errors while the letter remains on the computer screen.

_____ _____ _____ 11. Make corrections, proof again, and prepare a final copy for signature.

ENVELOPE

____/5 ____/5 ____/5 12. Prepare a No. 10 business envelope using the U.S. Postal Service's approved format.

_____ _____ _____ 13. Copy the letter and envelope.

_____ _____ _____ 14. Attach the original letter to the envelope.

_____ _____ _____ Complete within specified time.

____/40 ____/40 ____/40 **Total points earned** (To obtain a percentage score, divide the total points earned by the number of points possible.)

Comments:

Evaluator's Signature: _____ **Need to Repeat:** _____

National Curriculum Competency: CAAHEP: VII.C.3, 6; Psychomotor: VII.P.1, 4; Affective: VII.A.1	ABHES: 7.c, g

JOB SKILL 13-6
Complete a Financial Agreement

Name _____ Date _____ Score _____

Performance Objective

Task: Fill in a financial agreement with a schedule of payments.

Conditions: Need:

* Computer with Internet connection
* Online Form 54 (Financial Agreement) located at www.cengagebrain.com with student resources
* Calculator
* Pen or pencil

Refer to:

* *Textbook* Figure 13-11 for a visual example
* *Textbook* Procedure 13-3 for step-by-step directions

Standards: Complete all steps listed in this skill in _____ minutes with a minimum score of _____. (Time element and accuracy criteria may be given by instructor.)

Time: **Start:** _____ **Completed:** _____ **Total:** _____ minutes

Scoring: One point for each step performed satisfactorily unless otherwise listed or weighted by instructor.

Directions with Performance Evaluation Checklist

Mr. Biederman has received an itemization of all charges that are now overdue. He has no insurance and has agreed to a payment plan; there will be no financial charge.

1st Attempt	2nd Attempt	3rd Attempt	
_____	_____	_____	Gather materials (equipment and supplies) listed under *Conditions*.
_____/2	_____/2	_____/2	1. Enter patient's name, Alan Biederman, and telephone number, (555) 486-9093, on the financial agreement form.
_____/9	_____/9	_____/9	2. Mr. Biederman has incurred $3000 for medical services with Dr. Gerald Practon and has agreed to pay $600 as a down payment. Determine the unpaid balance and fill in Sections 1 through 9 on the agreement form.
_____/8	_____/8	_____/8	3. Mr. Biederman agrees to pay $200 on the first of every month starting August 1 (current year). Calculate the amount and number of monthly payments and fill in the lower section of the form.
_____	_____	_____	4. Have Mr. Biederman sign and date the form; it is July 1 (current year).
_____/3	_____/3	_____/3	5. On the Schedule of Payment, fill in the total amount owed, the down payment (DP), and the balance owed in the top right portion of the form.
___/24	___/24	___/24	6. Complete the Schedule of Payment by filling in all dates and the amount of each installment payment.
_____	_____	_____	7. Present the form to Dr. Practon for his signature.
_____	_____	_____	Complete within specified time.
_____/50	_____/50	_____/50	**Total points earned** (To obtain a percentage score, divide the total points earned by the number of points possible.)

JOB SKILL 13-6 (*continued*)

Comments:

Banking

STOP AND THINK CASE SCENARIOS

Refer to the end of Chapter 14 in the *textbook* for the following scenarios:

- Determine What Type of Checks to Write
- Answer Payment Question

EXAM-STYLE REVIEW QUESTIONS

Refer to the end of Chapter 14 in the *textbook*.

Abbreviation and Spelling Review

Read the patient's chart note and write the meanings for the abbreviations following the note. To decode any abbreviations you do not understand or that appear unfamiliar to you, refer to the list of abbreviations in Appendix B of this *Workbook*. Step-by-step directions for this exercise are found in Procedure 1-1 of Chapter 1 in the *textbook*. Medical terms in the chart note are italicized; study them for spelling. Use your medical dictionary to look up their definitions. Your instructor may give a spelling and definition test that includes these words and abbreviations.

Etta Chan

June 22, 20XX Pt was born with *cystic hydromas* and has had *epileptic seizures* without *vomiting* or *dyspnea*. Pt is on *Dilantin*. Pt is to be started on *phenobarbital* 100 mg t.i.d. i.e., 2 mg/kg per day. Ordered CT scan.

Gerald Practon, MD
Gerald Practon, MD

---

pt _____	i.e. _____
mg _____	kg _____
t.i.d. _____	CT _____

Note: *"i.e." is a Latin abbreviation and may be found in an English dictionary.*

Review Questions

Review the objectives, glossary, and chapter information before completing the following review questions.

1. Match the terms in the left column with the definitions in the right column by writing the letters in the blanks.

   _____ bearer

   _____ payee

   _____ voucher

   _____ ABA number

   _____ payer

   _____ currency

   a. a check stub

   b. paper money

   c. the person signing a check to pay out funds from a checking account

   d. person delivering an item for payment

   e. a fee assessed by a bank for processing transactions

   f. the person named on a check as the recipient of the amount shown

   g. bank or transit number

2. Write the meanings of the following abbreviations.

   a. NSF _____

   b. EFTS _____

   c. POS _____

   d. MICR _____

   e. ATM _____

3. Name the most common types of checking accounts.

   a. _____

   b. _____

4. Answer the following questions regarding inspecting a check presented for payment in a physician's office.

   a. What identification should be requested? _____

   _____

   b. What should you do if a patient presents an out-of-state check? _____

   _____

   c. What do you compare the information on the check to when verifying it? _____

5. What does ABA stand for and what is it used for? _____

   _____

   _____

   _____

6. What is the federal act that allows the use of electronic checks? _____

   _____

7. When using a pay-by-phone system, how is the caller verified so that the account can be accessed? _____

   _____

8. The following check endorsements are either blank, restrictive, or full. **Note:** *Next to each statement the type of endorsement.*

   a. For deposit only
      Jane Garner _____

   b. Ronald P. Yeager _____

   c. Pay to the order of
      Stationer's Corporation
      Betty T. White
      Harold M. Jeffers _____

9. To guard against embezzlement, what precaution needs to be taken in regards to bank deposits? _____

10. ATMs are open _____ hours a day and _____ days a week; a

    _____ card is typically used for ATM transactions.

11. Explain what procedures you should follow if an error is made in writing or typing a check. _____

    _____

    _____

12. Name three options you have when a check is missing the payer's signature.

    a. _____

    b. _____

    c. _____

13. If a check is written for an amount greater than the balance in the checkbook, it is referred to as

    an _____, which would be returned to the medical office stating the payer has

    _____.

14. In reconciling the monthly bank statement, refer to *textbook* Example 14-3 and indicate whether to *add* or *subtract* the following from (1) the balance appearing on the bank statement or (2) the balance in the checkbook.

    a. outstanding checks _____

    b. bank service charges _____

    c. deposits not shown on the bank statement _____

15. In adjusting the checkbook balance to obtain a reconciliation with the bank statement, what items, besides checks, might you list and subtract from the checkbook balance?

    a. _____

    b. _____

    c. _____

16. If an error is found when reconciling a bank statement, what number should be used to divide the amount of the difference by to find out if a transposition error has been made on the check stub

    register? _____

Critical Thinking Exercises

1. Compare electronic banking and traditional banking methods and summarize the differences between them.

   List features of electronic banking:

   a. _____

   b. _____

   c. _____

   d. _____

   List features of traditional banking:

   a. _____

   b. _____

2. State why you would choose to bank using either electronic banking or traditional banking.

   _____

   _____

   _____

   _____

JOB SKILL 14-1
Prepare a Bank Deposit

Name _____ Date _____ Score _____

Performance Objective

Task: Record checks on a bank deposit slip and calculate total.

Conditions: Need:

• Computer with Internet connection

• Online Form 55 (deposit slip) located at www.cengagebrain.com with student resources

• Pen or pencil

Refer to:

• *Textbook* Figure 14-3 for a visual example

• *Textbook* Procedure 14-1 for step-by-step directions

Standards: Complete all steps listed in this skill in _____ minutes with a minimum score of _____.
(Time element and accuracy criteria may be given by instructor.)

Time: Start: _____ Completed: _____ Total: _____ minutes

Scoring: One point for each step performed satisfactorily unless otherwise listed or weighted by instructor.

Directions with Performance Evaluation Checklist

You open today's mail and find six checks patients have sent to Practon Medical Group, Inc., to pay on their accounts. Record the date and amount of each check and the ABA routing number on a bank deposit slip, and then calculate the amount for deposit.

Keith Austin
7637 Concord Circle
Woodland Hills, XY 12345

16-21/1220   **6335**

Date *March 24, 20xx*

Pay to the order of *Gerald Practon, MD* $ *36.92*

Thirty six and 92/100 _____ Dollars

Santa Paula Interstate Bank

Memo *insurance balance*   *Keith Austin*

JOB SKILL 14-1 (*continued*)

Hope Wilburn
PO BOX 309
Woodland Hills, XY 12345

55-60/3222

1226

Date *March 26, 20xx*

Pay to the order of   *Fran Practon, MD* $ *250.00*

Two hundred and fifty dollars and no/100 ———— Dollars

Woodland Hills CITI Bank

Memo *April payment installment*   *Hope Wilburn*

Richard Rickman
444 Platte Place
Woodland Hills, XY 12345

154-20/440

410

Date *March 25, 20xx*

Pay to the order of   *Practon Medical Group* $ *15.00*

Fifteen and no/100 ———— Dollars

County Bank

Memo *Copay*   *R. Rickman*

Houshang Hutton
8989 Telegraph Rd
Woodland Hills, XY 12345

90-8030/2000

1229

Date *March 26, 20xx*

Pay to the order of   *Practon Medical Group, Inc.* $ *70.65*

Seventy dollars and 65/100 ———— Dollars

Westlake Bank & Trust

Memo *Noncovered services*   *Houshang Hutton*

JOB SKILL 14-1 *(continued)*

Carla M. Gafford
613 Redwood Avenue
Woodland Hills, XY 12345

90-4268/1222

4851

Date March 25, 20xx

Pay to the order of _Gerald Practon, MD_ $ 500.00

Five hundred and no/100 ———— Dollars

Intercommercial Bank

Memo _Outpatient surgery deductible_ Carla Gafford

Dick and Angie Hundley
109 Linden Drive
Woodland Hills, XY 12345

16-24/1220

8203

Date March 26, 20xx

Pay to the order of _Dr. Fran Practon_ $ 124.00

One hundred and twenty four dollars and no/100 ———— Dollars

Hillcrest Bank & Mortgage

Memo _Medicare deductible_ Angie Hundley

1st Attempt	2nd Attempt	3rd Attempt	
____	____	____	Gather materials (equipment and supplies) listed under *Conditions*.
____	____	____	1. Enter the date on the front of the deposit slip; use March 28 (current year).
____/2	____/2	____/2	2. Enter the first check from Keith Austin on the back of the deposit slip, recording the bank ABA number on the left and the amount on the right.
____/2	____/2	____/2	3. Enter the check from Hope Wilburn.
____/2	____/2	____/2	4. Enter the check from Richard Rickman.
____/2	____/2	____/2	5. Enter the check from Houshang Hutton.
____/2	____/2	____/2	6. Enter the check from Carla Gafford.
____/2	____/2	____/2	7. Enter the check from Angie Hundley.
____	____	____	8. Total the amounts from all checks and record.

JOB SKILL 14-1 *(continued)*

____/6 ____/6 ____/6 9. Total the check amounts written on the deposit slip and compare with the total of all checks. If the amounts match, write the total on the back of the deposit slip.

____ ____ ____ 10. Enter total of all checks from the reverse side on the front of the deposit slip.

____ ____ ____ 11. Enter the subtotal.

____ ____ ____ 12. Enter the total of the deposit, referred to as "net deposit."

____ ____ ____ Complete within specified time.

____/25 ____/25 ____/25 **Total points earned** (To obtain a percentage score, divide the total points earned by the number of points possible.)

Comments:

Evaluator's Signature: _____ **Need to Repeat:** _____

National Curriculum Competency: CAAHEP: Cognitive: II.C.1, Psychomotor: VII.P.2

JOB SKILL 14-2
Write Checks

Name _____ Date _____ Score _____

Performance Objective

Task: Handwrite or type two checks.

Conditions: Need:

- Computer with Internet connection
- Online Form 56 (two blank checks and two invoices) located at www.cengagebrain.com with student resources
- Pen

Refer to:

- *Textbook* Procedure 14-2 for step-by-step directions
- *Textbook* Figures 14-1A and 14-1B for visual illustrations

Standards: Complete all steps listed in this skill in _____ minutes with a minimum score of _____. (Time element and accuracy criteria may be given by instructor.)

Time: Start: _____ Completed: _____ Total: _____ minutes

Scoring: One point for each step performed satisfactorily unless otherwise listed or weighted by instructor.

Directions with Performance Evaluation Checklist

You have received two invoices for the Practon Medical Group. Handwrite or type two checks for Dr. Practon's signature to pay these bills. Note: The check stub is shown on the face of the check for this exercise but would actually appear as the "stub" shown in *textbook* Figure 14-1B or as a check register with consecutive lines for the date, check number, payee name, amount of check or deposit, and running balance.

1st Attempt	2nd Attempt	3rd Attempt	
_____	_____	_____	Gather materials (equipment and supplies) listed under *Conditions*.

CHECK NO 485

_____	_____	_____	1. Date the first check May 27 of the current year.
____/3	____/3	____/3	2. Make the check payable to Stationer's Corporation; include the company's address.
____/3	____/3	____/3	3. Make the check payable for the amount due indicated on the invoice.
____/3	____/3	____/3	4. Insert the balance forward from the checkbook on the check stub; the amount is $9,825.55.
____/3	____/3	____/3	5. Note the date, what the check is for, and the amount on the check stub.
____/2	____/2	____/2	6. Calculate a new balance and record.
____/3	____/3	____/3	7. Bring the balance forward to the next check, No. 486.

CHECK NO 486

_____	_____	_____	8. Date check May 27 of the current year.
____/3	____/3	____/3	9. Make the check payable to Randolph Electrical Supply; include the company's address.
____/3	____/3	____/3	10. Make the check payable for the amount due indicated on the invoice.

JOB SKILL 14-2 *(continued)*

____/3   ____/3   ____/3   11. Note the date, what the check is for, and the amount on the check stub.

____/2   ____/2   ____/2   12. Calculate a new balance and record.

INVOICE

____/6   ____/6   ____/6   13. Record the date paid, check number, and amount paid on each invoice.

____   ____   ____   Complete within specified time.

____/38   ____/38   ____/38   **Total points earned** (To obtain a percentage score, divide the total points earned by the number of points possible.)

Comments:

Evaluator's Signature: _____   **Need to Repeat:** _____

National Curriculum Competency: ABHES: 7.a, c

JOB SKILL 14-3
Endorse a Check

Name _____ Date _____ Score _____

Performance Objective

Task: Enter a restrictive endorsement on a check in the proper location.

Conditions: Need:
- Front and back of check from patient Jeffrey Brown (located following directions)
- Pen

Refer to:
- *Textbook* Figure 14-2 for an illustration
- Chapter material (Check Endorsements)

Standards: Complete all steps listed in this skill in _____ minutes with a minimum score of _____.
(Time element and accuracy criteria may be given by instructor.)

Time: Start: _____ Completed: _____ Total: _____ minutes

Scoring: One point for each step performed satisfactorily unless otherwise listed or weighted by instructor.

Directions with Performance Evaluation Checklist

Read chapter material on restrictive endorsements and complete the following steps.

Jeffrey Brown
7827 Minnow Street
Woodland Hills, XY 12345
Phone: 555-482-1976

90-7177₇₅₀
3222
7504003778

164

Date _____ June 3, 20xx _____

Pay to the order of _____ Practon Medical Group, Inc. _____ | $ | 199.03

One hundred ninety nine and 3/100 _____ Dollars

College National Bank
741 Main Street
Woodland Hills, XY 12345

Memo _____   _____ Jeffrey Brown _____   MP

⑆3222717⑆⑉:0164 ⑈750 40031641⑈

JOB SKILL 14-3 *(continued)*

```
┌─────────────────────────────────────────────────────────────────────────┐
│                                              │ │ │  ENDORSE HERE          │
│                                              │ │ │                        │
│                          DO NOT WRITE, STAMP,│ │ │                        │
│                          OR SIGN BELOW THIS  │ │ │                        │
│                          LINE RESERVED FOR   │ │ │                        │
│                          FINANCIAL           │ │ │                        │
│                          INSTITUTION USE     │ │ │                        │
│                                              │ │ │                        │
└─────────────────────────────────────────────────────────────────────────┘
```

1st Attempt	2nd Attempt	3rd Attempt	
_____	_____	_____	Gather materials (equipment and supplies) listed under *Conditions*.
____/6	____/6	____/6	1. Enter correct wording for a restrictive endorsement.
____/4	____/4	____/4	2. Place restrictive endorsement in proper location.
_____	_____	_____	Complete within specified time.
____/12	____/12	____/12	**Total points earned** (To obtain a percentage score, divide the total points earned by the number of points possible.)

Comments:

Evaluator's Signature: _____ **Need to Repeat:** _____

National Curriculum Competency: ABHES: 7.a, c

JOB SKILL 14-4
Inspect a Check

Name _____ Date _____ Score _____

Performance Objective

Task: Inspect a check and answer questions.

Conditions: Need:
• Pen or pencil

Refer to:
• Handwritten check from Rita Stevens (see following directions)

Standards: Complete all steps listed in this skill in _____ minutes with a minimum score of _____.
(Time element and accuracy criteria may be given by instructor.)

Time: Start: _____ Completed: _____ Total: _____ minutes

Scoring: One point for each step performed satisfactorily unless otherwise listed or weighted by instructor.

Directions with Performance Evaluation Checklist

As you learned after reading Chapter 14 in the *textbook*, a handwritten check has certain requirements that must be met to be valid. An established patient, Rita Stevens, wrote a check for a Level III office visit totaling $40.20 before leaving the office on May 21, 20XX. Inspect the check and answer the following questions.

RITA STEVENS
126 Sunset Lane
Woodland Hills, XY 12345

90-7177/750
3222
7504003778

164

Date *May 25, 20xx*

Pay to the order of *Practon Medical Group, Inc* $ 40.00

Forty and 20/100 Dollars

College National Bank
741 Main Street
Woodland Hills, XY 12345

Memo *Level III OV*   *Rita Stevens*   MP

⑈3222717 79⑈0164 ⑈750 4003778⑈

1st Attempt	2nd Attempt	3rd Attempt	
_____	_____	_____	Gather materials (equipment and supplies) listed under *Conditions*.
____/2	____/2	____/2	1. What two personal identification items should be obtained from the patient before accepting a check?
____/2	____/2	____/2	2. Does the check list the complete name, address, and telephone number of the patient? If not, what is missing?

JOB SKILL 14-4 (*continued*)

___/2	___/2	___/2	3. Is the check dated correctly? If not, what is the problem?
_____	_____	_____	4. Is the check made out to the correct payee?
_____	_____	_____	5. Did Mrs. Stevens make the check out for the proper amount?
___/2	___/2	___/2	6. If not, what is the problem?
___/2	___/2	___/2	7. How much will Dr. Practon receive?
_____	_____	_____	8. Is the check signed by Rita Stevens?
_____	_____	_____	Complete within specified time.
___/15	___/15	___/15	**Total points earned** (To obtain a percentage score, divide the total points earned by the number of points possible.)

Comments:

Evaluator's Signature: _____ **Need to Repeat:** _____

National Curriculum Competency: ABHES: 7.a, c

JOB SKILL 14-5
Reconcile a Bank Statement

Name _____ Date _____ Score _____

Performance Objective

Task: Reconcile a bank statement.

Conditions: Need:

- Computer with Internet connection
- Online Form 57 (Bank Reconciliation Worksheet) located at www.cengagebrain.com with student resources
- Pen or pencil

Refer to:

- Bank statement shown following this exercise
- *Textbook* Procedure 14-3 for step-by-step directions.

Standards: Complete all steps listed in this skill in _____ minutes with a minimum score of _____. (Time element and accuracy criteria may be given by instructor.)

Time: Start: _____ Completed: _____ Total: _____ minutes

Scoring: One point for each step performed satisfactorily unless otherwise listed or weighted by instructor.

Directions with Performance Evaluation Checklist

1st Attempt	2nd Attempt	3rd Attempt	
_____	_____	_____	Gather materials (equipment and supplies) listed under *Conditions*.
___/10	___/10	___/10	1. You compare and check off each transaction recorded in your checkbook with those listed in this statement and discover the following outstanding checks: No. 318 for $25, No. 337 for $60, No. 338 for $78, No. 340 for $15, and No. 341 for $18.20. Record these on the reconciliation form under "Outstanding Checks."
___/10	___/10	___/10	2. Add the total of outstanding checks and record on the reconciliation form.
___/4	___/4	___/4	3. Assume you made deposits of $3500 on June 30, 20XX, and $1800 on July 2, 20XX, which do not show on the statement. Record these on the reconciliation form under "Deposits Not Credited."
___/4	___/4	___/4	4. Add the total of deposits not credited and record on the reconciliation form.
___/2	___/2	___/2	5. Enter the ending statement balance on the reconciliation form.
___/2	___/2	___/2	6. Add the total of the deposits not credited to the ending statement balance and record (making a note of the subtotal).
___/2	___/2	___/2	7. Subtract the total of the outstanding checks from the figure determined in step 6 and record.

JOB SKILL 14-5 (*continued*)

_____ _____ _____   8. Verify the adjusted total you determined with the checkbook balance, which is $6807.89

_____ _____ _____   9. Do these figures match and does the checkbook balance? _____ If not, repeat the above steps, recalculating figures.

_____ _____ _____   Complete within specified time.

___/38 ___/38 ___/38   **Total points earned** (To obtain a percentage score, divide the total points earned by the number of points possible.)

Comments:

Evaluator's Signature: _____   **Need to Repeat:** _____

National Curriculum Competency: CAAHEP: Cognitive: II.C.1

JOB SKILL 14-5 (*continued*)

COLLEGE NATIONAL BANK
ACCOUNT ACTIVITY

College National Bank
700 West Main Street
Woodland Hills, XY 12345

(800) 540-5060

PRACTON MEDICAL GROUP, INC   140
4567 BROAD AVENUE
WOODLAND HILLS XY   12345

PAGE	1
ITEM COUNT	30

CHECKING — ACCOUNT 12345-6789

SUMMARY

BEGINNING STATEMENT BALANCE ON 20XX . . . . $		633.87
TOTAL OF 4 DEPOSITS/OTHER CREDITS		1414.75
TOTAL OF 15 CHECKS PAID.		271.53
5 WITHDRAWALS/OTHER CHARGES.		73.00
ENDING STATEMENT BALANCE ON 20XX		1704.09

CHECKS/ WITHDRAWALS/ OTHER CHARGES

CHECKS:

NUMBER	DATE	AMOUNT	NUMBER	DATE	AMOUNT
0317	06-08	17.40	0328	06-10	29.90
1319	05-25	30.00	0329	05-26	32.05
0320	05-30	7.59	0330	06-02	2.75
0321	05-27	9.00	0331	06-02	30.79
0322	05-24	1.00	0332	06-02	11.47
0323	06-03	6.13			
0324	05-30	1.78			
0325	06-02	67.50			
0326	05-25	21.92			
0327	06-03	2.25			

TOTAL OF 15 CHECKS PAID   271.53

WITHDRAWALS/OTHER CHARGES:

DATE	TRANSACTION DESCRIPTION	AMOUNT
06-10	SURGICAL SUPPLY PAYMENT AT ELECTRONIC BANKING	34.30
06-07	STAR FREE PRESS PAYMENT AT ELECTRONIC BANKING	2.00
06-07	MARINER'S MAIL PAYMENT AT ELECTRONIC BANKING	1.00
06-07	CELLULAR ONE PAYMENT AT ELECTRONIC BANKING	16.00
06-03	CLINT PHARMACY PAYMENT AT ELECTRONIC BANKING	19.70

DEPOSITS/ OTHER CREDITS

DEPOSITS:

DATE	TRANSACTION DESCRIPTION	AMOUNT
06-07	BRANCH DEPOSIT	250.24
06-09	BRANCH DEPOSIT	1000.00
06-15	BRANCH DEPOSIT	156.69
06-16	CHECK DEPOSIT AT BANK BY MAIL	7.82

DAILY BALANCES

DATE	BALANCE	DATE	BALANCE	DATE	BALANCE
05-24	632.87	06-02	418.02	06-09	1605.78
05-25	580.95	06-03	389.94	06-10	1573.88
05-26	548.90	06-07	623.18	06-15	1730.57
05-27	539.90	06-08	605.78	06-16	1704.09
05-30	530.53				

Bookkeeping

STOP AND THINK CASE SCENARIOS

Refer to the end of Chapter 15 in the textbook for the following scenarios:

- Determine an Accounting System
- Obtain Change for a Patient

EXAM-STYLE REVIEW QUESTIONS

Refer to the end of Chapter 15 in the *textbook*.

Abbreviation and Spelling Review

Read the patient's chart note and write the meanings for the abbreviations following the note. To decode any abbreviations you do not understand or that appear unfamiliar to you, refer to the list of abbreviations in Appendix B of this *Workbook*. Step-by-step directions for this exercise are found in Procedure 1-1 of Chapter 1 in the *textbook*. Medical terms in the chart note are italicized; study them for spelling. Use your medical dictionary to look up their definitions. Your instructor may give a spelling and definition test that includes these words and abbreviations.

Kevin T. Dusseau

June 30, 20XX. Pt has off and on problems with eye. Dx: Acute *bacterial conjunctivitis* L eye. Treat R eye at first sign of *symptoms*. Cold compresses L eye ad lib. for comfort. Retn p.r.n.

Fran Practon, MD
Fran Practon, MD

Pt _____   ad lib. _____

Dx _____   retn _____

L _____   p.r.n. _____

R _____

Review Questions

Review the objectives, glossary, and chapter information before completing the following review questions.

1. Match the terms in the left column with the definitions in the right column and write the letters in the blanks.

   _____ debit

   _____ post

   _____ accounts receivable ledger

   _____ asset

   _____ liability

   _____ daysheet

   _____ credit

   _____ proprietorship

   _____ accounts payable ledger

   a. bookkeeping entry that decreases assets and increases earnings

   b. register or checkbook that lists amounts paid out for expenses of the business practice

   c. the owner's net worth

   d. to record a charge, payment, or adjustment on a ledger or account

   e. register for recording all daily business transactions of patients

   f. that which is owned by the business

   g. monies that are owed for business expenditures

   h. record of all patients' outstanding accounts showing how much each one owes for services rendered

   i. a bookkeeping entry that records increases in assets and expenses and decreases liabilities

2. Name one or more advantages and disadvantages of each of the following accounting systems:

	Advantage	Disadvantage
a. single-entry	_____	_____
		_____
b. double-entry	_____	_____
c. pegboard	_____	_____
		_____
		_____
		_____
d. computerized	_____	_____
		_____
		_____
		_____

3. When using a computerized bookkeeping system, you would post charges, payments, and adjustments to a patient _____; in a manual system, you would post to a _____.

4. Charges are posted on the date _____; payments are posted on the date _____.

5. Circle the correct answer: In electronic accounting, the computer automatically adds all (debits or credits) and subtracts all (debits or credits) and computes a running balance.

6. When the insurance payment plus the patient responsibility is less than the amount of the charge, the amount over the "allowed amount" is written off the books. It is called a _____ for private insurance programs and a _____ for the Medicare program.

7. When an account is sent to a collection agency,

   a. what happens to the balance that is on the account?

   _____

   _____

   b. how do you post money sent by the collection agency to the physician's office?

   _____

   _____

8. Write the bookkeeping term that each of the following abbreviation stands for.

   a. B/F _____

   b. pd _____

   c. adj _____

   d. ROA _____

   e. recd _____

9. On the daysheet, the total of what patients have paid by cash and check must equal the total _____ for that day.

10. Explain what calculations need to be made to determine the new accounts receivable figure at the end of the month.

    a. _____

    b. _____

    c. _____

11. An amount evenly divisible by _____ may indicate a transposed figure, and an amount evenly divisible by _____ may indicate posting to the wrong column.

12. If a posting error occurs when writing 900 for 90, this type of error is called _____.

13. At the end of the day, to reconcile the cash and change drawer, the _____ should equal the cash amount on the _____, and the remaining amount in the change drawer should be the same as the beginning amount.

14. When is the petty cash fund replenished? _____ or _____, depending on the demand for funds.

15. When replenishing the petty cash fund, add the _____ to the _____ and compare this total to the amount established for the fund; they should equal.

16. Make a list of all forms required when using a pegboard bookkeeping system, and give a brief explanation of the function of each one.

Form   Function

a. _____   _____
                                                 _____

b. _____   _____
                                                 _____
                                                 _____

c. _____   _____
                                                 _____
                                                 _____

d. _____   _____
                                                 _____
                                                 _____

◥ Critical Thinking Exercises

1. Explain the purposes of a cash or change drawer and a petty cash fund, and tell why a medical practice needs both systems in place. _____

   _____

   _____

2. Mrs. Landry's account shows a delinquent balance of $30, and Dr. Practon wants the amount written off the books and the account closed. Explain what you would do.

   _____

   _____

BOOKKEEPING JOB SKILLS 15-1 THROUGH 15-13

Job Skills 15-1 through 15-13 take you through step-by-step procedures to gain experience in bookkeeping practices. Although these job skills utilize ledger cards and the pegboard bookkeeping system, the concepts learned apply to computerized bookkeeping and will help you understand posting steps needed in both systems as well as computations automatically done in electronic health record (EHR) systems.

Job Skill 15-1 presents a variety of posting scenarios including posting charges, adjustments, payments, a negative balance, and a returned check for nonsufficient funds (NSF). Refer to the figures and examples listed for illustrations and step-by-step directions found in Procedure 15-1.

Job Skill 15-2 involves setting up 28 ledger cards that will be used in the rest of the job skills.

Job Skills 15-3 through 15-6 (Day 1), 15-7 through 15-9 (Day 2), and 15-10 through 15-12 (Day 3) involve the daysheet and may be assigned individually; however, they must be done in order. Instead, the instructor may choose to assign these job skills as three projects to be done in class or as homework. Each grouping represents a different day in the medical practice that requires various posting, calculating, and balancing of financial records.

Job Skill 15-13 involves setting up a daysheet for a new month.

You will also be looking up procedure codes and using the fee schedule found in Appendix A of this *Workbook*. The selection of codes are arranged according to sections found in the 2017 *Current Procedural Terminology** code book. Locate the section and subsection as indicated, then find the description. Last, determine the patient's insurance and locate the fee according to the insurance type and categories listed. With each job skill, read it entirely before beginning.

---

*2017 Current Procedural Terminology © *2016 American Medical Association*. All rights reserved.

JOB SKILL 15-1
Post Entries to Ledger Cards and Calculate Balances

Name _____ Date _____ Score _____

Performance Objective

Task: Locate procedure codes and fees in the fee schedule, then post charges, adjustments, payments, a negative balance, a refund check, and a returned check for NSF; calculate percentages, send an account to a collection agency, and post a check from a collection agency making correct notations and calculating running balances.

Conditions: Need:

- Ledger cards (following directions)
- Calculator
- Pen or pencil

Refer to:

- *Workbook* Appendix A (mock fee schedule) for procedure codes and fees
- *Textbook* Figure 13-5 (Chapter 13) for illustration of a ledger card and posting entry labels with descriptions
- *Textbook* Figure 15-2 for ledger card with *posting illustrations*
- *Textbook* Example 15-3 for illustration of posting *contract adjustments*
- *Textbook* Example 15-4 for illustration of posting an account sent to and money received from a *collection agency*
- *Textbook* Example 15-5 for illustration of posting a *returned check*
- *Textbook* Example 15-6 for illustration of posting a *credit balance* and *refund adjustment*
- *Textbook* Procedure 15-1 for step-by-step directions

Standards: Complete all steps listed in this skill in _____ minutes with a minimum score of _____. (Time element and accuracy criteria may be given by instructor.)

Time: Start: _____ Completed: _____ Total: _____ minutes

Scoring: One point for each step performed satisfactorily unless otherwise listed or weighted by instructor.

Directions with Performance Evaluation Checklist

There are various types of posting exercises within this job skill. Post all transactions on the following ledger cards using the current date or date referred to. Enter appropriate references and descriptions to post all transactions, then calculate a running balance. **Note:** *Typically, when using a ledger card all transactions that occur on the same day are posted on one line. However, in this exercise (and when using a computerized system), each transaction is posted separately, line-by-line, to simplify the learning process and make sure that the addition of charges, subtraction of payments and adjustments, and the running balance are calculated correctly.*

JOB SKILL 15-1 (*continued*)

Star Collins

DATE	REFERENCE	DESCRIPTION	CHARGES	CREDITS		BALANCE	
				Pymnts	Adj		
		BALANCE FORWARD					

Elizabeth Hooper

DATE	REFERENCE	DESCRIPTION	CHARGES	CREDITS		BALANCE	
				Pymnts	Adj		
		BALANCE FORWARD					
6-1-20XX	99203	OV Level III NP	70 92				
6-1-20XX	99000	Handling Pap	5 00				
8-15-20XX	ck# 778	ROA ABC Ins.		69 00			

Maria Sanchez

DATE	REFERENCE	DESCRIPTION	CHARGES	CREDITS		BALANCE	
				Pymnts	Adj		
		BALANCE FORWARD					
7-6-20XX	99244	Consult Level IV	145 05				
7-20-20XX	ck# 432	ROA Pt		25 00			
8-15-20XX	ck# 451	ROA Pt		50 00			

JOB SKILL 15-1 (*continued*)

Jason Barnes

DATE	REFERENCE	DESCRIPTION	CHARGES		CREDITS				BALANCE	
					Pymnts		Adj			
		BALANCE FORWARD								

Brett Walker

DATE	REFERENCE	DESCRIPTION	CHARGES		CREDITS				BALANCE	
					Pymnts		Adj			
		BALANCE FORWARD								
7-1-20XX	99203	OV Level III NP	70	92						
7-15-20XX	45308	Proctosigmoidoscopy with removal polyp	135	34						
7-20-20XX	ck 2005	ROA Pt			50	00				
9-1-20XX	Voucher 4006	ROA Blue Cross			165	00				

Edna Hargrove

DATE	REFERENCE	DESCRIPTION	CHARGES		CREDITS				BALANCE	
					Pymnts		Adj			
		BALANCE FORWARD								
8-1-20XX	99213	OV Level III	40	20						
8-1-20XX	58300	IUD insertion	100	00						
8-14-20XX	ck 101	ROA Pt			100	00				

JOB SKILL 15-1 *(continued)*

Beth Jones

DATE	REFERENCE	DESCRIPTION	CHARGES	CREDITS		BALANCE	
				Pymnts	Adj		
		BALANCE FORWARD					

Helen Rice

DATE	REFERENCE	DESCRIPTION	CHARGES	CREDITS		BALANCE	
				Pymnts	Adj		
		BALANCE FORWARD					
1/16/XX	99205	NP OV level V	132 28			132	28
1/23/XX	99214	Est Pt OV level 4	61 51			193	79
1/30/XX	99213	Ext Pt OV level 3	40 20			233	99
2/1/XX	Billed pt	*Please pay balance due*				233	99
3/1/XX	Billed pt	*Account is overdue— please pay balance*				233	99
4/1/XX	Billed pt	*Final notice. If payment is not received in 5 days, your account will be sent to a collection agency*				233	99

1st Attempt	2nd Attempt	3rd Attempt	
_____	_____	_____	Gather materials (equipment and supplies) listed under *Conditions*.

POST CHARGES

____/7	____/7	____/7	1. **Star Collins**, a private pay new patient, saw Dr. Practon today for a Level V office visit. Locate the correct *CPT* code and corresponding charge in the fee schedule (Evaluation and Management section). Post the charge in the correct column with proper reference and description and indicate the running balance.
____/8	____/8	____/8	2. Star returned 1 week later for a follow-up office visit (Level II). Make the correct notations, post the charge, and calculate a running balance.

JOB SKILL 15-1 (*continued*)

POST ADJUSTMENT AND WRITE OFF BALANCE DUE

____/8 ____/8 ____/8 3. **Elizabeth Hooper** has a small uncollected balance due. Dr. Practon said he wishes to write off the balance. Use todays date and calculate the running balance, post the adjustment entry, and calculate the new balance.

POST PATIENT PAYMENT

____/8 ____/8 ____/8 4. **Maria Sanchez** was in for a consultation and has made two payments on her account. She makes another payment today in the amount of $25.00 (Ck No. 463). Post the current payment and calculate the running balance for each posting entry.

POST INSURANCE PAYMENT

____/7 ____/7 ____/7 5. **Jason Barnes** had a cholecystectomy performed on 4/3/XX. Locate the *CPT* code and Medicare participating charge in the fee schedule (Surgery Section: Mediastinum/Diaphragm/Digestive System). Post the charge using the proper reference and description.

____/4 ____/4 ____/4 6. On the day of the procedure Medicare was billed. Enter a notation on the ledger indicating this and bring down the current balance.

____/7 ____/7 ____/7 7. Two months later, Medicare paid 80% of the participating fee (Voucher No. 10032). Calculate and post this payment, then compute and post the current balance.

COMPUTE NEGATIVE BALANCE AND POST REFUND CHECK

____/9 ____/9 ____/9 8. **Brett Walker** paid on his account and his insurance also paid, resulting in an overpayment. The patient is to receive a refund. Use the current date and calculate the running balances then post the refund (check 2068) to clear the negative balance.

POST RETURN CHECK FOR NONSUFFICIENT FUNDS

____/12 ____/12 ____/12 9. **Edna Hargrove** issued a check for payment toward her last office visit, but it was returned today by XYZ Bank and marked NSF. Post a reversal of the payment for the returned check as well as the $10 bank charge on the ledger card and calculate the running balance for all postings.

POST CHARGES AND PAYMENTS, CALCULATE PERCENTAGES, AND COMPUTE A NEGATIVE BALANCE

____/7 ____/7 ____/7 10. **Beth Jones**, a private insurance patient, comes in today for a Level III new patient examination. She is complaining of fatigue, nausea, and dysuria. Locate the correct *CPT* code and charge in the fee schedule, then post the office visit and calculate the running balance.

____/7 ____/7 ____/7 11. Dr. Practon feels a laboratory test is needed for Beth (urinalysis, nonautomated without microscopy). Post this service and calculate the running balance.

____/7 ____/7 ____/7 12. The urinalysis was negative; however, Dr. Practon would like to run a urine pregnancy test. Post this service and calculate a running balance.

____/3 ____/3 ____/3 13. It is determined that she is pregnant with her first child. The medical assistant discusses maternity care and delivery and advises her of the obstetric fee for a routine vaginal delivery, which includes all antepartum and postpartum visits. Locate the correct *CPT* code; the fee is $ _____.

JOB SKILL 15-1 (*continued*)

___/10 ___/10 ___/10 14. Her insurance is verified, and it is determined that they will pay 85% of Dr. Practon's usual and customary fee for obstetric care. She pays by check (No. 798) for 15% of the total obstetric fee. Post this payment to her ledger card and calculate the running balance. Do not post the charge for the OB care; it will be posted at the time of delivery. Her ledger will indicate a negative balance until the obstetric fee is posted.

POST ON ACCOUNT SENT TO COLLECTION AGENCY AND MONEY RECEIVED FROM AGENCY

___/6 ___/6 ___/6 15. **Helen Rice** was seen as a new patient on 1/16/XX and came in for two follow-up office visits. She was billed three times and the patient has not responded so today you send the account to the Collect 4U Agency. Enter the proper reference and description on the ledger, then adjust the entire balance (subtract it from the running balance), circle it, and post a zero balance.

___/8 ___/8 ___/8 15. One month later the patient pays the collection agency $150 and the agency sends check No. 9876543 to the office. Post the agency check on the patient's ledger, reverse the adjustment by $150, and indicate, "account closed" in the balance column.

_____ _____ _____ Complete within specified time.

___/120 ___/120 ___/120 **Total points earned** (To obtain a percentage score, divide the total points earned by the number of points possible.)

Comments:

Evaluator's Signature: _____ **Need to Repeat:** _____

National Curriculum Competency: CAAHEP: Cognitive: II.C.1, 4 Psychomotor: VII.P.1   ABHES: 7.c

JOB SKILL 15-2
Prepare Ledger Cards

Name _____ Date _____ Score _____

Performance Objective

Task: Insert demographic information and post a balance forward to set up 28 ledger cards and arrange them in alphabetical sequence. These will be used for future job skills in this chapter.

Conditions: Need:

- Computer with Internet connection
- Online Forms 58 through 71 (ledger cards) located at www.cengagebrain.com with student resources
- Computer or pen

Refer to:

- *Textbook* Figure 15-2 (top portion for demographic input illustration)

Standards: Complete all steps listed in this skill in _____ minutes with a minimum score of _____. (Time element and accuracy criteria may be given by instructor.)

Time: Start: _____ Completed: _____ Total: _____ minutes

Scoring: One point for each step performed satisfactorily unless otherwise listed or weighted by instructor.

Directions with Performance Evaluation Checklist

Set up ledger cards for the following patients by keying or filling in their names, addresses, telephone numbers, dates of birth (DOB), and insurance information; each member of a family has a separate ledger. Indicate the current year in the first "DATE" column and post a balance forward on each ledger card as indicated. NOTE: If completing only Day 1 due to time constraints (Job Skills 15-3 through 15-6), you will set up 10 ledgers for patients listed in Steps 1, 3, 4, 5, 6, 7, 9, 10, 26, and 28.

1st Attempt	2nd Attempt	3rd Attempt	
_____	_____	_____	Gather materials (equipment and supplies) listed under *Conditions*.
___/10	___/10	___/10	1. Set up a ledger card for Mary Lou Chaney 4902 Saviers Road Woodland Hills, XY 12345-0000 Tel: 555-490-8755—home Tel: 555-490-5578—work DOB: 7/30/50 Ins: South West Ins. ID # 459-08-7655 Previous balance: new pt
___/10	___/10	___/10	2. Set up a ledger card for Russell P. Smith 2336 East Manly Street Woodland Hills, XY 12345-0000 Tel: 555-786-0123—home Tel: 555-786-3210—work DOB: 5/6/56 Ins: Blue Cross/Blue Shield Cert. # 58557AT Group #T84 Previous balance: zero

JOB SKILL 15-2 (*continued*)

____/10 ____/10 ____/10 3. Set up a ledger card for Jody F. Swinney
4300 Saunders Road
Woodland Hills, XY 12345-0000
Tel: 555-908-6605—home
DOB: 1/16/64
Ins: Aetna Casualty Company
Policy # 7821-11
Previous balance: $25.00

____/10 ____/10 ____/10 4. Set up a ledger card for Miss Adrienne Cane
6502 North J Street
Woodland Hills, XY 12345-0000
Tel: 555-498-2110—home
DOB: 7/29/46
Ins: R. L. Kautz & Company
Policy # 7821-1KBM
Previous balance: $85.00

____/10 ____/10 ____/10 5. Set up a ledger card for Mark B. Hanson
2560 South M Street
Woodland Hills, XY 12345-0000
Tel: 555-980-2210—home
Tel: 555-980-0122—work
DOB: 6/22/49
Ins: Prudential Insurance Co.
Policy # 4579
Previous balance: zero

____/10 ____/10 ____/10 6. Set up a ledger card for Robert T. Jenner
1300 Hampshire Road
Woodland Hills, XY 12345-0000
Tel: 555-986-6790—home
Tel: 555-986-0976—work
DOB: 2/28/68
Ins: Guarantee Insurance Company
Policy # 67021
Previous balance: zero

____/10 ____/10 ____/10 7. Set up a ledger card for Harold B. Mason
6107 Harcourt Street
Woodland Hills, XY 12345-0000
Tel: 555-615-0123—home
Tel: 555-615-3201—work
DOB: 8/20/46
Ins: Allstate Insurance Company
Policy # 7632111 BA
Previous balance: zero

JOB SKILL 15-2 (*continued*)

____/10 ____/10 ____/10   8. Set up a ledger card for J. B. Haupman
            15761 Dickens Street
            Woodland Hills, XY 12345-0000
            Tel: 555-457-0561—home
            DOB: 7/23/28
            Ins: Medicare
            Medicare ID # XXX-XX-0988A
            Previous balance: $1466.56

____/10 ____/10 ____/10   9. Set up a ledger card for Mrs. Betty K. Lawson
            6400 Best Way
            Woodland Hills, XY 12345-0000
            Tel: 555-450-9533—home
            DOB: 1/27/69
            Ins: TRICARE Extra ID # 5430982XX
            Previous balance: zero

____/10 ____/10 ____/10   10. Set up a ledger card for Miss Carol M. Wolf
            2765 Honey Lane Street
            Woodland Hills, XY 12345-0000
            Tel: 555-892-0651—home
            DOB: 8/25/76
            Ins: Blue Cross/Blue Shield
            Cert. # 76502 AT
            Group #T85
            Previous balance: zero

____/10 ____/10 ____/10   11. Set up a ledger card for Margaret Jenkins, RN
            5692 Rose Avenue
            Woodland Hills, XY 12345-0000
            Tel: 555-760-3211—home
            Tel: 555-760-1123—work
            DOB: 6/29/70
            Ins: Blue Cross/Blue Shield
            Cert. # 65923AT
            Group #T76
            Previous balance: new pt

____/10 ____/10 ____/10   12. Set up a ledger card for Roger T. Simpson
            792 Baker Street
            Woodland Hills, XY 12345-0000
            Tel: 555-549-0879—home
            Tel: 555-549-9780—work
            DOB: 11/2/52
            Ins: Farmers Insurance Group
            Policy # 56892
            Previous balance: $45.00

JOB SKILL 15-2 *(continued)*

___/10 ___/10 ___/10 13. Set up a ledger card for Joan Gomez
4391 Wooden Street
Woodland Hills, XY 12345-0000
Tel: 555-459-2399—home
Tel: 555-459-9932—work
DOB: 3/15/47
Ins: Fremont Indemnity Company
Policy # 56702111
Previous balance: $60.00

___/10 ___/10 ___/10 14. Set up a ledger card for Maria Bargioni
4892 Simpson Street
Woodland Hills, XY 12345-0000
Tel: 555-549-2344—home
Tel: 555-549-4432—work
DOB: 4/5/76
Ins: Fireman's Fund Insurance Companies
Policy # 568 MB 2111
Previous balance: $25.00

___/10 ___/10 ___/10 15. Set up a ledger card for Jack J. Johnson
5490 Olive Mill Road
Woodland Hills, XY 12345-0000
Tel: 555-857-9920—home
DOB: 5/27/59
Ins: Medicaid
Insurance ID # 458962016
Previous balance: zero

___/10 ___/10 ___/10 16. Set up a ledger card for Lois A. Conrad
8920 Canton Street
Woodland Hills, XY 12345-0000
Tel: 555-569-2201—home
Tel: 555-569-1022—work
DOB: 5/8/55
Ins: Gates, McDonald & Company
Policy # 4591 XT
Previous balance: $31.50

___/10 ___/10 ___/10 17. Set up a ledger card for Miss Marylou Conrad, c/o Lois Conrad
8920 Canton Street
Woodland Hills, XY 12345-0000
Tel: 555-569-2201—home
DOB: 4/22/95
Ins: Gates, McDonald & Company
Policy # 4591 XT
Previous balance: zero

JOB SKILL 15-2 *(continued)*

___/10 ___/10 ___/10 18. Set up a ledger card for Hannah F. Riley
459 Fifth Avenue
Woodland Hills, XY 12345-0000
Tel: 555-789-2201—home
Tel: 555-789-1022—work
DOB: 10/8/62
Ins: Hartford Insurance Group
Policy # 5601221
Previous balance: zero

___/10 ___/10 ___/10 19. Set up a ledger card for Stephen B. Riley Jr.
459 Fifth Avenue
Woodland Hills, XY 12345-0000
Tel: 555-789-2201—home
Tel: 555-789-1022—work
DOB: 6/29/62
Ins: Hartford Insurance Group
Policy # 5601221
Previous balance: new pt

___/10 ___/10 ___/10 20. Set up a ledger card for Rosa K. Okida
7900 Shatto Place
Woodland Hills, XY 12345-0000
Tel: 555-420-1121—home
Tel: 555-420-1211—work
DOB: 11/2/58
Ins: Home Insurance Company
Policy # 789-1191-21K
Previous balance: $201.00

___/10 ___/10 ___/10 21. Set up a ledger card for Howard S. Chan
3200 Shaw Avenue
Woodland Hills, XY 12345-0000
Tel: 555-660-3211—home
Tel: 555-660-1123—work
DOB: 8/3/58
Ins: Imperial Insurance Company
Policy # 21019KBM
Previous balance: zero

JOB SKILL 15-2 (*continued*)

___/10 ___/10 ___/10 22. Set up a ledger card for Rachel T. O'Brien
                  5598 East 17 Street
                  Woodland Hills, XY 12345-0000
                  Tel: 555-566-2199—home
                  Tel: 555-566-9912—work
                  DOB: 3/19/68
                  Ins: North America Health Net POS
                  Policy # 54901
                  Previous balance: $50.00

___/10 ___/10 ___/10 23. Set up a ledger card for Martin P. Owens
                  430 Herndon Place
                  Woodland Hills, XY 12345-0000
                  Tel: 555-542-2232—home
                  Tel: 555-542-2322—work
                  DOB: 12/3/73
                  Ins: John Deere Insurance Company
                  Policy # 67401 J
                  Previous balance: $25.00

___/10 ___/10 ___/10 24. Set up a ledger card for Joseph C. Smith
                  P.O. Box 4301
                  Woodland Hills, XY 12345-0000
                  Tel: 555-549-1124—home
                  Tel: 555-549-4211—work
                  DOB: 6/20/73
                  Ins: Home Insurance Company
                  Policy # 589102K
                  Previous balance: new pt

___/10 ___/10 ___/10 25. Set up a ledger card for Kathryn L. Hope
                  6680 Bascom Road
                  Woodland Hills, XY 12345-0000
                  Tel: 555-210-9980—home
                  Tel: 555-210-0899—work
                  DOB: 8/14/60
                  Ins: Met Life HMO
                  Policy # 8921
                  Previous balance: zero

JOB SKILL 15-2 (*continued*)

___/10   ___/10   ___/10   26. Set up a ledger card for Russell O. Smith

                       459 University Avenue

                       Woodland Hills, XY 12345-0000

                       Tel: 555-129-1980—home

                       Tel: 555-129-0891—work

                       DOB: 2/15/65

                       Ins: International Insurance Company

                       Policy # 8901

                       Previous balance: new pt

___/10   ___/10   ___/10   27. Set up a ledger card for Charlotte J. Brown

                       769 Sky Park Circle

                       Woodland Hills, XY 12345-0000

                       Tel: 555-780-2341—home

                       Tel: 555-780-1432—work

                       DOB: 9/5/66

                       Ins: Kemper Insurance Company

                       Policy # 5769

                       Previous balance: $35.00

___/3   ___/3   ___/3   28. Set up a ledger card with the heading "Miscellaneous Other Income" to be used to record charges and payments for lectures, published articles, and other miscellaneous items; previous balance zero.

___/28   ___/28   ___/28   29. Cut ledger cards apart and arrange them in alphabetical sequence with the "Miscellaneous Other Income" ledger at the end of the file.

_____   _____   _____   Complete within specified time.

___/303   ___/303   ___/303   **Total points earned** (To obtain a percentage score, divide the total points earned by the number of points possible.)

Comments:

Evaluator's Signature: _____ **Need to Repeat:** _____

National Curriculum Competency: CAAHEP: Cognitive: II.C.5   ABHES: 7.c

JOB SKILL 15-3
Bookkeeping Day 1—Post to Patient Ledger Cards and Prepare Cash Receipts

Name _____ Date _____ Score _____

Performance Objective

Task: Post charges and payments to patient ledger cards, calculate running balances, and prepare cash receipts.

Conditions: Need:

- Computer with Internet connection
- Online Forms 72 and 73 (five checks received by Practon Medical Group) located at www.cengagebrain.com with student resources
- Online Form 74 (cash receipts)
- Ledger cards, which have been alphabetized, from Job Skill 15-2
- Calculator
- Pencil

Refer to:

- *Workbook* Appendix A (Mock Fee Schedule)
- *Textbook* Figure 15-2 and Example 15-2 for posting illustrations
- *Textbook* Figure 15-7 for a cash receipt example

Standards: Complete all steps listed in this skill in _____ minutes with a minimum score of _____. (Time element and accuracy criteria may be given by instructor.)

Time: Start: _____ Completed: _____ Total: _____ minutes

Scoring: One point for each step performed satisfactorily unless otherwise listed or weighted by instructor.

Directions with Performance Evaluation Checklist

It is June 28, current year. Pull ledger cards for patients who are on today's schedule (they are highlighted in step-by-step instructions in **boldface**). Post all charges (line by line), referring to the "Mock Fee Schedule" (Figure A-1 in Appendix A of this *Workbook*) to obtain fees; calculate a running balance for each line of posting. For all commercial (private) insurance programs, Medicaid, and TRICARE, use figures from the "Mock Fees." Cut checks apart and post all payments after charges have been posted; calculate balance due. Complete a receipt for all patients who paid cash.

1st Attempt	2nd Attempt	3rd Attempt	
_____	_____	_____	Gather materials (equipment and supplies) listed under *Conditions*.
___/20	___/20	___/20	1. Post charges for patient **Mark B. Hanson**.
			Est Pt OV Level II (E/M Section)
			Post cash payment (patient paid in full); indicate receipt number in reference column.
			Complete cash receipt No. 147 (see Online Form 74).
___/5	___/5	___/5	2. Post charges for patient **Russell O. Smith**.
			NP Office Consult Level III (E/M Section).

JOB SKILL 15-3 (*continued*)

___/20 ___/20 ___/20 3. Post charges for patient **Betty K. Lawson**.

Est Pt Level I OV (E/M Section)

Therapeutic injection (IM—Medicine Section)

Vitamin B12 (medication supply—Special Services and Reports); fee $9.

Post copayment received by check (see Online Form 73).

___/10 ___/10 ___/10 4. Post charges for patient **Jody F. Swinney**.

Est Pt Level II OV (E/M Section)

Post copayment received by check (see Online Form 73).

___/30 ___/30 ___/30 5. Post charges for patient **Mary Lou Chaney**.

NP Level IV OV (E/M Section)

UA (nonautomated with microscopy—Laboratory Section)

Comprehensive audiometry (Medicine Section)

Post cash payment (patient paid in full) and indicate receipt number in reference column.

Complete cash receipt No. 148 (see Online Form 74).

___/15 ___/15 ___/15 6. Post charges for patient **Carol M. Wolf**.

Est Pt Level I OV (E/M Section)

Tetanus/Diphtheria Immunization Injection (vaccine product—Medicine Section) Immunization administration (Td—Medicine Section); fee $2.50

___/10 ___/10 ___/10 7. Post charges for patient **Harold B. Mason**.

Est Pt Level II OV (E/M Section)

ECG (Medicine Section)

___/5 ___/5 ___/5 8. Post charges for patient **Robert T. Jenner**.

Initial hospital care (30 minutes, Level I—E/M Section)

INCOMING MAIL: Several checks have been received in the mail today (see Online Form 72). Some will be posted to the "Miscellaneous Other Income" account. When payments are posted to this account, post the charges at the same time the check is received; this is standard office protocol.

___/6 ___/6 ___/6 9. Post check from ***Family Health Magazine*** for article written by Dr. Gerald Practon.

___/6 ___/6 ___/6 10. Post check from **Colony Boys School** for lecture by Dr. Fran Practon.

___/5 ___/5 ___/5 11. Post personal check from patient **Adrienne Cane**; payment on account.

_____ _____ _____ Complete within specified time.

___/134 ___/134 ___/134 **Total points earned** (To obtain a percentage score, divide the total points earned by the number of points possible.)

Comments:

Evaluator's Signature: _____ **Need to Repeat:** _____

National Curriculum Competency: CAAHEP: Cognitive: II.C.1, 4 Psychomotor: VII.P.1   ABHES: 7.c

JOB SKILL 15-4
Bookkeeping Day 1—Prepare the Daily Journal

Name _____ Date _____ Score _____

Performance Objective

Task: Set up the daily journal by inserting figures from the previous day's totals.

Conditions: Need:

- Computer with Internet connection
- Online Form 75 (daily journal—Day 1) located at www.cengagebrain.com with student resources
- Pencil
- Photocopy machine (optional) to enlarge daysheet to legal size
- *Textbook* Figure 15-6 for a daysheet illustration
- *Textbook* Procedure 15-1 for step-by-step directions

Standards: Complete all steps listed in this skill in _____ minutes with a minimum score of _____.
                 (Time element and accuracy criteria may be given by instructor.)

Time: Start: _____ Completed: _____ Total: _____ minutes

Scoring: One point for each step performed satisfactorily unless otherwise listed or weighted by instructor.

Directions with Performance Evaluation Checklist

1st Attempt	2nd Attempt	3rd Attempt	
_____	_____	_____	Gather materials (equipment and supplies) listed under *Conditions*.
____/2	____/2	____/2	1. It is June 28, current year. Enter this date on the top of the daysheet and in the "Record of Deposits" area and use it for all transactions that will occur today.
____/2	____/2	____/2	2. All transactions for June 28, 20XX, will fit on one daysheet; label it page 1 of 1.
____/2	____/2	____/2	3. Insert the daily journal (daysheet) previous page total charges ($14,336.60) for Column A from the previous day, June 27, 20XX.
____/2	____/2	____/2	4. Insert the daily journal previous page total payments ($8592.41) for Column B-1 from the previous day, June 27, 20XX.
____/2	____/2	____/2	5. Insert the daily journal previous page total adjustments ($450.00) for Column B-2 from the previous day, June 27, 20XX.
____/2	____/2	____/2	6. Insert the daily journal previous page total balance ($1387.56) for Column C from the previous day, June 27, 20XX.
____/2	____/2	____/2	7. Insert the daily journal previous page total ($980.00) for Column D from the previous day, June 27, 20XX.
____/2	____/2	____/2	8. At the bottom, enter the "Accounts Receivable Control," "Previous Day's Total" figure: $30,526.32.
____/2	____/2	____/2	9. Enter "Accounts Receivable Proof," "First of Month" figure: $25,232.13.
____/2	____/2	____/2	10. In the "Cash Control," enter the "Beginning Cash On Hand" figure: $50.00.
____/2	____/2	____/2	11. Insert your name at the bottom of the daysheet in the "Prepared by" area.

JOB SKILL 15-4 (*continued*)

_____ _____ _____ Complete within specified time.

___/24 ___/24 ___/24 **Total points earned** (To obtain a percentage score, divide the total points earned by the number of points possible.)

Comments:

Evaluator's Signature: _____ **Need to Repeat:** _____

National Curriculum Competency: ABHES: 7.c

JOB SKILL 15-5
Bookkeeping Day 1—Post Charges, Payments, and Adjustments Using a Daily Journal

Name _____ Date _____ Score _____

Performance Objective

Task: Post charges, payments, and adjustments on the daily journal; record payments on the bank deposit slip and in the cash control section; endorse checks and prepare the bank deposit.

Conditions: Need:

- Computer with Internet connection
- Ledgers used in Job Skill 15-3
- Daysheet prepared in Job Skill 15-4
- Checks (Online Forms 72 and 73) used in Job Skill 15-3
- Number 10 envelope (large)
- Calculator
- Pencil

Refer to:

- *Textbook* Figure 15-6 for daysheet posting illustrations
- *Textbook* Procedure 15-1 for step-by-step directions

Standards: Complete all steps listed in this skill in _____ minutes with a minimum score of _____. (Time element and accuracy criteria may be given by instructor.)

Time: Start: _____ Completed: _____ Total: _____ minutes

Scoring: One point for each step performed satisfactorily unless otherwise listed or weighted by instructor.

Directions with Performance Evaluation Checklist

Daily Journal Instructions

Post all charges, payments, and adjustments for each patient seen on a *single line* of the daysheet. Specific instructions follow:

COLUMNS:

Date: Enter date of posting in first column (e.g., 6/28/20XX).

Reference: This column may be used for various references. For this exercise, all charges and payments for each patient's professional services taking place today will be posted on *one line*; use this column to enter the patient's check number when payment is received (e.g., ck 123).

Description: Enter *CPT* code numbers for all professional services rendered. Enter abbreviation "ROA" and a reference to who paid when someone pays on an account. Enter "Miscellaneous Other Income" to designate the ledger you are posting to for checks received from other sources.

Charges: List *total* charge for *all* professional services rendered by each patient.

Credits—Payments: List payment amount.

Credits—Adjustments: List the amount to be written off the account.

Balance: Add the previous balance to charges and subtract credits (payments and adjustments) to obtain the current balance.

Previous Balance: Obtain and enter the amount extended from each patient's ledger card.

Name: Enter last name, first name, and middle initial.

Numbered Lines: Each line is numbered for reference to help with posting accuracy.

JOB SKILL 15-5 (*continued*)

Receipt Number: Enter the number from the cash receipt.

RECORD OF DEPOSITS: Make a photocopy of the "Record of Deposit" section of the daysheet to use as a bank deposit slip. At the top of the *deposit slip*, insert the name of the bank (The First National Bank) and checking account number (12345-6789).

  Date: Enter the current date on top of the daily journal form.

  ABA: Enter the bank ABA number listed on check.

  Cash: Enter amount of cash payment.

  Checks: Enter amount of check payment.

COPAY: Label and enter the copayment amount.

For posting information, refer to the ledgers used to post current charges and payments in Job Skill 15-3. In a pegboard bookkeeping system, journal entries will be automatically posted as they are written on ledgers by means of no carbon required (NCR) paper. In a computerized system, journal entries will be automatically posted as they are input into the patient's account.

1st Attempt	2nd Attempt	3rd Attempt	
_____	_____	_____	Gather materials (equipment and supplies) listed under *Conditions*.
____/7	____/7	____/7	1. Post charge and payment for **Mark B. Hanson**.
____/5	____/5	____/5	2. Post charge for **Russell O. Smith**.
____/10	____/10	____/10	3. Post charges and copayment for **Betty K. Lawson**.
____/10	____/10	____/10	4. Post charge and copayment for **Jody F. Swinney**.
____/7	____/7	____/7	5. Post charges and payment for **Mary Lou Chaney**.
____/5	____/5	____/5	6. Post charges for **Carol M. Wolf**.
____/5	____/5	____/5	7. Post charges for **Harold B. Mason**.
____/5	____/5	____/5	8. Post charge for **Robert T. Jenner**.
____/8	____/8	____/8	9. Post check (and charge) from ***Family Health Magazine***.
____/8	____/8	____/8	10. Post check (and charge) from **Colony Boys School**.
____/9	____/9	____/9	11. Post personal check from **Adrienne Cane**.
____/3	____/3	____/3	12. Add the proper endorsement for all checks received. Total the deposit and put them in an envelope with the bank slip.
_____	_____	_____	Complete within specified time.
____/84	____/84	____/84	**Total points earned** (To obtain a percentage score, divide the total points earned by the number of points possible.)

Comments:

Evaluator's Signature: _____ **Need to Repeat:** _____

National Curriculum Competency: CAAHEP: Cognitive: II.C.1, 4 Psychomotor: VI.P.1	ABHES: 7.C

JOB SKILL 15-6
Bookkeeping Day 1—Balance the Daysheet

Name _____ Date _____ Score _____

Performance Objective

Task: Total all columns on the daysheet, add previous page totals, and enter new figures in month-to-date areas.

Conditions: Need:
- Daysheet (Day 1) used in Job Skills 15-4 and 15-5
- Calculator
- Pencil

Refer to:
- *Textbook* Figure 15-6 for daysheet calculation examples
- *Textbook* Procedure 15-1 for step-by-step directions

Standards: Complete all steps listed in this skill in _____ minutes with a minimum score of _____. (Time element and accuracy criteria may be given by instructor.)

Time: Start: _____ Completed: _____ Total: _____ minutes

Scoring: One point for each step performed satisfactorily unless otherwise listed or weighted by instructor.

Directions with Performance Evaluation Checklist

1st Attempt	2nd Attempt	3rd Attempt	
_____	_____	_____	Gather materials (equipment and supplies) listed under *Conditions*.

DAYSHEET TOTALS

____/3	____/3	____/3	1. Total Column A, add "Previous Page" total, and enter the "Month-to-Date" figure.
____/3	____/3	____/3	2. Total Column B-1, add "Previous Page" total, and enter the "Month-to-Date" figure.
____/3	____/3	____/3	3. Total Column B-2, add "Previous Page" total, and enter the "Month-to-Date" figure.
____/3	____/3	____/3	4. Total Column C, add "Previous Page" total, and enter the "Month-to-Date" figure.
____/3	____/3	____/3	5. Total Column D, add "Previous Page" total, and enter the "Month-to-Date" figure.

PROOF OF POSTING

____/5	____/5	____/5	6. Transfer today's daysheet totals as directed in the "Proof of Posting" section and add or subtract as instructed. If the total does not equal Column C, recalculate and look for errors.

ACCOUNTS RECEIVABLE CONTROL

____/5	____/5	____/5	7. Enter figures from the "Proof of Posting" section to the "Accounts Receivable Control" section as indicated and add or subtract as instructed.

JOB SKILL 15-6 (*continued*)

ACCOUNTS RECEIVABLE PROOF

____/5 ____/5 ____/5   8. Enter "Month-to-Date" figures in the "Accounts Receivable Proof" section and add or subtract as instructed.

BALANCE DAYSHEET

____/10 ____/10 ____/10   9. Compare the dollar amount in the "Total Accounts Receivable" from the "Accounts Receivable Control" section with the dollar amount in the "Total Accounts Receivable" from the "Accounts Receivable Proof" section; they should match. If not, follow instructions on common posting problems to locate the error.

RECORD DEPOSIT AND BALANCE CASH CONTROL

____/3 ____/3 ____/3   10. Add all cash received in the "Record of Deposits" section and enter the amount in the "Total Cash" area at the bottom.

____/6 ____/6 ____/6   11. Add all checks received in the "Record of Deposits" section and enter the amount in the "Total Checks" area at the bottom.

____/3 ____/3 ____/3   12. Add total cash received and total checks received to obtain the total deposit amount and enter it in the "Total Deposit" area at the bottom; this amount should equal the total of today's payments found in Column B-1.

____/5 ____/5 ____/5   13. Balance cash on hand by following the steps listed in "Cash Control."

____ ____ ____   Complete within specified time.

____/59 ____/59 ____/59   **Total points earned** (To obtain a percentage score, divide the total points earned by the number of points possible.)

Comments:

Evaluator's Signature: _____ **Need to Repeat:** _____

National Curriculum Competency: CAAHEP: Cognitive: II.C.1	ABHES: 7.C

JOB SKILL 15-7
Bookkeeping Day 2—Prepare the Daily Journal

Name _____ Date _____ Score _____

Performance Objective

Task: Set up the daily journal by inserting figures from the previous day's totals.

Conditions: Need:

- Computer with Internet connection
- Online Form 72 (daily journal—Day 2) located at www.cengagebrain.com with student resources
- Pencil
- Photocopy machine (optional) to enlarge daysheet to legal size

Refer to:

- *Textbook* Procedure 15-1 for step-by-step directions

Standards: Complete all steps listed in this skill in minutes _____ with a minimum score of _____. (Time element and accuracy criteria may be given by instructor.)

Time: **Start:** _____ **Completed:** _____ **Total:** _____ minutes

Scoring: One point for each step performed satisfactorily unless otherwise listed or weighted by instructor.

Directions with Performance Evaluation Checklist

1st Attempt	2nd Attempt	3rd Attempt	
_____	_____	_____	Gather materials (equipment and supplies) listed under *Conditions*.
____/2	____/2	____/2	1. It is June 29, current year. Enter this date on the top of the daysheet and in the "Record of Deposits" area and use it for all transactions that will occur today.
____/2	____/2	____/2	2. All transactions for June 29, 20XX, will fit on one daysheet; label it page 1 of 1.
____/2	____/2	____/2	3. Insert the "Previous Page" totals at the bottom of the daily journal (daysheet) by picking up the figures from June 28, 20XX, "Month-to-Date" totals for Columns A, B-1, B-2, C, and D.
____/2	____/2	____/2	4. Insert the "Accounts Receivable Control" "Previous Day's Total" figure. This is the "Total Accounts Receivable" figure at the end of the previous day.
____/2	____/2	____/2	5. Carry forward the "Accounts Receivable Proof" "First of Month" figure as indicated on the previous daysheet.
____/2	____/2	____/2	6. Enter the "Beginning Cash On Hand" figure: $50.00.
____/2	____/2	____/2	7. Insert your name at the bottom of the daysheet in the "Prepared by" area.
_____	_____	_____	Complete within specified time.
____/16	____/16	____/16	**Total points earned** (To obtain a percentage score, divide the total points earned by the number of points possible.)

JOB SKILL 15-7 (*continued*)

Comments:

National Curriculum Competency: ABHES: 7.C

JOB SKILL 15-8

Bookkeeping Day 2—Post Charges, Payments, and Adjustments to Patient Ledger Cards and to the Daily Journal; Prepare Cash Receipts and the Bank Deposit

Name _____ Date _____ Score _____

Performance Objective

Task: Post charges and payments to patient ledger cards and calculate a running balance; prepare cash receipts. Duplicate posting entries on the daily journal (daysheet), record payments on the bank deposit slip, endorse checks, and prepare the bank deposit.

Conditions: Need:

- Computer with Internet connection
- Online Form 74 (cash receipts) located at www.cengagebrain.com with student resources
- Online Form 77 (three checks received by Practon Medical Group)
- Ledger cards, which have been alphabetized, from Job Skill 15-2
- Daysheet prepared in Job Skill 15-7
- Number 10 envelope (large)
- Calculator
- Pencil

Refer to:

- *Textbook* Figure 15-2 for ledger posting illustrations
- *Textbook* Figure 15-6 for daysheet posting illustrations
- Figure 15-7 for a cash receipt example
- *Workbook* Appendix A (Mock Fee Schedule)
- Procedure 15-1 for step-by-step directions

Standards: Complete all steps listed in this skill in _____ minutes with a minimum score of _____. (Time element and accuracy criteria may be given by instructor.)

Time: Start: _____ Completed: _____ Total: _____ minutes

Scoring: One point for each step performed satisfactorily unless otherwise listed or weighted by instructor.

Directions with Performance Evaluation Checklist

It is June 29, current year. For this job skill, you will be posting to the patient's ledger card and then to the daily journal (daysheet); refer to specific instructions in Job Skill 15- 5. Pull ledger cards for patients who are on today's schedule (they are highlighted in step-by-step instructions in **boldface)** and post entries as done in Job Skills 15-3 and 15-5. Post all charges (line by line) referring to the "Mock Fee Schedule" (Figure A-1 in Appendix A of this *Workbook*) to obtain fees; calculate a running balance for each line of posting. For all commercial (private) insurance programs, Medicaid, and TRICARE, use figures from the "Mock Fees" section. Cut checks apart and post all payments after charges have been posted, endorse checks, record on the deposit slip, total the bank deposit, and put into the envelope. Complete a receipt for all patients who paid cash; record all payments in the "Cash Control" section of the daily journal.

JOB SKILL 15-8 *(continued)*

1st Attempt	2nd Attempt	3rd Attempt	
_____	_____	_____	Gather materials (equipment and supplies) listed under *Conditions*.
___/11	___/11	___/11	1. Post charge on ledger for patient **Margaret Jenkins**.
			NP Office Consult Level IV (E/M Section)
			Post entry on daysheet.
___/21	___/21	___/21	2. Post charge on ledger for patient **Roger T. Simpson**.
			Est Pt OV Level IV (E/M Section)
			Post copayment received on ledger (see Online Form 77).
			Post entries on daysheet and record payment on bank deposit.
___/16	___/16	___/16	3. Post charges on ledger for patient **Joan Gomez**.
			ECG in office (Medicine Section)
			Admit to College Hospital; initial care—Level II (E/M Section)
			Post entries on daysheet.
___/11	___/11	___/11	4. Post charge on ledger for patient **Harold B. Mason**.
			Est Pt OV Level II (E/M Section)
			Post entry on daysheet.
___/11	___/11	___/11	5. Post charge on ledger for patient **Maria Bargioni**.
			Est Pt OV Level III (E/M Section)
			Post entry on daysheet.
___/31	___/31	___/31	6. Post charges on ledger for patient **Jack J. Johnson**.
			Est Pt OV Level I (E/M Section)
			Tetanus inj (Medicine Section)
			Immunization administration; IM (Medicine Section)
			Post Medicaid copayment (check) on ledger (see Online Form 77).
			Post entries on daysheet and record payment on bank deposit.
___/16	___/16	___/16	7. Post charges on ledger for patient **Lois A. Conrad**.
			Est Pt OV Level III (E/M Section)
			Pap smear collected and sent to laboratory. Note: The Pap smear is bundled into the office visit; however, there is a charge for the handling fee (Medicine Section—Special Services and Reports).
			Post entries on daysheet.
___/21	___/21	___/21	8. Post charges on ledger for patient **Marylou Conrad**.
			Est Pt OV Level II (E/M Section)
			Poliovirus vaccine; oral immunization (Medicine Section)
			Immunization administration (Medicine Section)
			Post entries on daysheet.
___/16	___/16	___/16	9. Post charges on ledger for patient **Hannah F. Riley**.
			Est Pt OV Level IV (E/M Section)
			IUD insertion (Male/Female Genital System)
			Post entries on daysheet.

JOB SKILL 15-8 (*continued*)

___/30 ___/30 ___/30 10. Post charge on ledger for patient **Stephen B. Riley Jr.**

Office Consult Level IV (E/M Section)

Post cash payment on ledger; $25.

Complete cash receipt No. 149 (see Online Form 74).

Post entries on daysheet; record payment on bank deposit and cash control.

___/16 ___/16 ___/16 11. Post charges on ledger for patient **Rosa K. Okida**.

Est Pt OV Level I (E/M Section)

X-ray R hip, single view (Radiology Section)

Post entries on daysheet.

___/11 ___/11 ___/11 12. Post charge on ledger for patient **Howard S. Chan**.

Est Pt OV Level IV (E/M Section)

Post entries on daysheet.

___/11 ___/11 ___/11 13. Post charge on ledger for patient **Robert T. Jenner**.

HV (subsequent) Level I (E/M Section)

Post entry on daysheet.

INCOMING MAIL: The morning mail contained a check from Prudential Insurance Company for processing a life insurance examination report (Online Form 77).

___/6 ___/6 ___/6 14. Post the check and charge on the ledger from **Prudential Insurance Company**. Post charge and payment on the daysheet and record on the bank deposit.

___/3 ___/3 ___/3 15. Add the proper endorsement for all checks received. Total the deposit and put them in an envelope with the bank slip.

_____ _____ _____ Complete within specified time.

___/233 ___/233 ___/233 **Total points earned** (To obtain a percentage score, divide the total points earned by the number of points possible.)

Comments:

Evaluator's Signature: _____ **Need to Repeat:** _____

National Curriculum Competency: CAAHEP: Cognitive: II.C.1, 4 Psychomotor: VII.P.1	ABHES: 7.c

JOB SKILL 15-9
Bookkeeping Day 2—Balance the Daysheet

Name _____ Date _____ Score _____

Performance Objective

Task: Total all columns on the daysheet, add previous page totals, and enter new figures in month-to-date areas.

Conditions: Need:
- Daysheet (Day 2) used in Job Skills 15-7 and 15-8
- Calculator
- Pencil

Refer to:
- *Textbook* Procedure 15-1 for step-by-step directions

Standards: Complete all steps listed in this skill in _____ minutes with a minimum score of _____. (Time element and accuracy criteria may be given by instructor.)

Time: **Start:** _____ **Completed:** _____ **Total:** _____ minutes

Scoring: One point for each step performed satisfactorily unless otherwise listed or weighted by instructor.

Directions with Performance Evaluation Checklist

1st Attempt	2nd Attempt	3rd Attempt	
_____	_____	_____	Gather materials (equipment and supplies) listed under *Conditions*.

DAYSHEET TOTALS

____/3	____/3	____/3	1. Total Column A, add "Previous Page" total, and enter the "Month-to-Date" figure.
____/3	____/3	____/3	2. Total Column B-1, add "Previous Page" total, and enter the "Month-to-Date" figure.
____/3	____/3	____/3	3. Total Column B-2, add "Previous Page" total, and enter the "Month-to-Date" figure.
____/3	____/3	____/3	4. Total Column C, add "Previous Page" total, and enter the "Month-to-Date" figure.
____/3	____/3	____/3	5. Total Column D, add "Previous Page" total, and enter the "Month-to-Date" figure.

PROOF OF POSTING

____/5	____/5	____/5	6. Transfer today's daysheet totals as directed in the "Proof of Posting" section and add or subtract as instructed. If the total does not equal Column C, recalculate and look for errors.

ACCOUNTS RECEIVABLE CONTROL

____/5	____/5	____/5	7. Enter figures from the "Proof of Posting" section to the "Accounts Receivable Control" section as indicated and add or subtract as instructed.

ACCOUNTS RECEIVABLE PROOF

____/5	____/5	____/5	8. Enter month-to-date figures in the "Accounts Receivable Proof" section and add or subtract as instructed.

JOB SKILL 15-9 (*continued*)

BALANCE DAYSHEET

____/10 ____/10 ____/10   9. Compare the dollar amount in the "Total Accounts Receivable" figure from the "Accounts Receivable Control" section with the dollar amount in the "Total Accounts Receivable" figure from the "Accounts Receivable Proof" section; they should match. If not, follow instructions on common posting problems to locate the error.

RECORD DEPOSIT AND BALANCE CASH CONTROL

____/3 ____/3 ____/3   10. Add all cash received in the "Record of Deposits" section and enter the amount in the "Total Cash" area at the bottom.

____/6 ____/6 ____/6   11. Add all checks received in the "Record of Deposits" section and enter the amount in the "Total Checks" area at the bottom.

____/3 ____/3 ____/3   12. Add total cash received and total checks received to obtain the total deposit amount and enter it in the "Total Deposit" area at the bottom; this amount should equal the total of today's payments found in Column B-1.

____/5 ____/5 ____/5   13. Balance cash on hand by following the steps listed in "Cash Control."

_____ _____ _____   Complete within specified time.

____/59 ____/59 ____/59   **Total points earned** (To obtain a percentage score, divide the total points earned by the number of points possible.)

Comments:

Evaluator's Signature: _____ **Need to Repeat:** _____

National Curriculum Competency: CAAHEP: Cognitive: II.C.1   ABHES: 7.c

JOB SKILL 15-10
Bookkeeping Day 3—Prepare the Daily Journal

Name _____ Date _____ Score _____

Performance Objective

Task: Set up the daily journal by inserting figures from the previous day's totals.

Conditions: Need:

   • Computer with Internet connection

   • Online Form 78 (daily journal—Day 3) located at www.cengagebrain.com with student
     resources

   • Pencil

   • Photocopy machine (optional) to enlarge daysheet to legal size

   Refer to:

   • *Textbook* Procedure 15-1 for step-by-step directions

Standards: Complete all steps listed in this skill in _____ minutes with a minimum score of _____.
                 (Time element and accuracy criteria may be given by instructor.)

Time: **Start:** _____ **Completed:** _____ **Total:** _____ minutes

Scoring: One point for each step performed satisfactorily unless otherwise listed or weighted by
                 instructor.

Directions with Performance Evaluation Checklist

1st Attempt	2nd Attempt	3rd Attempt	
_____	_____	_____	Gather materials (equipment and supplies) listed under *Conditions*.
_____/2	_____/2	_____/2	1. It is June 30, current year. Enter this date on the top of the daysheet and in the "Record of Deposits" area and use it for all transactions that will occur today.
_____/2	_____/2	_____/2	2. All transactions for June 30, 20XX, will fit on one daysheet; label it page number 1 of 1.
_____/2	_____/2	_____/2	3. Insert the "Previous Page" totals at the bottom of the daily journal (daysheet) by picking up the figures from June 29, 20XX, "Month-to-Date" totals for Columns A, B-1, B-2, C, and D.
_____/2	_____/2	_____/2	4. Insert the "Accounts Receivable Control" "Previous Day's Total" figure. This is the "Total Accounts Receivable" figure at the end of the previous day.
_____/2	_____/2	_____/2	5. Carry forward the "Accounts Receivable Proof" "First of Month" figure as indicated on the previous daysheet.
_____/2	_____/2	_____/2	6. Enter the "Beginning Cash On Hand" figure: $50.00.
_____/2	_____/2	_____/2	7. Insert your name at the bottom of the daysheet in the "Prepared by" area.
_____	_____	_____	Complete within specified time.
____/16	___/16	___/16	**Total points earned** (To obtain a percentage score, divide the total points earned by the number of points possible.)

JOB SKILL 15-10 (*continued*)

Comments:

JOB SKILL 15-11

Bookkeeping Day 3—Post Charges, Payments, and Adjustments to Patient Ledger Cards and to the Daily Journal; Prepare Cash Receipts and the Bank Deposit

Name _____ Date _____ Score _____

Performance Objective

Task: Post charges and payments to patient ledger cards and calculate a running balance; prepare cash receipts. Duplicate posting entries on the daily journal (daysheet), record payments on the bank deposit slip, endorse checks, and prepare the bank deposit.

Conditions: Need:

- Computer with Internet connection
- Online Form 79 (two checks received by Practon Medical Group) located at www.cengagebrain.com with student resources
- Online Form 74 (cash receipts)
- Ledger cards, which have been alphabetized, from Job Skill 15-2
- Daysheet prepared in Job Skill 15-10
- Number 10 envelope (large)
- Calculator
- Pencil

Refer to:

- *Textbook* Figure 15-2 for ledger posting illustrations
- *Textbook* Figure 15-6 for daysheet posting illustrations
- *Textbook* Figure 15-7 for cash receipt example
- *Workbook* Appendix A (Mock Fee Schedule)
- Procedure 15-1 for step-by-step directions

Standards: Complete all steps listed in this skill in _____ minutes with a minimum score of _____. (Time element and accuracy criteria may be given by instructor.)

Time: Start: _____ Completed: _____ Total: _____ minutes

Scoring: One point for each step performed satisfactorily unless otherwise listed or weighted by instructor.

Directions with Performance Evaluation Checklist

It is June 30, current year. For this job skill, you will be posting to the patient's ledger card and then to the daily journal (daysheet); refer to specific instructions in Job Skill 15-5. Pull ledger cards for patients who are on today's schedule (they are highlighted in step-by-step instructions in **boldface)** and post entries as done in Job Skills 15-3, 15-5, and 15-8. Post all charges (line by line), referring to the "Mock Fee Schedule" (Figure A-1 in Appendix A of this *Workbook*) to obtain fees; calculate a running balance for each line of posting.

Doctors Fran and Gerald Practon are participating physicians in the Medicare program and bill using the "Medicare Participating" provider fee schedule. For all other insurance types, use figures from the "Mock Fees" column. Cut checks apart and post all payments after charges have been posted, endorse checks, record on the deposit slip, total the deposit, and put into an envelope. Complete a receipt for all patients who paid cash; record all payments in the "Cash Control" section of the daily journal.

JOB SKILL 15-11 (*continued*)

1st Attempt	2nd Attempt	3rd Attempt	
_____	_____	_____	Gather materials (equipment and supplies) listed under *Conditions*.
___/11	___/11	___/11	1. Post charge on ledger for patient **J. B. Haupman**. Est Pt OV Level II (E/M Section) Post entry on daysheet.
___/21	___/21	___/21	2. Post charge on ledger for patient **Rachel T. O'Brien**. Est Pt OV Level II (E/M Section) Post copayment received (check) from managed care plan on ledger (see Form Online 79). Post entries on daysheet and record payment on bank deposit.
___/16	___/16	___/16	3. Post charges on ledger for patient **Martin P. Owens**. Est Pt OV Level II (E/M Section) Diathermy (Medicine Section—Physical Medicine) Post entries on daysheet.
___/25	___/25	___/25	4. Post charges on ledger for patient **Joseph C. Smith**. NP OV Level III (E/M Section) Esophageal motility with interpretation and report (Medicine Section—Gastroenterology) Post payment (check) on ledger (see Online Form 79). Post entries on daysheet.
___/20	___/20	___/20	5. Post charge on ledger for patient **Kathryn L. Hope**. Est Pt OV Level II (E/M Section) Post HMO copayment on ledger; $10 cash. Complete cash receipt No. 150 (see Online Form 74). Post entries on daysheet.
___/11	___/11	___/11	6. Post charges on ledger for patient **Russell P. Smith**. Est Pt OV Level II (E/M Section) Post entry on daysheet.
___/21	___/21	___/21	7. Post charge on ledger for patient **Charlotte J. Brown**. Est Pt OV Level III (E/M Section) Post entry on daysheet.
___/11	___/11	___/11	8. Post charge on ledger for patient **Joan Gomez**. HV (subsequent) Level I (E/M Section) Post entry on daysheet.
___/11	___/11	___/11	9. Post charge on ledger for patient **Robert T. Jenner**. Hospital discharge (E/M Section) Post entry on daysheet.

TELEPHONE CALL: Mr. Howard S. Chan telephoned and said he was unable to pay his bill because he lost his job. You spoke with Dr. Practon and he told you to cancel the patient's debt.

JOB SKILL 15-11 (*continued*)

___/12　___/12　___/12　10. Post an adjustment on the ledger for patient **Howard S. Chan.**

　　　　　　　　　　　　　Reference Dr. G. Practon's name on the ledger.

　　　　　　　　　　　　　Describe the adjustment as a "hardship."

　　　　　　　　　　　　　Post entry on daysheet.

_____　_____　_____　Complete within specified time.

___/161　___/161　___/161　**Total points earned** (To obtain a percentage score, divide the total points earned by the number of points possible.)

Comments:

Evaluator's Signature: _____　**Need to Repeat:** _____

National Curriculum Competency: CAAHEP: Cognitive: II.C.1, 4 Psychomotor: VII.P.1　　　　ABHES: 7.c

JOB SKILL 15-12
Bookkeeping Day 3—Balance the Daysheet

Name _____ Date _____ Score _____

Performance Objective

Task: Total all columns on the daysheet, add previous page totals, and enter new figures in month-to-date areas.

Conditions: Need:
- Daysheet (Day 3) used in Job Skills 15-10 and 15-11
- Calculator
- Pencil

Refer to:
- *Textbook* Procedure 15-1 for step-by-step directions

Standards: Complete all steps listed in this skill in _____ minutes with a minimum score of _____. (Time element and accuracy criteria may be given by instructor.)

Time: Start: _____ Completed: _____ Total: _____ minutes

Scoring: One point for each step performed satisfactorily unless otherwise listed or weighted by instructor.

Directions with Performance Evaluation Checklist

1st Attempt	2nd Attempt	3rd Attempt	
_____	_____	_____	Gather materials (equipment and supplies) listed under *Conditions*.

DAYSHEET TOTALS

____/3	____/3	____/3	1. Total Column A, add "Previous Page" total, and enter the "Month-to-Date" figure.
____/3	____/3	____/3	2. Total Column B-1, add "Previous Page" total, and enter the "Month-to-Date" figure.
____/3	____/3	____/3	3. Total Column B-2, add "Previous Page" total, and enter the "Month-to-Date" figure.
____/3	____/3	____/3	4. Total Column C, add "Previous Page" total, and enter the "Month-to-Date" figure.
____/3	____/3	____/3	5. Total Column D, add "Previous Page" total, and enter the "Month-to-Date" figure.

PROOF OF POSTING

____/5	____/5	____/5	6. Transfer today's daysheet totals as directed in the "Proof of Posting" section and add or subtract as instructed. If the total does not equal Column C, recalculate and look for errors.

ACCOUNTS RECEIVABLE CONTROL

____/5	____/5	____/5	7. Enter figures from the "Proof of Posting" section to the "Accounts Receivable Control" section as indicated and add or subtract as instructed.

ACCOUNTS RECEIVABLE PROOF

____/5	____/5	____/5	8. Enter month-to-date figures in the "Accounts Receivable Proof" section and add or subtract as instructed.

JOB SKILL 15-12 (*continued*)

BALANCE DAYSHEET

___/10   ___/10   ___/10   9. Compare the dollar amount in the "Total Accounts Receivable" figure from the "Accounts Receivable Control" section with the dollar amount in the "Total Accounts Receivable" figure from the "Accounts Receivable Proof" section; they should match. If not, follow instructions on common posting problems to locate the error.

RECORD DEPOSIT AND BALANCE CASH CONTROL

___/3   ___/3   ___/3   10. Add all cash received in the "Record of Deposits" section and enter the amount in the "Total Cash" area at the bottom.

___/6   ___/6   ___/6   11. Add all checks received in the "Record of Deposits" section and enter the amount in the "Total Checks" area at the bottom.

___/3   ___/3   ___/3   12. Add total cash received and total checks received to obtain the total deposit amount and enter it in the "Total Deposit" area at the bottom; this amount should equal the total of today's payments found in Column B-1.

___/5   ___/5   ___/5   13. Balance cash on hand by following the steps listed in "Cash Control."

___   ___   ___   Complete within specified time.

___/59   ___/59   ___/59   **Total points earned** (To obtain a percentage score, divide the total points earned by the number of points possible.)

Comments:

Evaluator's Signature: _____   **Need to Repeat:** _____

National Curriculum Competency: CAAHEP: Cognitive: II.C.1	ABHES: 7.c

JOB SKILL 15-13
Bookkeeping Day 4—Set Up the Daysheet for a New Month

Name _____ Date _____ Score _____

Performance Objective

Task: Set up the daily journal for a new month by inserting figures from the previous month totals.

Conditions: Need:

  • Computer with Internet connection

  • Online Form 80 (header and bottom section of daily journal) located at
    www.cengagebrain.com with student resources

  • Pencil

  Refer to:

  • Daysheet from previous day/month (Day 3—Job Skill 15-12)

Standards: Complete all steps listed in this skill in _____ minutes with a minimum score of _____.
         (Time element and accuracy criteria may be given by instructor.)

Time: Start: _____ Completed: _____ Total: _____ minutes

Scoring: One point for each step performed satisfactorily unless otherwise listed or weighted by
         instructor.

Directions with Performance Evaluation Checklist

1st Attempt	2nd Attempt	3rd Attempt	
_____	_____	_____	Gather materials (equipment and supplies) listed under *Conditions*.
____/3	____/3	____/3	1. It is July 1, current year. Enter this date on the top of the daysheet and label it page 1 of 1.
____/5	____/5	____/5	2. Because it is the first of the month, there will be no "Previous Page" totals in Columns A, B-1, B-2, C, and D at the bottom of the daily journal; this area is used to calculate month-to-date figures. Enter zeros in the "Previous Page" columns.
____/2	____/2	____/2	3. Insert the "Accounts Receivable Control" figure at the bottom of the daysheet. This is the "Total Accounts Receivable" figure at the end of the previous day.
____/2	____/2	____/2	4. Insert the end-of-month total accounts receivable from June 30, 20XX, in the "Accounts Receivable Proof" "Accounts Receivable First of Month" area, found in the ending "Total Accounts Receivable" section. This will be the same total as the previous day's total (i.e., end-of-month total) entered into the "Accounts Receivable Control" section.
_____	_____	_____	5. The daysheet is now set up to record the day's and month-to-date totals, along with the total accounts receivable to date. Insert your name at the bottom of the daysheet in the "Prepared by" area.
_____	_____	_____	Complete within specified time.
____/15	____/15	____/15	**Total points earned** (To obtain a percentage score, divide the total points earned by the number of points possible.)

JOB SKILL 15-13 (*continued*)

Comments:

National Curriculum Competency: CAAHEP: Cognitive: II.C.1   ABHES: 7.c

Procedure Coding

STOP AND THINK CASE SCENARIOS

Refer to the end of Chapter 16 in the *textbook* for the following scenarios:

- Match the Correct Section of *Current Procedural Terminology* (*CPT*) with Specific Procedures and Services
- Determine Where to Look for Codes

EXAM-STYLE REVIEW QUESTIONS

Refer to the end of Chapter 16 in the *textbook*.

Abbreviation and Spelling Review

Read the patient's chart note and write the meanings for the abbreviations following the note. To decode any abbreviations you do not understand or that appear unfamiliar to you, refer to the list of abbreviations in Appendix B of this *Workbook*. Step-by-step directions for this exercise are found in Procedure 1-1 of Chapter 1 in the *textbook*. Medical terms in the chart note are italicized; study them for spelling. Use your medical dictionary to look up their definitions. Your instructor may give a spelling and definition test that includes these words and abbreviations.

Julie Odegard

March 31, 20XX Wendy Smith, CMA (AAMA) accompanied me to 679 Chapel Street, Woodland Hills, XY this afternoon for a HC on pregnant pt Julie Odegard; G III, Para I. She has been at bed rest for 3 wks due to HBP. She is in her third *trimester*; LMP 7/1/XX, approx EDC 4/7/XX. Pt lying on L side, BP 170/92. Pt seems to be in good spirits. Collected sample for a UA, FHS strong. Perf. a PE, C/O abd discomfort, has not started to *dilate*. Will come into ofc in 3 days for a *non-stress test*. Adv to call if any concerns arise.

CMA (AAMA)	_____	L	_____
HC	_____	BP	_____
Pt	_____	UA	_____
G III	_____	FHS	_____
Para I	_____	perf.	_____
wks	_____	PE	_____
HBP	_____	C/O	_____
LMP	_____	abd	_____
approx	_____	ofc	_____
EDC	_____	adv	_____

Review Questions

Review the objectives, glossary, and chapter information before completing these review questions.

1. When coding insurance claims, the _____ code will determine whether the physician gets paid, and the _____ code will determine how much the practice receives.

2. When completing health insurance claims electronically, list the types of codes required on the claim according to the Standard Code Set.

    a. _____

    b. _____

    c. _____

3. An automated system that uses language processing software and can assign codes to clinical procedures and services is called _____

    _____

4. What is the commonly used code system called for coding workers' compensation claims? _____

    _____

5. What is the codebook called used for complementary and alternative medicine? _____

    _____

    _____

6. For coding purposes, the definition of *new patient* is _____

    _____

7. True or False. Critical care must always be provided in some type of critical care unit.

8. Explain the difference between a consult and a patient referral.

    a. Consult: _____

    _____

    b. Referral: _____

    _____

9. Write the definition of these three symbols that appear in the *CPT** codebook.

   a. + _____

   b. ● _____

   c. ▲ _____

10. Write the definition of a "bundled code." _____

    _____

11. Procedure codes consist of _____ -digit numbers with _____ -digit modifiers.

12. In what section of *CPT* are office visits and hospital visits found? _____

13. To code from the Evaluation and Management (E/M) section of *CPT*, what three things must be determined?

    a. _____

    b. _____

    c. _____

14. What is the largest section of *CPT*, which has the most subsections? _____

15. Surgical package rules are established by _____, and global

    package rules are established by _____.

16. Repairs of lacerations are coded according to:

    a. _____

    b. _____

    c. _____

17. When coding fractures, name two things that need to be determined.

    a. _____

    b. _____

18. Endoscopes should always reflect the _____ area of visualization.

19. What is the less-invasive surgical approach called when coding abdominal procedures? _____

    _____

20. True or False. When coding lesion removals on male or female genitalia, always select codes from the Integumentary subsection of the Surgery section in *CPT*.

21. The documentation required in a patient's medical record when an injection is given includes the following:

    a. _____

    b. _____

    c. _____

    d. _____

22. A two-digit code used in addition to the procedure code to indicate circumstances in which the

    procedure differs in some way from that described is called a _____ code, and a five-digit code that cannot stand alone but is designed to be used with primary procedure codes,

    known as "parent codes" are _____ codes.

Critical Thinking Exercises

You desire to communicate to the physician the importance of the relationship between correct coding and reimbursement. Role-play a meeting in which you emphasize various aspects of accurate procedure and diagnostic coding.

JOB SKILL 16-1
Review *Current Procedural Terminology* Codebook Sections

Name _____ Date _____ Score _____

Performance Objective

Task: Locate procedure codes in various sections of the *CPT** codebook.

Conditions: Need:
- *CPT* codebook
- Pen or pencil

Standards: Complete all steps listed in this skill in _____ minutes with a minimum score of _____.
(Time element and accuracy criteria may be given by instructor.)

Time: **Start:** _____ **Completed:** _____ **Total:** _____ minutes

Scoring: One point for each step performed satisfactorily unless otherwise listed or weighted by instructor.

Directions with Performance Evaluation Checklist

Insert the section of *CPT* where each of the following codes is located. If they are found in the Surgery section, name the subsection.

1st Attempt	2nd Attempt	3rd Attempt	
_____	_____	_____	Gather materials (equipment and supplies) listed under *Conditions*.
_____	_____	_____	1. 99202 _____
_____	_____	_____	2. 27500 _____
_____	_____	_____	3. 73501 _____
_____	_____	_____	4. 00500 _____
_____	_____	_____	5. 80055 _____
_____	_____	_____	6. 90713 _____
_____	_____	_____	7. 75970 _____
_____	_____	_____	8. 41872 _____
_____	_____	_____	9. 86805 _____
_____	_____	_____	10. 95004 _____
_____	_____	_____	11. 99281 _____
_____	_____	_____	12. 01810 _____
_____	_____	_____	Complete within specified time.
___/14	___/14	___/14	**Total points earned** (To obtain a percentage score, divide the total points earned by the number of points possible.)

Current Procedural Terminology codes, descriptions, and two-digit numeric modifiers only are from *CPT 2017*. ©2016, American Medical Association. All rights reserved.

JOB SKILL 16-1 (*continued*)

Comments:

National Curriculum Competency: CAAHEP: Cognitive: IX.C.1 Affective: IX.A.1 | ABHES: 7.d

JOB SKILL 16-2
Code Evaluation and Management Services

Name _____ Date _____ Score _____

Performance Objective

Task: Locate evaluation and management codes in various subsections of the E/M section of *CPT*.

Conditions: Need:
- *CPT* codebook
- Pen or pencil

Refer to:
- *Evaluation and Management Services Guidelines* found at the beginning of the E/M section
- *CPT* notes that appear prior to the subsections and within categories of the E/M section
- *Textbook* section, "Coding for Professional Services"
- *Textbook* Procedure 16-1 for step-by-step directions

Standards: Complete all steps listed in this skill in _____ minutes with a minimum score of _____.
(Time element and accuracy criteria may be given by instructor.)

Time: **Start:** _____ **Completed:** _____ **Total:** _____ minutes

Scoring: One point for each step performed satisfactorily unless otherwise listed or weighted by instructor.

Directions with Performance Evaluation Checklist

The following divisions in this job skill are designed to acquaint you with various subsections in the E/M section of *CPT*. The problems become more difficult as you progress.

E/M codes are used by physicians to report a significant portion of their services. Some physicians rank E/M codes on a scale of 1 to 5, with 5 as the highest, most complex level, and 1 as the lowest, least-complex level. This terminology appears on multipurpose billing forms. The levels are determined by the last digit and are broken down as follows:

	OFFICE VISITS		CONSULTATIONS	
	New	Established	Office	Hospital
Level 1	99201	99211	99241	99251
Level 2	99202	99212	99242	99252
Level 3	99203	99213	99243	99253
Level 4	99204	99214	99244	99254
Level 5	99205	99215	99245	99255

Remember, it is the physician's responsibility to assign E/M codes, and this job skill is for familiarization purposes. The problems will acquaint you with terminology for this section of the *CPT* codebook.

1st Attempt	2nd Attempt	3rd Attempt	
_____	_____	_____	Gather materials (equipment and supplies) listed under *Conditions*.

NEW PATIENT OFFICE OR OTHER OUTPATIENT SERVICES: Select by level of service and key components.

_____ _____ _____ 1. This is a level 2 case:

Expanded problem-focused history

Expanded problem-focused examination   _____

Straightforward medical decision making

JOB SKILL 16-2 (*continued*)

_____ _____ _____ 2. This is a level 4 case:

Comprehensive examination _____

Comprehensive history

Moderate complexity medical decision making

_____ _____ _____ 3. This is a level 1 case: _____

Problem-focused history

Problem-focused examination

Straightforward decision making

ESTABLISHED PATIENT OFFICE OR OTHER OUTPATIENT SERVICES: Select by level of service and key components, taking into consideration the rule that states you need "two out of three" key components to assign a code for an established patient.

_____ _____ _____ 4. This is a level 2 case:

Problem-focused history _____

Problem-focused examination

Straightforward medical decision making

_____ _____ _____ 5. This is a level 4 case:

Detailed history _____

Detailed examination

Moderate-complexity medical decision making

_____ _____ _____ 6. This is a level 5 case:

Comprehensive history _____

Comprehensive examination

High-complexity decision making

CODE RANGE 99201 TO 99239—Services provided in physician's office, hospital inpatient/outpatient, or other ambulatory facility. Select codes according to key components.

_____/3 _____/3 _____/3 7. Office visit for a 4-year-old male, established patient, _____ with an expanded problem-focused history and physical examination for earache and dyshidrosis of feet and low-complexity medical decision making.

_____/3 _____/3 _____/3 8. Office visit for a 35-year-old male, established patient, with _____ a detailed history and examination for a new-onset right lower quadrant (RLQ) pain. Medical decision making is of moderate complexity.

_____/3 _____/3 _____/3 9. Initial hospital visit for a 15-year-old male with a detailed _____ history and examination for infectious mononucleosis and dehydration. Medical decision making is of low complexity.

_____/3 _____/3 _____/3 10. Subsequent hospital visit for a 9-year-old female admitted for _____ lobar pneumonia with vomiting and dehydration. A problem-focused interval history is taken because she is becoming afebrile but tolerates oral fluids. An expanded problem-focused examination is done, with straightforward decision making.

_____/3 _____/3 _____/3 11. Office visit for a 9-year-old male, established patient, _____ who has been taking swimming lessons and now presents with a two-day history of left ear pain with purulent drainage. This visit requires a problem-focused history and examination, with straightforward decision making.

JOB SKILL 16-2 (*continued*)

CODE RANGE 99241 TO 99255—Consultation services provided in the physician's office, hospital inpatient/outpatient, or other ambulatory facility. Select codes according to key components.

____/3 ____/3 ____/3   12. Office consultation for a 67-year-old male with chronic low-back pain radiating to the left leg requiring a detailed history and examination and low-complexity decision making.   _____

____/3 ____/3 ____/3   13. Initial office consultation for a 21-year-old female with acute upper respiratory tract symptoms that require an expanded problem-focused history and examination with straightforward decision making.   _____

____/3 ____/3 ____/3   14. Office consultation for a 30-year-old female with chronic pelvic inflammatory disease, who now has left lower quadrant pain with a palpable pelvic mass. This visit requires a comprehensive history and examination and moderate-complexity decision making.   _____

____/3 ____/3 ____/3   15. Initial office consultation for a 60-year-old carpenter with olecranon bursitis requiring a problem-focused history and examination. Medical decision making is straightforward.   _____

____/3 ____/3 ____/3   16. Hospital consultation for a highly functional 70-year-old male to review laboratory studies. A problem-focused history and examination is performed. Medical decision making is straightforward.   _____

CODE RANGE 99281 TO 99498—Services provided in a hospital emergency or critical care department, nursing facility, rest home or custodial care facility, and patient's home as well as prolonged physician standby, case management, care plan, and preventive medicine services. Select codes according to key components or time.

____/3 ____/3 ____/3   17. First hour of critical care of a 16-year-old male with acute respiratory failure from asthma.   _____

____/3 ____/3 ____/3   18. A child is seen in the emergency department with a rash on both legs after exposure to poison ivy. This visit requires an expanded problem-focused history and examination but low-complexity medical decision making.   _____

____/3 ____/3 ____/3   19. Initial nursing facility visit to evaluate a 70-year-old male found confused and wandering, admitted by Adult Protective Services without a qualifying stay or inpatient diagnostic workup. Patient lives alone and has no relatives in the area. A comprehensive history and examination is performed. Medical decision making is of moderate complexity.   _____

____/3 ____/3 ____/3   20. Subsequent visit in a skilled nursing facility to a female with controlled dementia, hypertension, and diabetes. During the visit, she seems to exhibit flu symptoms. An expanded problem-focused interval history and examination is performed. Medical decision making is straightforward.   _____

____/3 ____/3 ____/3   21. Emergency department visit for a female who received an abrasion and needs a tetanus toxoid immunization. A problem-focused history and examination is performed, and medical decision making is straightforward.   _____

____/3 ____/3 ____/3   22. A 16-year-old patient presents for her yearly physical examination.   _____

JOB SKILL 16-2 (*continued*)

___/3   ___/3   ___/3   23. Rest home visit for the evaluation and management of a new 86-year-old patient with a detailed history and examination and moderate-complexity medical decision making.   _____

___/3   ___/3   ___/3   24. Complex interval history and examination done during a home visit for an established patient; high-complexity medical decision making.   _____

___/3   ___/3   ___/3   25. A 26-year-old new patient presents for an initial comprehensive preventive medicine visit. The physician performs a history and examination, then counsels the patient regarding birth control.   _____

_____   _____   _____   Complete within specified time.

___/65   ___/65   ___/65   **Total points earned** (To obtain a percentage score, divide the total points earned by the number of points possible.)

Comments:

Evaluator's Signature: _____   **Need to Repeat:** _____

National Curriculum Competency: CAAHEP: Psychomotor: IX.P. 1 Affective: IX.A.1   ABHES: 7.d

JOB SKILL 16-3
Code Surgical Procedures and Services

Name _____ Date _____ Score _____

Performance Objective

Task: Locate the correct procedure code within the Surgery section of *CPT* for each description listed.

Conditions: Need:
- *CPT* codebook
- Pen or pencil

Refer to:
- *Surgery Guidelines* found at the beginning of the Surgery section
- *CPT* notes that appear prior to and within the subsections and categories of the Surgery section
- *Textbook* section, "How to Code from the Surgery Section"
- *Textbook* section, "Coding for Professional Services"
- *Textbook* Procedure 16-1 for step-by-step directions

Standards: Complete all steps listed in this skill in _____ minutes with a minimum score of _____. (Time element and accuracy criteria may be given by instructor.)

Time: Start: _____ Completed: _____ Total: _____ minutes

Scoring: One point for each step performed satisfactorily unless otherwise listed or weighted by instructor.

Directions with Performance Evaluation Checklist

Surgery codes 10021 to 69990 are divided according to body systems, then anatomic parts of the body. Use the *CPT* codebook to obtain the correct code number for each descriptor given. Critical thinking enters this job skill as you use your judgment to determine the correct code, since some cases do not contain full details. Read each case and code descriptions carefully.

1st Attempt	2nd Attempt	3rd Attempt		
_____	_____	_____	Gather materials (equipment and supplies) listed under *Conditions*.	

INTEGUMENTARY SYSTEM 10021–19499

____/5	____/5	____/5	1. Excision, benign lesion, face, 0.5 cm	_____
____/5	____/5	____/5	2. Repair layered closure of lt leg 2.7 cm laceration	_____

MUSCULOSKELETAL SYSTEM 20005–29999

____/5	____/5	____/5	3. Closed reduction of rt humeral shaft fracture, no manipulation	_____
____/5	____/5	____/5	4. Subsequent application of long leg cast (walker)	_____

RESPIRATORY SYSTEM 30000–32999

____/5	____/5	____/5	5. Remove fried potato from left nostril of child	_____
____/5	____/5	____/5	6. Simple excision of small nasal polyp	_____

CARDIOVASCULAR SYSTEM 33010–37799

____/5	____/5	____/5	7. Introduction of catheter into superior vena cava	_____
____/5	____/5	____/5	8. Coronary artery bypass using single arterial graft	_____

JOB SKILL 16-3 (*continued*)

HEMIC/LYMPHATIC & MEDIASTINUM/DIAPHRAGM 38100–39599

____/5 ____/5 ____/5   9. Biopsy of cervical lymph nodes; open, deep   _____

____/5 ____/5 ____/5 10. Open excision for removal of total spleen   _____

DIGESTIVE SYSTEM 40490–49999

____/5 ____/5 ____/5 11. Liver biopsy; needle; percutaneous   _____

____/5 ____/5 ____/5 12. Open excision to remove gallbladder (cholecystectomy)   _____

URINARY SYSTEM 50010–53899

____/5 ____/5 ____/5 13. Drainage of deep periurethral abscess   _____

____/5 ____/5 ____/5 14. Aspiration of bladder by needle   _____

MALE GENITAL/INTERSEX/FEMALE GENITAL/MATERNITY CARE AND DELIVERY 54000–60699

____/5 ____/5 ____/5 15. Removal of IUD   _____

____/5 ____/5 ____/5 16. Cesarean delivery including obstetric   _____
    /antepartum/postpartum care

ENDOCRINE/NERVOUS SYSTEMS 60000–64999

____/5 ____/5 ____/5 17. Complete thyroidectomy   _____

____/5 ____/5 ____/5 18. Cervical laminoplasty with decompression of   _____
    spinal cord; two segments

EYE AND OCULAR ADNEXA/AUDITORY/OPERATING MICROSCOPE 65091–69990

____/5 ____/5 ____/5 19. Subconjunctival injection   _____

____/5 ____/5 ____/5 20. Removal of temporal bone tumor   _____

_____   Complete within specified time.

___/102 ___/102 ___/102   **Total points earned** (To obtain a percentage score, divide the total points earned by the number of points possible.)

Comments:

Evaluator's Signature: _____ **Need to Repeat:** _____

National Curriculum Competency: CAAHEP: Psychomotor: IX.P. 1 Affective: IX.A.1	ABHES: 7.d

JOB SKILL 16-4
Code Radiology and Laboratory Procedures and Services

Name _____ Date _____ Score _____

Performance Objective

Task: Locate the correct procedure code in the Radiology and Pathology/Laboratory section of *CPT* for each description.

Conditions: Need:

  • *CPT* codebook

  • Pen or pencil

  Refer to:

  • Radiology and Pathology/Laboratory Guidelines found at the beginning of those sections in *CPT*

  • *CPT* notes that appear prior to and within the subsections and categories

  • *Textbook* section, "Coding for Professional Services"

  • *Textbook* Procedure 16-1 for step-by-step directions

Standards: Complete all steps listed in this skill in _____ minutes with a minimum score of _____. (Time element and accuracy criteria may be given by instructor.)

Time: Start: _____ Completed: _____ Total: _____ minutes

Scoring: One point for each step performed satisfactorily unless otherwise listed or weighted by instructor.

Directions with Performance Evaluation Checklist

1st Attempt	2nd Attempt	3rd Attempt		
_____	_____	_____	Gather materials (equipment and supplies) listed under *Conditions*.	

RADIOLOGY 70010–79999 AND PATHOLOGY/LABORATORY 80047–89398

1st Attempt	2nd Attempt	3rd Attempt		
___/5	___/5	___/5	1. X-rays of hand, four views	_____
___/5	___/5	___/5	2. Internal mammary angiography; radiological supervision and interpretation	_____
___/5	___/5	___/5	3. Computed tomography of the abdomen with contrast material	_____
___/5	___/5	___/5	4. Retrograde urethrocystography with supervision and interpretation	_____
___/5	___/5	___/5	5. Lipid panel	_____
___/5	___/5	___/5	6. Bacterial culture quantitative, urine	_____
___/5	___/5	___/5	7. Bone marrow (blood cells) tissue culture for neoplastic disorders	_____
___/5	___/5	___/5	8. Surgical pathology examination of the gallbladder	_____
_____	_____	_____	Complete within specified time.	
___/42	___/42	___/42	**Total points earned** (To obtain a percentage score, divide the total points earned by the number of points possible.)	

JOB SKILL 16-4 (*continued*)

Comments:

Evaluator's Signature: _____   **Need to Repeat:** _____

National Curriculum Competency: CAAHEP: Psychomotor: IX.P. 1 Affective: IX.A.1   ABHES: 7.d

JOB SKILL 16-5
Code Procedures and Services in the Medicine Section

Name _____ Date _____ Score _____

Performance Objective

Task: Locate the correct procedure code from the Medicine section of *CPT* for each scenario.

Conditions: Need:

  • *CPT* codebook

  • Pen or pencil

  Refer to:

  • Medicine Guidelines found at the beginning of the Medicine section

  • *CPT* notes that appear prior to and within the subsections and categories of the Medicine section

  • *Textbook* section, "Coding for Professional Services"

  • *Textbook* Procedure 16-1 for step-by-step directions

Standards: Complete all steps listed in this skill in _____ minutes with a minimum score of _____. (Time element and accuracy criteria may be given by instructor.)

Time: **Start:** _____ **Completed:** _____ **Total:** _____ minutes

Scoring: One point for each step performed satisfactorily unless otherwise listed or weighted by instructor.

Directions with Performance Evaluation Checklist

1st Attempt	2nd Attempt	3rd Attempt	
_____	_____	_____	Gather materials (equipment and supplies) listed under *Conditions*.

MEDICINE SECTION 90281—99607

___/10	___/10	___/10	1. Immune globulin injection, botulism, intravenous push

  Product: _____

  Administration: _____

___/10	___/10	___/10	2. Influenza virus vaccine, trivalent (split virus) intramuscular injection (IM), to a 62-year-old patient

  Product: _____

  Administration: _____

___/5	___/5	___/5	3. Replacement of contact lens _____
___/5	___/5	___/5	4. Cardiovascular stress test (treadmill) with continuous electrocardiographic monitoring with supervision, interpretation, and report _____
___/5	___/5	___/5	5. Handling of specimen for transfer from the office to a laboratory _____
_____	_____	_____	Complete within specified time.
___/37	___/37	___/37	**Total points earned** (To obtain a percentage score, divide the total points earned by the number of points possible.)

JOB SKILL 16-5 (*continued*)

Comments:

Evaluator's Signature: _____ **Need to Repeat:** _____

National Curriculum Competency: CAAHEP: Psychomotor: IX.P.1 Affective: IX.A.1	ABHES: 7.d

JOB SKILL 16-6
Code Clinical Examples

Name _____ Date _____ Score _____

Performance Objective

Task: Read each scenario; select the correct *CPT* or *Healthcare Common Procedure Coding System (HCPCS) Level II* procedure code.

Conditions: Need:

- *CPT* codebook or *textbook* Tables 16-3 and 16-4
- Pen or pencil

Refer to:

- *Workbook*, Appendix A, Mock Fee Schedule
- *Workbook*, Appendix A, *HCPCS Level II* codes

Standards: Complete all steps listed in this skill in _____ minutes with a minimum score of _____. (Time element and accuracy criteria may be given by instructor.)

Time: **Start:** _____ **Completed:** _____ **Total:** _____ minutes

Scoring: One point for each step performed satisfactorily unless otherwise listed or weighted by instructor.

Directions with Performance Evaluation Checklist

This job skill will familiarize you with parts of the CMS-1500 claim form where you will insert procedure codes. You will also be coding from SOAP chart notes and selecting *HCPCS Level II* codes. All sections of *CPT* will be used. Answer the questions and insert data in Field 24 of the CMS-1500 claim form.

1st Attempt	2nd Attempt	3rd Attempt	
_____	_____	_____	Gather materials (equipment and supplies) listed under *Conditions*.

CMS-1500 CLAIM FORM—SCENARIO A: On February 3, current year, a private insurance patient is taken to an ambulatory surgery center with effusion of fluid (hydrarthrosis) of the right knee. The physician does an arthrocentesis and aspirates. A dressing is applied and patient is to return to office in one week.

____/7	____/7	____/7	1. What is the date of the service or procedure? Indicate the eight-digit date in the unshaded area of Field 24A (left portion only).
____/7	____/7	____/7	2. What is the correct procedure code? Insert this in the unshaded area of Field 24D (*CPT/HCPCS*).
____/7	____/7	____/7	3. What is the mock fee for this service? Insert this in the unshaded area of Field 24F.
____/7	____/7	____/7	4. How many times was this procedure performed? Indicate this in the unshaded area of Field 24G (DAYS OR UNITS).

24. A.	DATE(S) OF SERVICE				B.	C.	D. PROCEDURES, SERVICES, OR SUPPLIES		E.	F.	G.	H.	I.	J.
	From		To		PLACE OF		(Explain Unusual Circumstances)		DIAGNOSIS		DAYS OR	EPSDT Family	ID.	RENDERING
MM	DD	YY	MM	DD	YY	SERVICE	EMG	CPT/HCPCS	MODIFIER	POINTER	$ CHARGES	UNITS	Plan	QUAL.	PROVIDER ID. #
														NPI	

Courtesy of the Centers for Medicare and Medicaid Services

JOB SKILL 16-6 (*continued*)

CMS-1500 CLAIM FORM—SCENARIO B: On May 6, a new private insurance patient is seen in the office of an otologist after referral by a family physician to evaluate and treat diminished hearing in the right ear. The physician performs an expanded problem-focused history and examination. A comprehensive audiometry threshold evaluation and speech recognition test is performed, revealing a conductive right ear low-frequency loss of hearing. Patient is referred to an audiologist for hearing aid examination and selection. Decision making is straightforward. Patient is asked to return in one month.

____/7   ____/7   ____/7   5. What is the date of the service for each procedure?
Indicate the eight-digit date in the unshaded area of Field 24A
(left portion only).

____/14   ____/14   ____/14   6. What are the correct procedure codes?
Insert these in the unshaded area of Field 24D (*CPT/HCPCS*).

____/14   ____/14   ____/14   7. What are the mock fees for these services?
Insert these in the unshaded area of Field 24F.

____/7   ____/7   ____/7   8. How many times were these procedures performed?
Indicate this in the unshaded area of Field 24G (DAYS OR UNITS).

24. A. DATE(S) OF SERVICE						B. PLACE OF SERVICE	C. EMG	D. PROCEDURES, SERVICES, OR SUPPLIES (Explain Unusual Circumstances) CPT/HCPCS	MODIFIER	E. DIAGNOSIS POINTER	F. $ CHARGES	G. DAYS OR UNITS	H. EPSDT Family Plan	I. ID. QUAL.	J. RENDERING PROVIDER ID. #
From MM	DD	YY	To MM	DD	YY										
														NPI	
														NPI	

Courtesy of the Centers for Medicare and Medicaid Services

SOAP CHART NOTE A:

4/15/XX Maria Gomez

S: A 35-year-old female established patient is seen for a new complaint of left lower quadrant pain; 1 wk. duration. Symptoms: mild fever, decreased appetite, and mild constipation for 1 wk. Pt denies abdominal injury, change in urination, or abnormal menstruation. LMP: 3/12/XX.

O: Temp: 100.2°F; BP 130/80, HR 80; RR 18.

Lungs: Clear.

Abdomen: Both sides mildly hyperactive, flat, mild guarding LLQ, rebound neg; fullness LLQ; no discrete masses; no HSM.

Rectal: Normal tone; no masses; guaiac positive.

Pelvic: Cervix closed, uterus and ovaries normal, fullness lt lat adnexa c̄ tenderness.

Lab: CBC, elevated. WBC c̄ mild lt shift; UA, normal; HCG, pregnancy test negative.

A: Probable diverticulitis of sigmoid colon based on clinical picture.

P: Obtain barium enema to R/O diverticulitis. Begin antibiotics and dietary restriction during acute phase and follow up in three days.

____/8   ____/8   ____/8   9. Read the SOAP note and select the correct E/M code.   _____

CHART NOTE B:

A physician does a history and examination on an established patient for 5 minutes, performs acne surgery (code 10040), and counsels the patient on skin care and diet for 10 minutes.

____/8   ____/8   ____/8   10. Read the chart note and select the correct E/M code.   _____

JOB SKILL 16-6 *(continued)*

HCPCS LEVEL II CODES

____/3 ____/3 ____/3   11. Select the correct *HCPCS* Level II code for one   _____
                            sterile eye pad.

____/3 ____/3 ____/3   12. Select the correct *HCPCS* Level II code for   _____
                            metal underarm crutches.

____/3 ____/3 ____/3   13. Select the correct *HCPCS* Level II code for 1 cc   _____
                            gamma globulin inj IM.

____/3 ____/3 ____/3   14. Select the correct *HCPCS* Level II code for the   _____
                            physician interpretation of a screening Pap smear.

_____ _____ _____   Complete within specified time.

__/100 __/100 __/100   **Total points earned** (To obtain a percentage score, divide the total points
earned by the number of points possible.)

Comments:

Evaluator's Signature: _____ **Need to Repeat:** _____

National Curriculum Competency: CAAHEP: Psychomotor: IX.P. 1 Affective: IX.A.1	ABHES: 8.c.3

Diagnostic Coding

STOP AND THINK CASE SCENARIOS

Refer to the end of Chapter 17 in the *textbook* for the following scenarios:
- Practice Code Linkage
- Verify Diagnosis

EXAM-STYLE REVIEW QUESTIONS

Refer to the end of Chapter 17 in the *textbook*.

Abbreviation and Spelling Review

Read the patient's chart note and write the meanings for the abbreviations following the note. To decode any abbreviations you do not understand or that appear unfamiliar to you, refer to the list of abbreviations in Appendix B of this *Workbook*. Step-by-step directions for this exercise are found in Procedure 1-1 of Chapter 1 in the *textbook*. Medical terms in the chart note are italicized; study them for spelling. Use your medical dictionary to look up their definitions. Your instructor may give a spelling and definition test that includes these words and abbreviations.

Vance Romanelli

July 17, 20XX
A 30-year-old diabetic WM, referred by Dr. Marshall, presents for an init CON for a skin inf in his RLQ at an injection site. He has been on AB for 1 week but there is still slt inflam approximately 3 by 4 inches and the area is still quite painful. Proceeded with BI for *pathologic* interpret and a C & S. Results in approx 3 to 4 days. Cleaned and redressed the wound and adv patient to take OTC Advil, 3 every 6 hours for pain. Patient to report if any temperature over 100 degrees presents. RTO in 1 wk.

WM _____   BI _____

init _____   interpret _____

CON _____   C & S _____

inf _____   approx _____

RLQ _____   adv _____

AB _____   OTC _____

slt _____   RTO _____

inflam _____   wk _____

Review Questions

Review the objectives, glossary, and chapter information before completing these review questions.

1. The first Classification of Causes of Death was introduced by the French physician Jacques Bertillon in the year _____.

2. What was the compliance implementation date for using *ICD-10-CM* codes? _____

3. Name five benefits of using *ICD-10-CM* over *ICD-9-CM*?

   a. _____

   b. _____

   c. _____

   d. _____

   e. _____

4. Computer-assisted coding uses _____ and _____ to read and analyze the medical record.

5. What guidelines does the medical assistant need to become familiar with to assign correct diagnostic codes? _____

6. In an outpatient setting, the condition, problem, or other reason for the health encounter that is chiefly responsible for the services provided is called the _____ or the _____.

7. Explain code linkage. _____

8. What is the abbreviation for the coding edits that were implemented by the Centers for Medicare and Medicaid Services (CMS) to promote correct coding and control inappropriate reimbursement? _____

9. A single code used to describe two diagnoses is called a _____.

_____

10. Explain a "qualified diagnosis," and state what terms (descriptions) to code instead.

    _____

    _____

    _____

    _____

    _____

11. In your own words, describe what the following terms mean.

    a. NEC: _____

    b. NOS: _____

12. When coding an underlying cause of a disease, along with the disease that resulted, name the rule to follow and state which is coded first and second.

    a. Rule: _____

    b. Code first: _____

    c. Code second: _____

13. Explain what the following terms mean that are found in the diagnostic codebook:

    a. Excludes 1: _____

    b. Excludes 2: _____

    c. Initial encounter (injury): _____

    d. Laterality: _____

    e. Sequela: _____

14. List the various categories to look under when searching for a "main term" in the Alphabetic Index (Volume II).

    a. _____

    b. _____

    c. _____

    d. _____

    e. _____

    f. _____

    g. _____

    h. _____

    i. _____

    j. _____

15. To code diagnoses, start in Volume _____ and verify the code in Volume

    _____.

16. Diagnostic codes using *ICD-10-CM* can vary from _____ to

    _____ digits.

17. The character "x" used in the fourth, fifth, or sixth digit with certain character codes to allow for future

    expansion is called a _____.

18. The code B20 (human immunodeficiency virus [HIV] disease) can only be used in _____
_____.

19. When coding neoplasms, name the five titles that codes are listed under and give a brief definition of each term.

    a. _____

    b. _____

    c. _____

    d. _____

    e. _____

20. Diabetes codes are combination codes that include the _____
_____

_____.

21. True or False. Routine postoperative pain should not be coded.

22. True or False. Essential hypertension does not include high blood pressure.

23. The abbreviation "STEMI" stands for _____.

24. True or False. When you code for a specific type of influenza documented in the medical record, it does not need to be verified by positive laboratory serology.

25. List the time frames for the following trimesters in pregnancy:

    First Trimester: _____

    Second Trimester: _____

    Third Trimester: _____

26. True or False. If documentation does not specify if a fracture is *displaced* or *not displaced*, code as *not displaced*.

27. When coding burns, name the three elements in which burns are classified and give a brief description of each term.

    a. _____

    b. _____

    c. _____

28. Codes for external causes of morbidity start with the letters ___, ___, ___, and ___. Codes for factors that

    influence health status, and contact with health services start with the letter ___.

Critical Thinking Exercises

Underline the "main term" in the following diagnostic statements. When determining the main term, do not forget to ask, "What is wrong with the patient?"

a. The patient received an insect bite on the index finger of her right hand.

b. The newborn baby is experiencing spasmodic colic.

c. The patient is suffering from gastrointestinal anthrax.

d. The patient experienced lung edema due to flying at a high altitude.

 e. After having a vaginal hysterectomy, the patient developed a vaginoperineal fistula.

 f. The patient has all the symptoms of Bright's disease.

 g. The patient had an infection during labor.

 h. The baby has jaundice due to preterm delivery.

 i. The patient has bilateral glaucoma with increased episcleral venous pressure.

 j. The patient is a drug addict and has drug-induced Korsakoff's with an amnesic disorder.

 k. The patient has lymphoid leukemia but is in remission.

 l. The patient is experiencing an acute post-traumatic headache.

m. The patient is suffering from acute purulent otitis media in the right ear.

 n. The patient was hospitalized with acute alcohol-induced hemorrhagic pancreatitis.

 o. The baby was born with facial neuritis.

 p. The patient has myocarditis due to streptococcus.

 q. After childbirth, the patient developed an incomplete rectocele with uterine prolapse.

 r. The patient has gangrenous quinsy.

 s. The patient is seen today for gonococcal urethritis with a periurethral abscess.

 t. The patient has postmenopausal atrophic vaginitis.

 u. After a bone scan, the patient was diagnosed with hereditary bone xanthoma.

 v. The patient has rhinocerebral zygomycosis.

w. The patient was hospitalized with thrombosis due to a breast implant.

 x. The patient is experiencing psychogenic yawning.

 y. The patient was hospitalized with a penetrating wound in the abdominal cavity.

 z. The patient returned from Palm Springs, where it was 110 degrees, and is still experiencing lower limb swelling in both legs.

JOB SKILL 17-1
Code Diagnoses from Chapters 1, 2, 3, 4, and 5 in *ICD-10-CM*

Name _____ Date _____ Score _____

Performance Objective

Task: Code diagnoses from the first five chapters of *ICD-10-CM*, Volumes 1 and 2.

Conditions: Need:
                • *International Classification of Diseases, 10th Revision, Clinical Modification**, Volumes 1 and 2
                • Pen or pencil
                Refer to:
                • *Textbook* Procedure 17-1 for step-by-step directions

Standards: Complete all steps listed in this job skill in _____ minutes with a minimum score of _____.
                (Time element and accuracy criteria may be given by instructor.)

Time: Start: _____ Completed: _____ Total: _____ minutes

Scoring: One point for each step performed satisfactorily unless otherwise listed or weighted by
                instructor.

Directions with Performance Evaluation Checklist

Read the following statements, look up main terms in Volume 2—the Alphabetic Index of the diagnostic codebook, select a code and confirm the code selection in Volume 1, the Tabular List.

1st Attempt	2nd Attempt	3rd Attempt		
_____	_____	_____	Gather materials (equipment and supplies) listed under *Conditions*.	
____/5	____/5	____/5	1. Code human immunodeficiency virus.	_____
____/5	____/5	____/5	2. Code blackwater fever malaria.	_____
____/5	____/5	____/5	3. Code malignant melanoma in situ of the shoulder and left upper arm.	_____
____/5	____/5	____/5	4. Code benign neoplasm of the right testes.	_____
____/5	____/5	____/5	5. Code hereditary hemolytic anemia.	_____
____/5	____/5	____/5	6. Code primary thrombocytopenia.	_____
____/5	____/5	____/5	7. Code type 2 diabetes mellitus without complications.	_____
____/5	____/5	____/5	8. Code active rickets.	_____
____/5	____/5	____/5	9. Code anxiety.	_____
____/5	____/5	____/5	10. Code mild mental retardation.	_____
_____	_____	_____	Complete within specified time.	
____/52	____/52	____/52	**Total points earned** (To obtain a percentage score, divide the total points earned by the number of points possible.)	

International Classification of Diseases, 10th Revision, Clinical Modification codes in this chapter are from the 2017 *ICD-10-CM* codebook.

JOB SKILL 17-1 (*continued*)

Comments:

JOB SKILL 17-2
Code Diagnoses from Chapters 6, 7, 8, 9, and 10 in *ICD-10-CM*

Name _____ Date _____ Score _____

Performance Objective

Task: Code diagnoses from Chapters 6 through 10 of *ICD-10-CM*, Volumes 1 and 2.

Conditions: Need:

- *International Classification of Diseases, 10th Revision, Clinical Modification,* Volumes 1 and 2
- Pen or pencil

Refer to:

Textbook Procedure 17-1 for step-by-step directions

Standards: Complete all steps listed in this job skill in _____ minutes with a minimum score of _____.
(Time element and accuracy criteria may be given by instructor.)

Time: Start: _____ Completed: _____ Total: _____ minutes

Scoring: One point for each step performed satisfactorily unless otherwise listed or weighted by instructor.

Directions with Performance Evaluation Checklist

Read the following statements, look up main terms in Volume 2—the Alphabetic Index of the diagnostic codebook, select a code and then confirm the code selection in Volume 1, the Tabular List.

1st Attempt	2nd Attempt	3rd Attempt		
_____	_____	_____	Gather materials (equipment and supplies) listed under *Conditions*.	
____/5	____/5	____/5	1. Code epileptic seizure.	_____
____/5	____/5	____/5	2. Code pneumococcal meningitis.	_____
____/5	____/5	____/5	3. Code borderline glaucoma.	_____
____/5	____/5	____/5	4. Code right, lower eyelid sebaceous cyst.	_____
____/5	____/5	____/5	5. Code bilateral otorrhea.	_____
____/5	____/5	____/5	6. Code acute eustachian salpingitis of the right ear.	_____
____/5	____/5	____/5	7. Code malignant hypertension.	_____
____/5	____/5	____/5	8. Code nontraumatic cerebral hemorrhage; brain stem.	_____
____/5	____/5	____/5	9. Code viral pneumonia.	_____
____/5	____/5	____/5	10. Code chronic bronchitis.	_____
_____	_____	_____	Complete within specified time.	
____/52	____/52	____/52	**Total points earned** (To obtain a percentage score, divide the total points earned by the number of points possible.)	

Comments:

Evaluator's Signature: _____ **Need to Repeat:** _____

National Curriculum Competency: CAAHEP: Cognitive: IX.C.2 Psychomotor: IX.P.2	ABHES: 7.d

JOB SKILL 17-3
Code Diagnoses from Chapters 11, 12, 13, 14, and 15 in *ICD-10-CM*

Name _____ Date _____ Score _____

Performance Objective

Task: Code diagnoses from Chapters 11 through 15 of *ICD-10-CM*, Volumes 1 and 2.

Conditions: Need:

- *International Classification of Diseases, 10th Revision, Clinical Modification,* Volumes 1 and 2
- Pen or pencil

Refer to:

- *Textbook* Procedure 17-1 for step-by-step directions

Standards: Complete all steps listed in this job skill in _____ minutes with a minimum score of _____. (Time element and accuracy criteria may be given by instructor.)

Time: Start: _____ Completed: _____ Total: _____ minutes

Scoring: One point for each step performed satisfactorily unless otherwise listed or weighted by instructor.

Directions with Performance Evaluation Checklist

Read the following statements, look up main terms in Volume 2—the Alphabetic Index of the diagnostic codebook, select a code and then confirm the code selection in Volume 1, the Tabular List.

1st Attempt	2nd Attempt	3rd Attempt		
_____	_____	_____	Gather materials (equipment and supplies) listed under *Conditions*.	
____/5	____/5	____/5	1. Code ulcerative stomatitis.	_____
____/5	____/5	____/5	2. Code acute peptic ulcer with hemorrhage.	_____
____/5	____/5	____/5	3. Code impetigo.	_____
____/5	____/5	____/5	4. Code dermatitis due to cold weather.	_____
____/5	____/5	____/5	5. Code Kaschin-Beck disease affecting multiple sites.	_____
____/5	____/5	____/5	6. Code spondylosis of the lumbar spine without myelopathy or radiculopathy.	_____
____/5	____/5	____/5	7. Code stage II chronic renal disease.	_____
____/5	____/5	____/5	8. Code fibroadenosis of the left breast.	_____
____/5	____/5	____/5	9. Code excessive vomiting in early pregnancy causing dehydration.	_____
____/5	____/5	____/5	10. Code postpartum condition of retained placenta without hemorrhage.	_____
_____	_____	_____	Complete within specified time.	
____/52	____/52	____/52	**Total points earned** (To obtain a percentage score, divide the total points earned by the number of points possible.)	

JOB SKILL 17-3 (*continued*)

Comments:

Evaluator's Signature: _____   **Need to Repeat:** _____

National Curriculum Competency: CAAHEP: Cognitive: IX.C.2 Psychomotor: IX.P.2	ABHES: 7.d

JOB SKILL 17-4
Code Diagnoses from Chapters 16, 17, 18, 19, and 20 in *ICD-10-CM*

Name _____ Date _____ Score _____

Performance Objective

Task: Code diagnoses from Chapters 16 through 20 of *ICD-10-CM*, Volumes 1 and 2.

Conditions: Need:

* *International Classification of Diseases, 10th Revision, Clinical Modification*, Volumes 1 and 2
* Pen or pencil

Refer to:

* *Textbook* Procedure 17-1 for step-by-step directions

Standards: Complete all steps listed in this job skill in _____ minutes with a minimum score of _____. (Time element and accuracy criteria may be given by instructor.)

Time: **Start:** _____ **Completed:** _____ **Total:** _____ minutes

Scoring: One point for each step performed satisfactorily unless otherwise listed or weighted by instructor.

Directions with Performance Evaluation Checklist

Read the following statements, look up main terms in Volume 2—the Alphabetic Index of the diagnostic codebook, select a code and then confirm the code selection in Volume 1, the Tabular List.

1st Attempt	2nd Attempt	3rd Attempt		
_____	_____	_____	Gather materials (equipment and supplies) listed under *Conditions*.	
____/5	____/5	____/5	1. Code bradycardia in a neonate.	_____
____/5	____/5	____/5	2. Code neonatal diabetes mellitus.	_____
____/5	____/5	____/5	3. Code bilateral cleft lip and palate (hard and soft).	_____
____/5	____/5	____/5	4. Code accessory toe on right foot.	_____
____/5	____/5	____/5	5. Code frequent urination.	_____
____/5	____/5	____/5	6. Code microcalcification found on mammogram.	_____
____/5	____/5	____/5	7. Code fracture of two ribs, right side; initial encounter.	_____
____/5	____/5	____/5	8. Code left ankle sprain; subsequent encounter.	_____
____/5	____/5	____/5	9. Code drowning due to an overturned sailboat.	_____
____/5	____/5	____/5	10. Code an initial encounter for exposure to excessive natural heat.	_____
_____	_____	_____	Complete within specified time.	
____/52	____/52	____/52	**Total points earned** (To obtain a percentage score, divide the total points earned by the number of points possible.)	

Comments:

Evaluator's Signature: _____ **Need to Repeat:** _____

National Curriculum Competency: CAAHEP: Cognitive: IX.C.2 Psychomotor: IX.P.2   ABHES: 7.d

JOB SKILL 17-5

Code Diagnoses from Chapter 21 and the Table of Drugs and Chemicals in *ICD-10-CM*

Name _____ Date _____ Score _____

Performance Objective

Task: Code diagnoses from Chapter 21 and the Table of Drugs and Chemicals of *ICD-10-CM*, Volumes 1 and 2.

Conditions: Need:

- *International Classification of Diseases, 10th Revision, Clinical Modification,* Volumes 1 and 2
- Pen or pencil

Refer to:

- *Textbook* Procedure 17-1 and 17-3 for step-by-step directions

Standards: Complete all steps listed in this job skill in _____ minutes with a minimum score of _____. (Time element and accuracy criteria may be given by instructor.)

Time: **Start:** _____ **Completed:** _____ **Total:** _____ minutes

Scoring: One point for each step performed satisfactorily unless otherwise listed or weighted by instructor.

Directions with Performance Evaluation Checklist

Read the following statements, look up main terms in Volume 2—the Alphabetic Index of the diagnostic codebook, select a code and then confirm the code selection in Volume 1, the Tabular List. Use the Table of Drugs and Chemicals, found at the end of Volume 2 when selecting "X" codes.

1st Attempt	2nd Attempt	3rd Attempt		
_____	_____	_____	Gather materials (equipment and supplies) listed under *Conditions*.	
____/5	____/5	____/5	1. Code supervision of first normal pregnancy.	_____
____/5	____/5	____/5	2. Code personal history of blood disease.	_____
____/5	____/5	____/5	3. Code encounter for influenza vaccination.	_____
____/5	____/5	____/5	4. Code encounter for patient with positive HIV test result with no symptoms.	_____
____/5	____/5	____/5	5. Code rattlesnake bite reaction.	_____
____/5	____/5	____/5	6. Code accidental poisoning using tranquilizers.	_____
_____	_____	_____	Complete within specified time.	
____/32	____/32	____/32	**Total points earned** (To obtain a percentage score, divide the total points earned by the number of points possible.)	

Comments:

Evaluator's Signature: _____ **Need to Repeat:** _____

National Curriculum Competency: CAAHEP: Cognitive: IX.C.2 Psychomotor: IX.P.2	ABHES: 7.d

JOB SKILL 17-6
Code Diagnoses from Chart Notes Using *ICD-10-CM*

Name _____ Date _____ Score _____

Performance Objective

Task: Code diagnoses from chart notes using *ICD-10-CM*, Volumes 1 and 2.

Conditions: Need:

- *International Classification of Diseases, 10th Revision, Clinical Modification,* Volumes 1 and 2
- Pen or pencil

Refer to:

- *Textbook* Procedure 17-1, 17-2, and 17-3 for step-by-step directions

Standards: Complete all steps listed in this job skill in _____ minutes with a minimum score of _____. (Time element and accuracy criteria may be given by instructor.)

Time: Start: _____ Completed: _____ Total: _____ minutes

Scoring: One point for each step performed satisfactorily unless otherwise listed or weighted by instructor.

Directions with Performance Evaluation Checklist

Review the coding guidelines for specific areas of *ICD-10-CM*. Then, read the following chart notes, look up main terms in Volume 2—the Alphabetic Index of the diagnostic codebook, select a code and then confirm the code selection in Volume 1, the Tabular List.

1st Attempt	2nd Attempt	3rd Attempt		
_____	_____	_____	Gather materials (equipment and supplies) listed under *Conditions*.	
___/10	___/10	___/10	1. Susan Roth presents in the office today for a follow-up visit. She had a breast biopsy performed and the pathology report indicates she has a primary malignant neoplasm in the lower-inner quadrant of her right breast.	_____
___/10	___/10	___/10	2. Susan Roth's secondary complaint is that of acute pain in the area of the primary neoplasm.	_____
___/10	___/10	___/10	3. Houshang Deniston is seen today as a new patient. On his routine electrocardiogram (ECG) it was discovered that he has had a myocardial infarction sometime in the past. He currently has no symptoms.	_____
___/10	___/10	___/10	4. Bloyd Wade brings in his son, three-year-old Gavin who fell off a swing and hurt his right arm. An x-ray was performed and a fracture of the lower end of the humerus was diagnosed involving the lateral condyle.	_____
___/10	___/10	___/10	5. Arwin Johnsen burned her lips on a hot cup of cocoa. Dr. Practon examined her initially and determined that she had second degree burns, which were treated.	_____
_____	_____	_____	Complete within specified time.	
___/52	___/52	___/52	**Total points earned** (To obtain a percentage score, divide the total points earned by the number of points possible.)	

JOB SKILL 17-6 (continued)

Comments:

Evaluator's Signature: _____ **Need to Repeat:** _____

National Curriculum Competency: CAAHEP: Cognitive: IX.C.2 Psychomotor: IX.P.2	ABHES: 8.c.3

Health Insurance Systems and Claim Submission

STOP AND THINK CASE SCENARIOS

Refer to the end of Chapter 18 in the *textbook* for the following scenarios:

- Submission of a Late Medicare Claim
- Determine TRICARE Coverage and Benefits
- Determine the Responsible Party in an Injury Case

EXAM-STYLE REVIEW QUESTIONS

Refer to the end of Chapter 18 in the *textbook*.

Abbreviation and Spelling Review

Read the patient's chart note and write the meanings for the abbreviations following the note. To decode any abbreviations you do not understand or that appear unfamiliar to you, refer to the list of abbreviations in Appendix B of this *Workbook*. Step-by-step directions for this exercise are found in Procedure 1-1 of Chapter 1 in the *textbook*. Medical terms in the chart note are italicized; study them for spelling. Use your medical dictionary to look up their definitions. Your instructor may give a spelling and definition test that includes these words and abbreviations.

Brad Chieu

May 5, 20XX Pt came into the hosp c̄ a CC of *dyspnea* & pain in the RUQ. He was seen in the ED. Pt has had *diabetes* since childhood/hypertension for 3 years. Smoker. Increasing *malaise, nausea, anorexia* for past 5 days. *Polyuria, polydipsia*. The RN took his FH & vitals & recorded his TPR of 96.5°F & BP of 120/70 on the chart. After exam, the Dr. verified that the pt was suffering from COPD & scheduled him for an IPPB TX b.i.d. AP chest x-rays, a TB test and O2 therapy.

Gerald Practon, MD
Gerald Practon, MD

Pt	_____	BP	_____
hosp	_____	Dr.	_____
c̄	_____	COPD	_____
CC	_____	IPPB	_____
RUQ	_____	TX	_____
ED	_____	b.i.d.	_____
RN	_____	AP	_____
FH	_____	TB	_____
TPR	_____	O2	_____
F	_____		

Review Questions

Review the objectives, glossary, and chapter information before completing these review questions.

1. Match the terms in the left column with the definitions in the right column by writing letters in the blanks.

   _____ adjudicate

   _____ third-party payer

   _____ indemnity

   _____ deductible

   _____ carrier

   _____ adjuster

   _____ fiscal intermediary

   _____ elimination period

   _____ premium

   _____ partial disability

   a. employee of a workers' compensation insurance carrier with whom a case is assigned and who follows the case until it is settled

   b. contractor that processes payments to providers on behalf of state or federal agencies or insurance companies

   c. insurance carrier that intervenes to pay hospital or medical expenses on behalf of beneficiaries or recipients

   d. benefits paid in a predetermined amount in the event of a covered loss

   e. periodic payment made to keep an insurance policy in force

   f. organization that offers protection against losses in exchange for a premium

   g. determination for monetary settlement or payment

   h. period of time after the beginning of a disability for which no benefits are payable

   i. illness or injury preventing the insured from performing one or more functions of his or her occupation

   j. amount the insured must pay in a calendar or fiscal year before an insurance company will begin the payment of benefits

2. Name and give a brief definition of three types of commercial (private) health insurance plans.

   a. _____

   b. _____

   c. _____

3. The abbreviation for an insurance plan that has a high annual deductible is a/an:

    a. HSA

    b. HFSA

    c. HDHP

    d. UCR

    e. COB

4. The insured is also known as a/an _____, _____, _____, or _____.

5. An elimination period written in an insurance policy may also be known as a/an _____

    _____ or _____.

6. An attachment to a policy excluding certain illnesses or disabilities is called a/an _____

    _____

7. What is the source document used to verify insurance coverage? _____

8. When a child is covered by both parent's health insurance, what is the rule that most states honor to

    determine which plan is primary? _____

9. What are two important aspects to remember when treating managed care patients in the office?

    a. _____

    b. _____

10. True or False. Each state operates its own Medicaid program.

11. True or False. Medicaid coverage benefits are the same across all states.

12. There are several parts that indicate different types of coverage in the Medicare program (A, B, C, D).

    Which part is used to bill for services in a physician's office? _____

13. At what age is a person eligible for Medicare health insurance? _____

14. Circle the correct answer. Medicare Part D is (voluntary or involuntary) prescription drug coverage
    offered by (government or private) insurance carriers.

15. What is the name of the regulation that prohibits a physician or any member of a physician's family
    who has a financial relationship with an outside ancillary facility or service (e.g., laboratory, physical

    therapy office) from referring patients to that facility or service? _____

16. A patient who qualifies for both Medicare and Medicaid is often referred to as a _____
    patient.

17. Medigap insurance policies are offered by _____ and controlled by the

    _____.

18. True or False. Medicare secondary payer is the same as Medigap.

19. Name and define the three types of TRICARE coverage:

    a. _____

    b. _____

    c. _____

20. CHAMPVA is a military service benefit program for _____.

21. Define the following terms in relation to disability insurance.

    a. Temporary disability: _____

    _____

    b. Partial disability: _____

    _____

    c. Total disability: _____

    _____

22. After an initial workers' compensation report, insurance carriers want progress reports submitted on the injured worker each time the patient is seen, or every _____ to _____ days.

23. Name the four main stages of the life cycle of an insurance claim.

    a. _____

    b. _____

    c. _____

    d. _____

24. The paper insurance claim form that is accepted by most commercial (private) insurance companies, Medicare, Medicaid, and TRICARE is called the _____.

25. Indicate whether the following statements are true (T) or false (F).

    a. _____ Only an original CMS-1500 claim form may be optically scanned.

    b. _____ It is preferable to type data in lowercase for claims being optically scanned.

    c. _____ When entering data on a claim that is to be optically scanned, dates are keyed in using six digits.

    d. _____ Staples and paper clips may be used for attachments when sending insurance claims.

26. The standard unique health identifier that all health care providers use when submitting claims is called the _____.

27. A service that receives insurance claims, edits and sorts them, and then electronically transmits them to insurance companies is called a/an _____.

28. When Medicare is not likely to pay for a service or procedure because of medical necessity parameters, a/an _____ needs to be obtained by the provider and signed by the patient.

29. What is the time limit for submission of a Medicare claim? _____

    _____

30. A claim processed by Medicare and automatically processed by Medicaid is referred to as a/an _____ _____ claim.

31. The TRICARE fiscal year is from _____ to _____.

    _____

32. If payment is not received after inquires have been made, a/an _____ may need to be filed.

Critical Thinking Exercises

The following scenario is designed for students to role-play to gain experience interacting with insurance carriers and patients. Students should honor confidentiality, be courteous and demonstrate sensitivity, and display assertiveness and confidence while communicating with the provider and patient.

Divide students into groups of three—one can play a medical assistant, the second the insurance company employee, and the third can be the patient.

SCENARIO: An insurance claim for a biopsy has evidently been lost. You think that it has been billed but cannot find a copy of the claim. A statement has been sent to the patient for the full charge, $383.34, and she is now in the office wanting an explanation. Call the insurance carrier to see if they received it and determine the status of the claim. Advise the patient of your findings.

JOB SKILL 18-1
Complete a Managed Care Authorization Form

Name _____ Date _____ Score _____

Performance Objective

Task: Complete a managed care authorization form, coding the diagnosis and requested procedure.

Conditions: Need:

- Computer with Internet connection
- Online Form 81 (Managed Care Plan Treatment Authorization Request) located at www.cengagebrain.com with student resources
- *International Classification of Diseases, 10th Revision, Clinical Modification,* Volumes 1 and 2
- *Current Procedural Terminology* codebook
- Computer or typewriter

Refer to:

- *Textbook* Figure 2-3 in Chapter 2 for a visual example
- *Textbook* Appendix A, Medical Practice Reference Material

Standards: Complete all steps listed in this skill in _____ minutes with a minimum score of _____. (Time element and accuracy criteria may be given by instructor.)

Time: Start: _____ Completed: _____ Total: _____ minutes

Scoring: One point for each step performed satisfactorily unless otherwise listed or weighted by instructor.

Directions with Performance Evaluation Checklist

Read the following scenario and complete the Managed Care Authorization Form: On August 3, (current year), Antoyan Gagonian comes into Dr. Gerald Practon's office complaining of low back pain of 2 weeks' duration. He has difficulty walking, moving to a sitting position, and standing from a sitting position. Mr. Gagonian, born on October 10, 1963, lives at 2345 West Bath Street, Woodland Hills, XY 12345-0324; telephone number (555) 765-0720.

After taking a history and complete physical examination, Dr. Practon orders x-rays of the lower back and determines a working diagnosis of lumbago due to displacement of lumbar intervertebral disc. However, Mr. Gagonian's symptoms exceed typical criteria for this diagnosis. The patient is given a prescription for pain medication and muscle relaxant for muscle spasm. Dr. Practon recommends a magnetic resonance imaging (MRI) scan of the lumbar spine (without contrast) to investigate the problem further. The scan is to be done at College Hospital outpatient radiology.

Dr. Practon is the primary care physician for the managed care program, Health Net, of which Mr. Gagonian is a member. Dr. Practon's state license number is his member identification number with the insurance company. An authorization must be obtained for this study; the patient's insurance eligibility is verified today.

1st Attempt	2nd Attempt	3rd Attempt	
_____	_____	_____	Gather materials (equipment and supplies) listed under *Conditions.*
____/6	____/6	____/6	1. Complete the patient's demographic information on the authorization form.
____/5	____/5	____/5	2. Complete the information for the primary care physician, referring physician, and managed care plan.
____/8	____/8	____/8	3. Look up the code for the diagnosis, record it and list the description.
____/3	____/3	____/3	4. Indicate the treatment plan.

JOB SKILL 18-1 (*continued*)

___/8   ___/8   ___/8   5. Look up the code for the requested procedure, record it and list the description.

___/3   ___/3   ___/3   6. Indicate the facility information.

_____ _____ _____   7. Obtain the physician's signature.

___/4   ___/4   ___/4   8. Have Dr. Practon complete the primary care physician portion of the form.

_____ _____ _____   Complete within specified time.

___/40 ___/40 ___/40   **Total points earned** (To obtain a percentage score, divide the total points earned by the number of points possible.)

Comments:

Evaluator's Signature: _____   **Need to Repeat:** _____

National Curriculum Competency: CAAHEP: Psychomotor: VIII.P.21, 3	ABHES: 7.a, c

JOB SKILL 18-2
Complete a Health Insurance Claim Form for a Commercial Case

Name _____ Date _____ Score _____

Performance Objective

Task: Abstract information from a patient record and progress note to complete a health insurance claim form for a commercial case. Code diagnoses and procedures then determine fees and post the information to the patient's ledger card.

Conditions: Need:
- Computer with Internet connection
- Online Form 82 (health insurance claim form) located at www.cengagebrain.com with student resources
- *International Classification of Diseases, 10th Revision, Clinical Modification,* Volumes I and II
- *Current Procedural Terminology* codebook
- Pen or pencil

   Refer to:
- Workbook Figure 18-1, Cathy B. Maywood's patient record and progress notes
- *Workbook* Figure 18-2 (ledger card)
- *Workbook* Appendix A (physician information and fee schedule).
- *Textbook* Appendix A (CMS-1500 field instructions for commercial insurance)
- *Textbook* Appendix A (Figure A-1, visual example of template for commercial [private] insurance claim form)
- *Textbook* Procedure 18-2 for step-by-step instructions

Standards: Complete all steps listed in this skill in _____ minutes with a minimum score of _____. (Time element and accuracy criteria may be given by instructor.)

Time: **Start:** _____ **Completed:** _____ **Total:** _____ minutes

Scoring: One point for each step performed satisfactorily unless otherwise listed or weighted by instructor.

Directions with Performance Evaluation Checklist

1st Attempt	2nd Attempt	3rd Attempt	
_____	_____	_____	Gather materials (equipment and supplies) listed under *Conditions*.

CMS-1500 CLAIM FORM

Day 1

____/3	____/3	____/3	1. Address the claim form to the insurance carrier in the top right corner to indicate where the claim is being sent.
____/17	____/17	____/17	2. Obtain patient and insured information from the patient record, and complete the top portion of the claim form—Fields 1 through 11.
____/3	____/3	____/3	3. On the initial date of service, obtain the patient's signature on the claim form in Field 12 indicating the date and authorization to release medical information to the insurance carrier and in Field 13 to assign benefits to the physician.
_____	_____	_____	4. Answer the question in Field 20 and mark the correct box.
____/10	____/10	____/10	5. Look up the diagnostic codes and insert in Fields 21.A and 21.B.

JOB SKILL 18-2 (*continued*)

_____/2 _____/2 _____/2   6. Insert the eight-digit date for the first line of service in Field 24-1A and indicate the place of service code in Field 24-1B.

_____/7 _____/7 _____/7   7. Look up and insert the *CPT* code for the office consult in Field 24-1D and link the diagnostic code(s) with an indicator in Field 24-1E.

_____/4 _____/4 _____/4   8. Look up and insert the charge for the office consult in Field 24-1F and indicate the number of times it was done in Field 24-1G.

_____/2 _____/2 _____/2   9. Look up and insert the attending physician's National Provider Identifier (NPI) number in Field 24-1J.

_____/15 _____/15 _____/15   10. Look up and insert the *CPT* code for the handling of two specimens and complete the second line of service. Note: Multiply the charge by the number of times the service was done (2 units) and list the total in Field 24F. Indicate 2 units in Field 24G.

Day 2

_____/13 _____/13 _____/13   11. Look up and insert the *CPT* code and complete the third line of service for the procedure on June 9, 20XX.

Day 3

_____/13 _____/13 _____/13   12. Look up and insert the *CPT* code and complete the fourth line of service for the procedure on June 12, 20XX.

_____/18 _____/18 _____/18   13. Total the claim and complete Fields 25 through 33 on the claim form; date the claim June 30, current year.

LEDGER CARD

_____/4 _____/4 _____/4   14. List procedure codes in the Reference column on ledger card.

_____/4 _____/4 _____/4   15. List charges in the Charge column on ledger card.

_____/4 _____/4 _____/4   16. Calculate and record running balance for each charge posted.

_____/4 _____/4 _____/4   17. Indicate when the insurance company has been billed and bring down the balance.

_____ _____ _____   Complete within specified time.

_____/125 _____/125 _____/125   **Total points earned** (To obtain a percentage score, divide the total points earned by the number of points possible.)

Comments:

Evaluator's Signature: _____ **Need to Repeat:** _____

National Curriculum Competency: CAAHEP: Cognitive: II.C.1 Psychomotor: VII.P.1, VIII.P.4   ABHES: 7.d

JOB SKILL 18-2 (*continued*)

No. 1612

PATIENT RECORD

Maywood	Cathy	B.		11-24-62	F	(555) 592-1841
LAST NAME	**FIRST NAME**	**MIDDLE NAME**		**BIRTH DATE**	**SEX**	**HOME PHONE**
384 Gary Street		Woodland Hills		XY		12345
ADDRESS		**CITY**		**STATE**		**ZIP CODE**
(555) 206-7788				Cmaywood@EM.com		
CELL PHONE	**PAGER NO.**	**FAX NO.**		**E-MAIL ADDRESS**		
XXX-XX-2601				CP22498X		
PATIENT'S SOC. SEC. NO.				**DRIVER'S LICENSE**		
public relations secretary		St. Joseph's Hospital				
PATIENT'S OCCUPATION		**NAME OF COMPANY**				
4501 Main Street Woodland Hills, XY 1234						(555) 581-2600
ADDRESS OF EMPLOYER						**PHONE**
Robert M. Maywood			supervisor			
SPOUSE OR PARENT			**OCCUPATION**			
United Parcel			261 Jeffers Street, Woodland Hills, XY 12345			(555) 521-8011
EMPLOYER			**ADDRESS**			**PHONE**
Colonial Health Ins. Co. 11 Royal St. Woodland Hills, 12345				self		
NAME OF INSURANCE			**INSURED OR SUBSCRIBER**			
265012B			687SJ			
POLICY/CERTIFICATE NO.			**GROUP NO.**			

REFERRED BY: Bert B. Evans, MD, NPI 00065411XX

DATE	PROGRESS
6/2/20XX	New patient was referred for consultation (comprehensive history and examination with moderate medical decision making) with complaints of irregular vaginal bleeding after intercourse. Pelvic exam showed cervicitis and cervical erosion. Pap smear and cervical mucosa smear taken and sent to outside laboratory. Patient to return in one week for possible cauterization of cervix. llf *Fran Practon, MD*
6/9/20XX	Lab results indicate Class IIB PAP. Patient has cryocauterization of cervix performed. Recommend endometrial biopsy. Pt. scheduled for outpatient surgery at College Hospital on June 12, 20XX. llf *Fran Practon, MD*
6/12/20XX	Pt reports to outpatient surgery at College Hospital at 5:30 a.m. Endometrial biopsy performed. Diagnosis: Postcoital bleeding. llf *Fran Practon, MD*

FIGURE 18-1

JOB SKILL 18-2 (*continued*)

STATEMENT

PRACTON MEDICAL GROUP, INC.

4567 Broad Avenue

Woodland Hills, XY 12345-4700

Tel. 555-486-9002

Fax No. 555-488-7815

Cathy B. Maywood
384 Gary Street
Woodland Hills, XY 12345

Phone No.(H) 555-592-1841 (W) 555-581-2600 Birthdate 11-24-62

Insurance Co. *Colonial Health Ins. Co.* Policy No. 265012B / 687SJ

DATE	REFERENCE	DESCRIPTION	CHARGES	CREDITS		BALANCE
				Pymnts	Adj	
		BALANCE FORWARD				
6-2-XX		Consult NP				
6-2-XX		Handling of Specimens				
6-9-XX		Cauterization of Cervix				
6-12-XX		Endometrial Bx				

Pay last amount in balance column

FIGURE 18-2

JOB SKILL 18-3
Complete a Health Insurance Claim Form for a Medicare Case

Name _____ Date _____ Score _____

Performance Objective

Task: Abstract information from a patient record and progress note and complete a health insurance claim form for a Medicare case. Code diagnoses and procedures then determine fees and post the information to the patient's ledger card.

Conditions: Need:

- Computer with Internet connection
- Online Form 83 (health insurance claim form) located at www.cengagebrain.com with student resources
- *International Classification of Diseases, 10th Revision, Clinical Modification,* Volumes I and II
- *Current Procedural Terminology* codebook

Refer to:

- *Workbook* Figure 18-3, Michael T. Donlevy's patient record and progress notes
- *Workbook* Figure 18-4 (ledger card)
- *Workbook* Appendix A (physician information and fee schedule)
- *Textbook* Appendix A (CMS-1500 field instructions for the Medicare program)
- *Textbook* Figure 18-15, visual example of template for a Medicare claim
- *Textbook* Procedure 18-2 for step-by-step instructions

Standards: Complete all steps listed in this skill in _____ minutes with a minimum score of _____. (Time element and accuracy criteria may be given by instructor.)

Time: Start: _____ Completed: _____ Total: _____ minutes

Scoring: One point for each step performed satisfactorily unless otherwise listed or weighted by instructor.

Directions with Performance Evaluation Checklist

Dr. Gerald Practon is a participating physician with the Medicare program, so he accepts assignment; bill using the participating physician fees. After completing the claim form and ledger card, refer to the Mock Fee Schedule in Appendix A of this *Workbook* and answer the fee-related questions.

1st Attempt	2nd Attempt	3rd Attempt	
_____	_____	_____	Gather materials (equipment and supplies) listed under *Conditions*.

CMS-1500 CLAIM FORM

____/3	____/3	____/3	1. Address the claim form to the Medicare Administrative Contractor in the top right corner to indicate where the claim is being sent.
____/14	____/14	____/14	2. Obtain patient and insured information from the patient record and complete the top portion of the claim form.
____/2	____/2	____/2	3. On the initial date of service, obtain the patient's signature on the claim form indicating authorization to release medical information to the insurance carrier and assignment of benefits to the physician.
____/2	____/2	____/2	4. Fill in Field 14 and answer the question in Field 20; mark the correct box.
____/5	____/5	____/5	5. Look up the diagnostic code and insert it in Field 21.A.
____/13	____/13	____/13	6. Look up the *CPT* code for the emergency room visit and complete the first line of service for June 3, 20XX.

JOB SKILL 18-3 (*continued*)

___/13   ___/13   ___/13   7. Look up the *CPT* code for the laceration repair and complete the second line of service for June 3, 20XX.

___/2   ___/2   ___/2   8. Link the diagnostic code to the procedure codes in Field 24E with the correct indicator.

_____   _____   _____   9. Determine whether or not you would bill for the follow-up office visit on 6/7/XX, and state the logic for your answer. _____
_____

___/16   ___/16   ___/16   10. Total the claim and complete Fields 25 through 33 on the claim form.

_____   _____   _____   11. Date the claim June 30, current year.

LEDGER CARD

___/2   ___/2   ___/2   12. List procedure codes in the Reference column on the ledger card.

___/2   ___/2   ___/2   13. List charges in the Charge column on the ledger card.

___/2   ___/2   ___/2   14. Calculate and record running balance for each charge posted.

___/4   ___/4   ___/4   15. Indicate when the insurance company has been billed and bring down the balance.

FEE SCHEDULE

___/6   ___/6   ___/6   16. If Dr. Practon is *participating* in the Medicare program, how much will he receive for the emergency room visit?

From Medicare: $ _____

From the patient: $ _____

___/3   ___/3   ___/3   17. If Dr. Practon is *not participating* in the Medicare program, how much will he receive for the emergency room visit from Medicare? $ _____

___/12   ___/12   ___/12   18. If Dr. Practon is *not participating* in the Medicare program and charges the maximum *limiting charge*, how much will he receive for the emergency room visit?

From Medicare: $ _____

From the patient: $ _____

_____   _____   _____   Complete within specified time.

___/105   ___/105   ___/105   **Total points earned** (To obtain a percentage score, divide the total points earned by the number of points possible.)

Comments:

Evaluator's Signature: _____   **Need to Repeat:** _____

National Curriculum Competency: CAAHEP: Cognitive: VII.C.1; Psychomotor: VII.P.1, VIII.P.4   ABHES: 7.d

JOB SKILL 18-3 (*continued*)

PATIENT RECORD

No. 1613

Donlevy	Michael	T.	3/10/37	M	(555) 421-0015
LAST NAME	**FIRST NAME**	**MIDDLE NAME**	**BIRTH DATE**	**SEX**	**HOME PHONE**
282 Georgia Street		Woodland Hills	XY		12345
ADDRESS		**CITY**	**STATE**		**ZIP CODE**

CELL PHONE	**PAGER NO.**	**FAX NO.**	**E-MAIL ADDRESS**	
XXX-XX-9003			D033123X	
PATIENT'S SOC. SEC. NO.			**DRIVER'S LICENSE**	
Retired truck driver				
PATIENT'S OCCUPATION		**NAME OF COMPANY**		
ADDRESS OF EMPLOYER				**PHONE**
Patricia M. Donlevy			retired	
SPOUSE OR PARENT		**OCCUPATION**		
EMPLOYER		**ADDRESS**		**PHONE**
Medicare Administrator Contractor PO Box 123, Anytown, XY 12345			self	
NAME OF INSURANCE		**INSURED OR SUBSCRIBER**		
XXX-XX-9003A				
POLICY/CERTIFICATE NO.		**GROUP NO.**		

REFERRED BY: Harry Donlevy (brother)

DATE	PROGRESS
6/3/20XX	Called to ER at the request of patient who fell at home and cut his head (EPF HX & PX, LC MDM). Sutured a 3.5 cm scalp wound (intermediate repair laceration). RTO in 4 days for dressing change.
	llf *Gerald Practon, MD*
6/7/20XX	Dressing changed. Wound healing well, no signs of infection. Pt RTO next week for suture removal.
	llf *M. Athims, CMA(AAMA)*

FIGURE 18-3

JOB SKILL 18-3 *(continued)*

STATEMENT
PRACTON MEDICAL GROUP, INC.
4567 Broad Avenue
Woodland Hills, XY 12345-4700
Tel. 555-486-9002
Fax No. 555-488-7815

Michael T. Donlevy
282 Georgia Street
Woodland Hills, XY 12345

Phone No.(H) 555-421-0015 (W)_____ Birthdate 3/10/17

Insurance Co. Medicare_____ Policy No. xxx-xx-9003A

DATE	REFERENCE	DESCRIPTION	CHARGES	CREDITS Pymnts	Adj	BALANCE
		BALANCE FORWARD				
6-3-XX		ER Visit				
6-3-XX		Laceration repair				

Pay last amount in balance column

FIGURE 18-4

JOB SKILL 18-4
Complete a Health Insurance Claim Form for a TRICARE Case

Name _____ Date _____ Score _____

Performance Objective

Task: Abstract information from a patient record and progress note and complete a health insurance claim form for a TRICARE case. Code diagnoses and procedures then determine fees and post the information to the patient's ledger card.

Conditions: Need:

- Computer with Internet connection
- Online Form 84 (health insurance claim form) located at www.cengagebrain.com with student resources
- *International Classification of Diseases, 10th Revision, Clinical Modification,* Volumes I and II
- *Current Procedural Terminology* codebook

Refer to:

- *Workbook* Figure 18-5, Frances O. Davidson's patient record and progress notes.
- *Workbook* Figure 18-6 (ledger card)
- *Workbook* Appendix A (physician information and fee schedule)
- *Textbook* Appendix A (CMS-1500 field instructions for the TRICARE program)
- *Textbook* Figure 18-18, visual example of a completed TRICARE claim form

Standards: Complete all steps listed in this skill in _____ minutes with a minimum score of _____.
(Time element and accuracy criteria may be given by instructor.)

Time: Start: _____ Completed: _____ Total: _____ minutes

Scoring: One point for each step performed satisfactorily unless otherwise listed or weighted by instructor.

Directions with Performance Evaluation Checklist

Dr. Gerald Practon is a participating physician with the TRICARE program, so he accepts assignment; bill using the mock fees.

1st Attempt	2nd Attempt	3rd Attempt	
_____	_____	_____	Gather materials (equipment and supplies) listed under *Conditions*.

CMS-1500 CLAIM FORM

____/3	____/3	____/3	1. Address the claim form to TRICARE in the top right corner to indicate where the claim is being sent.
____/24	____/24	____/24	2. Obtain patient and insured information from the patient record, and complete the top portion of the claim form.
____/2	____/2	____/2	3. On the initial date of service, obtain the patient's signature on the claim form indicating authorization to release medical information to the insurance carrier and assignment of benefits to the physician.
____/2	____/2	____/2	4. Fill in Field 14 and answer the question in Field 20; mark the correct box.
____/5	____/5	____/5	5. Look up the diagnostic code and insert it in Field 21.A.
____/13	____/13	____/13	6. Look up the *CPT* code and complete the first line of service for the office visit for June 4, 20XX.

JOB SKILL 18-4 (*continued*)

___/13 ___/13 ___/13   7. Look up the *CPT* code and complete the second line of service for the electrocardiogram for June 4, 20XX.

___/13 ___/13 ___/13   8. Look up the *CPT* code and complete the third line of service for the spirometry for June 4, 20XX.

___/13 ___/13 ___/13   9. Look up the *CPT* code and complete the fourth line of service for the blood draw on June 4, 20XX.

___/13 ___/13 ___/13 10. Look up the *CPT* code and complete the fifth line of service for the specimen handling fee for June 4, 20XX.

___/13 ___/13 ___/13 11. Look up the *CPT* code and complete the sixth line of service for the urinalysis for June 4, 20XX.

_____ _____ _____ 12. Link the diagnostic code indicator to each line of service on the claim form.

___/16 ___/16 ___/16 13. Total the claim and complete Fields 25 through 33 on the claim form; date the claim June 30, current year.

LEDGER CARD

___/6 ___/6 ___/6 14. List procedure codes in the Reference column on the ledger card.

___/6 ___/6 ___/6 15. List charges in the Charge column on the ledger card.

___/6 ___/6 ___/6 16. Calculate and record running balance for each charge posted.

___/4 ___/4 ___/4 17. Indicate when the insurance company has been billed and bring down the balance.

_____ _____ _____ Complete within specified time.

___/155 ___/155 ___/155 **Total points earned** (To obtain a percentage score, divide the total points earned by the number of points possible.)

Comments:

Evaluator's Signature: _____ **Need to Repeat:** _____

National Curriculum Competency: CAAHEP: Cognitive: VII.C.1; Psychomotor: VII.P.1, VIII.P.4   ABHES: 7.d

JOB SKILL 18-4 *(continued)*

No. 1614

PATIENT RECORD

Davidson	Frances	O.	4/10/60	F	(555) 217-8105
LAST NAME	**FIRST NAME**	**MIDDLE NAME**	**BIRTH DATE**	**SEX**	**HOME PHONE**
128 Watson Street		Woodland Hills	XY		12345
ADDRESS		**CITY**	**STATE**		**ZIP CODE**
(555) 324-0088		(555) 217-8105	Fdavidson@EM.com		
CELL PHONE	**PAGER NO.**	**FAX NO.**	**E-MAIL ADDRESS**		
XXX-XX-1651			D034963X		
PATIENT'S SOC. SEC. NO.			**DRIVER'S LICENSE**		
tailor		Sampson Department Store			
PATIENT'S OCCUPATION		**NAME OF COMPANY**			
7841 Broadway St. Woodland Hills, XY 12345				(555) 289-7811	
ADDRESS OF EMPLOYER				**PHONE**	
Lieutenant William C. Davidson		U.S. Navy Lieutenant/Active Status NY		DOB 11/4/61	
SPOUSE OR PARENT		**OCCUPATION**			
USN		PO Box 1878, APO New York, NY 09194			
EMPLOYER		**ADDRESS**		**PHONE**	
TRICARE Standard, PO Box 444, Anytown, XY 12345			husband/sponsor		
NAME OF INSURANCE			**INSURED OR SUBSCRIBER**		
Social Security No. XXX-XX-2601		DOD No. 4445566777			
POLICY/CERTIFICATE NO.		**GROUP NO.**			

REFERRED BY: Martha B. Emory (friend)

DATE	PROGRESS
6/4/20XX	New patient comes in with CC of chest pain (moderate to severe), difficulty breathing, weakness, fatigue, & dizziness (Level 4 E/M). Performed ECG; normal sinus rhythm. Performed spirometry total and timed capacity; reduced lung capacity. Took blood specimen and sent to outside lab for CBC and basic metabolic panel. UA (non-automated with microscopy neg.) Edema throughout lower extremities. Dx: congestive heart failure. Start patient on diuretic; may need hospitalization. RTO tomorrow. llf *Gerald Practon, MD*

FIGURE 18-5

JOB SKILL 18-4 *(continued)*

STATEMENT

PRACTON MEDICAL GROUP, INC.
4567 Broad Avenue
Woodland Hills, XY 12345-4700
Tel. 555 -486-9002
Fax No. 555 -488-7815

Frances O. Davidson
128 Watson Street
Woodland Hills, XY 12345

Phone No.(H) 555-217-8105 (W) 555-289-7811 Birthdate 4/10/50
Insurance Co. TRICARE Standard Policy No. xxx-xx-2601

DATE	REFERENCE	DESCRIPTION	CHARGES	CREDITS		BALANCE
				Pymnts	**Adj**	
		BALANCE FORWARD				
6-4-XX		OV NP				
6-4-XX		ECG				
6-4-XX		Spirometry				
6-4-XX		Venipuncture				
6-4-XX		Handling Spec				
6-4-XX		UA				

Pay last amount in balance column

FIGURE 18-6

C H A P T E R **19**

Office Managerial Responsibilities

STOP AND THINK CASE SCENARIOS

Refer to the end of Chapter 19 in the *textbook* for the following scenarios:
- Determine the Agenda for a Staff Meeting
- Calculate Prices for an Order Form

EXAM-STYLE REVIEW QUESTIONS

Refer to the end of Chapter 19 in the *textbook*.

Abbreviation and Spelling Review

Read the patient's chart note and write the meanings for the abbreviations following the note. To decode any abbreviations you do not understand or that appear unfamiliar to you, refer to the list of abbreviations in Appendix B of this *Workbook*. Step-by-step directions for this exercise are found in Procedure 1-1 of Chapter 1 in the *textbook*. Medical terms in the chart note are italicized; study them for spelling. Use your medical dictionary to look up their definitions. Your instructor may give a spelling and definition test that includes these words and abbreviations.

DATE	PROGRESS
12-14-20XX	Helen P. Craig CC: Back pain originating in the *flank* + radiating across the *abdomen*. Pt complains of *abdominal distention* & difficulty *urinating*. Exam reveals increased *sensitivity* in lumbar & *groin* areas. Considerable discomfort c̄ marked *urethral stenosis*. U/A: 5-10 RBC, occ wbc, sp gr 1.012; X: KUB & IVP revealed small *calculus* in R UPJ dilat to 24F c̄ Brev. Inc fluid intake, low *calcium* diet. RX *Aluminum hydroxide* gel 60 ml q.i.d. RTC 1 wk for FU + decision on whether to operate.
	G Practon, MD G Practon, MD

CC	_____	UPJ	_____
Pt	_____	dilat	_____
c̄	_____	F	_____
U/A	_____	Brev	_____
RBC	_____	inc	_____
occ	_____	RX	_____
wbc	_____	ml	_____
sp gr	_____	q.i.d.	_____
X	_____	RTC	_____
KUB	_____	Wk	_____
IVP	_____	FU	_____
R	_____		

Review Questions

Review the objectives, glossary, and chapter information before completing the following review questions.

1. Why is it important for the office manager to be a mentor and coach? _____

_____

2. What two mechanisms can be put into place in a medical office to help patient relations, promote

patient satisfaction, and learn what policies and procedures need improvement? _____

_____

3. To boost job performance, what three things should be emphasized during a staff meeting?

a. _____

b. _____

c. _____

4. As a new employee, where would you look to find your job description? _____

_____

5. What is the purpose of an office policies and procedures manual? _____

_____

6. List one federal agency that administers statutes and regulations that employers must adhere to, and name a resource it publishes that can be used to determine which statutes apply to your office.

_____

_____

7. What is the name of the act that covers most benefit plans in the private sector? _____

_____

_____

8. What laws prohibit job discrimination based on race, color, religion, sex, or national origin? _____

_____

9. How would you know if the Family and Medical Leave Act applies to your job in a medical office?

_____

_____

10. As an office manager, what two questions will you be expected to answer if a case of sexual harassment goes to court? _____

_____

_____

11. When hiring a new employee, what are the four responsibilities of an office manager? What would you do first, second, third, and fourth? _____

_____

12. After an employee has been hired and before he or she is expected to perform all tasks, what are the two responsibilities of the office manager? _____

13. What observations should be included when an office manager evaluates a new employee? _____

_____

_____

14. Before selecting a housecleaning service, what must be done? _____

_____

15. When selecting a new piece of equipment for the medical office, what are some things to consider?

   a. _____

   b. _____

   c. _____

   d. _____

   e. _____

   f. _____

   g. _____

16. What are the three important points to consider when selecting a vendor from which to order office or medical supplies?

   a. _____

   b. _____

   c. _____

17. State four reasons why it may be unsatisfactory to order supplies in bulk.

   a. _____

   b. _____

   c. _____

   d. _____

18. When an order for merchandise arrives, what steps should be taken after the package is opened? _____

_____

_____

19. Name three items that must appear on a running-inventory card.

    a. _____

    b. _____

    c. _____

20. If the physician is planning to attend a medical convention, at what point should the office manager

    start making the arrangements? _____

    _____

Critical Thinking Exercises

1. As an office manager, what strategy would you use to correct an employee who is a gossip and spreads

    a harmful rumor about another employee? _____

    _____

    _____

    _____

    _____

    _____

2. List some methods that an office manager might implement to promote open and honest
    communication.

    _____

    _____

    _____

    _____

    _____

    _____

3. As an office manager, describe how you would make a new employee feel more relaxed during his or

    her first week at work. _____

    _____

    _____

    _____

    _____

    _____

4. During team meetings and staff meetings, a team member always comes in late. Often, the attention is turned to this person and derogatory remarks are said by other employees—like, "Glad you could join us," "Nice of you to show up," or "The meeting started 10 minutes ago." State how you would you

handle this situation. _____

_____

_____

_____

_____

_____

5. When interacting with an employee, or when witnessing an employee interacting with other employees, you notice that the employee always has something negative to say. This saps the listener's energy and can be very wearing; it can affect the entire office environment. How would you handle

this situation? _____

_____

_____

_____

_____

_____

_____

JOB SKILL 19-1
Document Patient Complaints and Determine
Actions to Resolve Problems

Name _____ Date _____ Score _____

Performance Objective

Task: Document two patient complaints, and then determine the action to take to resolve each problem.

Conditions: Need:

- Computer with Internet connection
- Online Forms 85 and 86 (Patient Complaint Documents) located at www.cengagebrain.com with student resources
- Pen or pencil

Refer to:

- Scenario A and Scenario B listed within exercise
- *Textbook* Figure 19-1 for a visual example
- *Textbook* Procedure 19-1 for step-by-step directions

Standards: Complete all steps listed in this job skill in _____ minutes with a minimum score of _____. (Time element and accuracy criteria may be given by instructor.)

Time: **Start:** _____ **Completed**: _____ **Total:** _____ minutes

Scoring: One point for each step performed satisfactorily unless otherwise listed or weighted by instructor.

Directions with Performance Evaluation Checklist

Scenario A: You are working as the receptionist and patient Margaret Williams walks in and is very upset. She requested and received a copy of her medical records last week and while reading them discovered several errors. She wants to cancel her appointment later today and is thinking of changing doctors. Mrs. Williams' account number is 987-23A and her account balance is $132.28.

1st Attempt	2nd Attempt	3rd Attempt	
_____	_____	_____	Gather materials (equipment and supplies) listed under *Conditions*.
_____	_____	_____	1. Use Online Form 85 and fill in the current date.
_____	_____	_____	2. Record the patient's account number.
_____	_____	_____	3. Record the patient's name.
_____	_____	_____	4. List the account balance.
____/5	____/5	____/5	5. Document the patient's complaint, using quotation marks when writing her exact words; demonstrate empathy and use active listening skills.
____/10	____/10	____/10	6. Determine what action you would take and document the plan.

Scenario B. It is 4:00 p.m. and patient Susan Robles (account 689-41A, balance $250.00) calls and starts complaining to you about how she is never able to get through to Dr. Practon when she needs him. She says, "The telephone lines are always busy, busy, busy!" You ask how many times she has called, and she indicates her telephone has been on automatic dialing on and off for 2 hours.

_____	_____	_____	7. Use Online Form 86 and fill in the current date.
_____	_____	_____	8. Record the patient's account number.

JOB SKILL 19-1 (*continued*)

_____	_____	_____	9.	Record the patient's name.
_____	_____	_____	10.	List the account balance.
___/5	___/5	___/5	11.	Document the patient's complaint, using quotation marks when writing her exact words; demonstrate empathy and use active listening skills.
___/10	___/10	___/10	12.	Determine what action you would take and document the plan.
_____	_____	_____		Complete within specified time.
___/40	___/40	___/40		**Total points earned** (To obtain a percentage score, divide the total points earned by the number of points possible.)

Comments:

Evaluator's Signature: _____   **Need to Repeat:** _____

National Curriculum Competency: ABHES: 7.a

JOB SKILL 19-2
Write an Agenda for an Office Meeting

Name _____ Date _____ Score _____

Performance Objective

Task: Assemble information and key or type an outline for an office meeting agenda.

Conditions: Need:

• One sheet of white paper

• Computer with printer

Refer to:

• *Textbook* Figure 19-4 (example of an agenda outlining items covered in the previous staff meeting)

• *Workbook* Figure 19-1 (agenda suggestions posted on a bulletin board)

• *Textbook* Procedure 19-3 for step-by-step directions

Standards: Complete all steps listed in this skill in _____ minutes with a minimum score of _____.
(Time element and accuracy criteria may be given by instructor.)

Time: **Start:** _____ **Completed:** _____ **Total:** _____ minutes

Scoring: One point for each step performed satisfactorily unless otherwise listed or weighted by instructor.

Directions with Performance Evaluation Checklist

Refer to *textbook* Figure 19-4 to learn what occurred at the previous meeting and to determine unfinished business. Study the notes in *Workbook* Figure 19-1, gathered from members of the staff, indicating actions they wish to introduce at the meeting and when the meeting is scheduled. List all subject matter for the agenda in rough draft outline form.

1st Attempt	2nd Attempt	3rd Attempt	
_____	_____	_____	Gather materials (equipment and supplies) listed under *Conditions*.
____/2	____/2	____/2	1. Key a heading for the staff meeting agenda.
____/3	____/3	____/3	2. Indicate when the meeting will take place.
_____	_____	_____	3. Indicate that the office manager, Jane Paulsen, will act as the chairperson and will call the meeting to order.
_____	_____	_____	4. Indicate that the minutes from the previous meeting will be read.
_____	_____	_____	5. Indicate who is present at the meeting (i.e., staff members).
____/5	____/5	____/5	6. Under Committee Reports, indicate that staff members Amy Fluor (transcription) and Mike O'Shea (bookkeeping) will be reporting as committee chairpersons.
____/5	____/5	____/5	7. Indicate that Jane Paulsen and Dr. Fran Practon will be reporting unfinished business.
____/5	____/5	____/5	8. Indicate that Dr. Gerald Practon and Carla Haskins will be reporting new business.
_____	_____	_____	9. Note that the next meeting is scheduled at 8:30 a.m. on March 20, 20XX.
_____	_____	_____	10. Indicate that the meeting is adjourned.

JOB SKILL 19-2 (*continued*)

_____ _____ _____ Complete within specified time.

____/27 ____/27 ____/27 **Total points earned** (To obtain a percentage score, divide the total points earned by the number of points possible.)

Mon.

I want to discuss possibility of moving transcription station to Rm. A, which is away from reception room interruptions.

Amy Fluor

---

from the desk of Gerald Practon...

I will present summer vacation schedule for sign-ups.

G.P.

Staff meeting scheduled for 2/25/XX in conference room at 12 noon. Lunch will be provided. Please make plans to attend.

Jane Paulsen-OM

I PLAN TO INTRODUCE GARY KLEIN, FROM MEDICAL ARTS PRESS, WHO WILL PRESENT THE ADVANTAGES OF ALPH/COLOR FILING SYSTEM. (I THINK HIS REPORT SHOULD BE SCHEDULED LAST ON THE AGENDA.)

CARLA HASKINS

F.P. and G.P.

At our last meeting I was asked to investigate cleaning services. I'm going to recommend we hire Todd's Cleaning to begin on March 15, and I'll make a motion to this effect.

Also, someone needs to notify Martha's Maids soon that we are terminating their services. Would you like me to do this?

Jane Paulsen-OM

I am going to suggest hiring an accting firm to audit the books yearly on Jan. 1.

Mike O'Shea
bookkeeper

From the desk of Fran Practon...

I will suggest that since flex-time is to be initiated in May, a committee should be named to spell out scheduling, compensation, and benefits for the staff and incorporate it into the office procedures manual; also there should be a discussion of circumstances under which an alternative work schedule will be used.

FIGURE 19-1

Comments:

Evaluator's Signature: _____ **Need to Repeat:** _____

National Curriculum Competency: ABHES: 7.g

JOB SKILL 19-3
Prepare Material for an Office Procedures Manual

Name _____ Date _____ Score _____

Performance Objective

Task: Assemble information on office appointments for Practon Medical Group, Inc., and key or type a sample reference sheet for an office procedures manual.

Conditions: Need:

- One or two sheets of white paper
- Computer with printer

Refer to:

- *Workbook* Appendix A (*Appointment* section of *Office Policies*)
- Chapter 7 (general appointment guidelines)
- *Textbook* Figure 19-6 (example of appointment reference sheet)
- *Textbook* Procedure 19-6 for step-by-step directions

Standards: Complete all steps listed in this skill in _____ minutes with a minimum score of _____. (Time element and accuracy criteria may be given by instructor.)

Time: **Start:** _____ **Completed:** _____ **Total:** _____ minutes

Scoring: One point for each step performed satisfactorily unless otherwise listed or weighted by instructor.

Directions with Performance Evaluation Checklist

Doctors Gerald and Fran Practon have asked you to prepare a reference sheet for the office procedures manual detailing appointment procedures. Create a page listing information regarding appointments that is easy for all employees to follow.

1st Attempt	2nd Attempt	3rd Attempt	
_____	_____	_____	Gather materials (equipment and supplies) listed under *Conditions*.
_____	_____	_____	1. Key a heading for the reference sheet.
_____	_____	_____	2. Key a heading for "Appointment Office Hours."
____/5	____/5	____/5	3. List appointment days and times as well as office policy for routine appointments.
____/5	____/5	____/5	4. List appointment days and times as well as office policy for emergency appointments, work-ins, callbacks, and dictation.
____/5	____/5	____/5	5. List hospital surgery days and times for doctors Gerald and Fran Practon.
____/2	____/2	____/2	6. List the appropriate times for house calls.
____/7	____/7	____/7	7. Create a heading for time allotment for office visits and procedures and state office scheduling policy.
_____	_____	_____	8. List the time allotment for initial office visits.
_____	_____	_____	9. List the time allotment for consultations.
_____	_____	_____	10. List the time allotment for follow-up office visits.
____/6	____/6	____/6	11. List the time allotment for brief office visits for such things as suture removal; name various procedures that fit into this category.

JOB SKILL 19-3 (*continued*)

_____ _____ _____ 12. List the time allotment for office procedures.

_____ _____ _____ 13. List the office policy for house calls.

_____ _____ _____ 14. Create a heading for questions to be asked when an appointment is made over the telephone.

___/5 ___/5 ___/5 15. List five basic questions to ask when an appointment is made over the telephone.

a. _____

b. _____

c. _____

d. _____

e. _____

_____ _____ _____ Complete within specified time.

___/45 ___/45 ___/45 **Total points earned** (To obtain a percentage score, divide the total points earned by the number of points possible.)

Comments:

Evaluator's Signature: _____ **Need to Repeat:** _____

National Curriculum Competency: ABHES: 7.a

JOB SKILL 19-4
Perform Inventory Control and Keep an Equipment Maintenance Log

Name _____ Date _____ Score _____

Performance Objective

Task: List office equipment on an inventory control sheet and track the maintenance of each piece of equipment.

Conditions: Need:

- Computer with Internet connection
- Online Form 87 (Inventory Control Sheet/Maintenance Log) located at www.cengagebrain .com with student resources
- Pen or pencil

Refer to:

- List of office equipment with manufacturer, model number, length of warranty, date of purchase, and purchase price—listed within exercise

Standards: Complete all steps listed in this job skill in _____ minutes with a minimum score of _____. (Time element and accuracy criteria may be given by instructor.)

Time: Start: _____ Completed: _____ Total: _____ minutes

Scoring: One point for each step performed satisfactorily unless otherwise listed or weighted by instructor.

Directions with Performance Evaluation Checklist

Scenario: You have just been promoted to office manager and Dr. Practon has asked you to look in your file cabinet and locate the warranties for each piece of office equipment. He presents you with an inventory control sheet with a maintenance log and asks you to record the file information so that you can make sure the equipment undergoes routine maintenance; it has been neglected in the past. You have located files for the equipment; their contents are listed in steps 2 through 7. Read the information about each piece of equipment, then abstract and record the pertinent data.

1st Attempt	2nd Attempt	3rd Attempt	
_____	_____	_____	Gather materials (equipment and supplies) listed under *Conditions*.
_____	_____	_____	1. Using the Inventory Control Sheet/Maintenance Log (Online Form 87), record information for the equipment listed in the following steps; list each in alphabetical order by name (e.g., fax machine), recording data in each section of the form.
____/7	____/7	____/7	2. Macintosh iMac computer (3.2 GHz) with a 27-inch screen, bought October 3, 2011, for $1699. There is a warranty for 3 years, and it went through a routine service on October 12, 2012. You cannot find the serial number so you look it up on the computer (W88000XZX00) and record it on the warranty.
____/6	____/6	____/6	3. There is a file for the office stereo with two speakers. It has a CD player with FM/AM radio. The brand is "Denon," Model M37. It has a 2-year warranty and was purchased December 2, 2014, for $369.
____/12	____/12	____/12	4. You locate a file under "Philips" that includes a couple of items. A Desktop Dictaphone Cassette Transcriber/Recorder machine and a Dictaphone SpeechMike III. They were both purchased on June 20, 2008, and each has a 5-year warranty; it does not look like either has been serviced. The machine (model 3742) cost $440.98 and the handheld "mike" (model LFH3215) cost $70.

JOB SKILL 19-4 (*continued*)

___/13 ___/13 ___/13 5. There is a big file for the Sharp copy machine but that is not the one in the office; it is a Xerox machine. After sifting through all the papers you locate the sales receipt—it was purchased on February 11, 2008, and cost $4299. You have to look at the machine to find the model number (5225); it is called a "Xerox WorkCentre." You locate paperwork that says it has a 3-year warranty, so it has run out. There is a service book that lists service calls on the following dates: 2/15/09, 3/1/10, 3/12/11, 3/14/12, 2/25/13, 3/3/14, and 1/15/15.

___/6 ___/6 ___/6 6. The Panasonic fax machine (model UF-4000) was purchased on February 12, 2015, for $517. It has a 1-year warranty.

___/7 ___/7 ___/7 7. You cannot find a record for the Hewlett Packard LaserJet printer, model P2035, so you look in the check register and find that it was purchased on September 14, 2010, for $1476. You call Hewlett Packard and give them the serial number and find out it has a 3-year warranty. Dr. Practon says it was serviced around the middle of March 2012.

_____ _____ _____ 8. You cannot find any more paperwork for the other equipment in the office, so you will have to go to each piece of equipment and record the pertinent data.

_____ _____ _____ Complete within specified time.

___/55 ___/55 ___/55 **Total points earned** (To obtain a percentage score, divide the total points earned by the number of points possible.)

Comments:

Evaluator's Signature: _____ **Need to Repeat:** _____

National Curriculum Competency: CAAHEP: Cognitive: II.C.12, 2 IV.C.9, 10 Psychomotor: VI.P.8, 9   ABHES: 7. f

JOB SKILL 19-5
Abstract Data from a Catalog and Key an Order Form

Name _____ Date _____ Score _____

Performance Objective

Task: Abstract information from catalog data sheets, determine charges, accurately key or type an order form, calculate discounts and sales tax, and compute a total.

Conditions: Need:

* Computer with Internet connection
* Online Form 88 (order form) located at www.cengagebrain.com with student resources
* Calculator
* Pen or pencil

Refer to:

* *Workbook* Figure 19-2 and Figure 19-3 (catalogue sheets)
* *Workbook* Appendix A (Medical Practice Reference Material)
* *Textbook* Figure 19-8 (illustration of order form)
* *Textbook* Example 19-5 (calculating sales tax example)
* *Textbook* Procedure 19-10 for step-by-step directions

Standards: Complete all steps listed in this skill in _____ minutes with a minimum score of _____. (Time element and accuracy criteria may be given by instructor.)

Time: Start: _____ Completed: _____ Total: _____ minutes

Scoring: One point for each step performed satisfactorily unless otherwise listed or weighted by instructor.

Directions with Performance Evaluation Checklist

Doctors Fran and Gerald Practon want to order some printed letterhead, second sheets, and envelopes from Medical Arts Press. Study and abstract the correct information from the catalog sheets, noting the discount offered for second sheets. Then, complete the order form using the name, address, and so forth of Practon Medical Group, Inc. Determine the cost for each item, calculate discounts, and insert this information on the order form.

1st Attempt	2nd Attempt	3rd Attempt	
_____	_____	_____	Gather materials (equipment and supplies) listed under *Conditions*.
____/6	____/6	____/6	1. Complete the "Bill to" information on the order form.
_____	_____	_____	2. Fill in the email address for Practon Medical Group, Inc. (PMGI@aol.com).
_____	_____	_____	3. Indicate "SAME" in the "Ship to" location on the order form.
____/2	____/2	____/2	4. Fill in the customer order number (0001002345) and the source code (BTGF) from the catalog.
____/2	____/2	____/2	5. List your name as the person to call for questions and the office telephone number; you are at extension 12.
_____	_____	_____	6. List the practice specialty and number of doctors.
_____	_____	_____	7. Indicate the method of shipping as UPS 2nd Day.
____/7	____/7	____/7	8. List the first item ordered: 2000 raised-printed 25% rag content bond paper (8½" by 11"; black ink, type style NR, product color ivory, order number PNB-530.

JOB SKILL 19-5 (*continued*)

___/5 ___/5 ___/5 9. List the second item ordered: 1000 Hammermill bond unprinted second sheets (8½" by 11"), color ivory. See pricing under "Hammermill Bond Stock-Raised Printed" and apply the discount.

___/7 ___/7 ___/7 10. List the third item ordered: 1000 raised-printed 25% rag content bond envelopes (number 10); black ink, type style NR, color ivory.

_____ _____ _____ 11. Total the merchandise order and insert figure.

_____ _____ _____ 12. Calculate 7% sales tax and insert figure.

_____ _____ _____ 13. Add the sales tax to the total of the order and insert figure.

_____ _____ _____ Complete within specified time.

___/38 ___/38 ___/38 **Total points earned** (To obtain a percentage score, divide the total points earned by the number of points possible.)

Comments:

Evaluator's Signature: _____   **Need to Repeat:** _____

National Curriculum Competency: CAAHEP: Cognitive: II.C.1, 2   ABHES: 7. f

JOB SKILL 19-5 *(continued)*

letterheads

555 896 1114

RAYMOND S. STRONG, M.D.
SUITE 315 PROFESSIONAL BUILDING

1616 SHERIDAN WAY   LAKESIDE CITY XY 12345-0000

Distinctive. Dignified. Four popular sizes in your choice of paper stocks with flat or raised printing. Select either Hammermill Bond, an extremely popular paper noted for its bright white, smooth surface or 25% Rag Content Bond with its cockle surface and crisp finish. We take an intense pride in these papers and the craftsmanship of the printing. All copy in black ink.

Raymond S. Strong, M.D.
1616 Sheridan Way
Suite 315, Professional Building
Lakeside City, XY 12345-0000
(555) 896-1114

SECOND SHEETS
Unprinted. Available at 60% of the Hammermill Bond price. Choice of onlonskin or Hammermill.

Raymond S Strong MD
1616 Sheridan Way
Suite 315 Professional Building
Lakeside City XY 12345-0000
555-896-1114

555/896-1114   Suite 315 Professional Bldg

Raymond S. Strong
1616 Sheridan Way
Lakeside City XY 12345-0000

5½ 8½ inches   **6¼ 9¼ inches**   **7¼ 10½ inches**   **8½ 11 inches**

HAMMERMILL BOND STOCK

		5½×8½	6¼×9¼	7¼×10½	8½×11
	Quantity	HB-407	HB-690	HB-403	HB-401
FLAT-PRINTED	500	$9.85	$12.25	$13.55	$15.95
	1000	13.95	18.35	20.70	23.10
	2000	24.95	30.65	34.95	39.60
	5000	58.15	70.60	80.10	83.65
		5½×8½	6¼×9¼	7¼×10½	8½×11
	Quantity	PE-144	PE-695	PE-146	PE-140
RAISED-PRINTED	500	$11.70	$14.50	$16.00	$17.65
	1000	16.45	20.45	22.75	25.25
	2000	28.35	35.40	40.65	45.15
	5000	56.30	75.15	86.90	99.65

25% RAG CONTENT BOND

		5½×8½	6¼×9¼	7¼×10½	8½×11
	Quantity	NB-675	NB-69	NB-70	NB-81
	500	$11.35	$13.55	$16.40	$18.65
	1000	16.25	22.00	24.55	26.80
	2000	27.25	37.55	42.10	48.60
	5000	59.55	82.15	93.25	113.50
		5½×8½	6¼×9¼	7¼×10½	8½×11
	Quantity	PNB-560	PNB-695	PNB-540	PNB-530
	500	$13.15	$16.00	$17.60	$21.50
	1000	18.70	22.15	26.15	29.65
	2000	32.80	40.75	45.50	51.15
	5000	71.90	92.50	104.65	114.40

FIGURE 19-2

JOB SKILL 19-5 *(continued)*

envelopes

RAYMOND S. STRONG, M.D.

SUITE 315 PROFESSIONAL BUILDING
1616 SHERIDAN WAY
LAKESIDE CITY XY 12345-0000

SIZE 10 ENVELOPES: 4½×9½ inches. For 8½×11-inch letterheads.

SIZE 7½ ENVELOPES: 3½×7½ inches. For 7¼×10½-inch letterheads.

Raymond S. Strong, M.D.

1616 Sheridan Way Suite 315
Lakeside City, XY 12345-0000

Raymond S Strong MD

1616 Sheridan Way Ste 315
Lakeside City XY 12345-0000

SIZE 6¼ ENVELOPES: 3½×6½ inches.
For 6¼×9¼-inch letterheads.

Unless specified, we print your copy in the upper left-hand corner on the front of the envelope. Flat-printed envelopes can be imprinted on the back flap as shown.

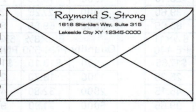

Raymond S. Strong
1616 Sheridan Way, Suite 315
Lakeside City XY 12345-0000

Envelopes are produced on the same fine stocks as our letterheads. Hammermill Bond is a bright white, smooth-surfaced paper. 25% Rag Content Bond is a crisp paper with a cockle finish —a most distinctive stationery. Both available in either flat or raised printing with your copy in 3 or 4 lines in the upper left-hand corner or on their back flap (flat-printed only). All printing in black ink.

HAMMERMILL BOND FLAT-PRINTED

Quantity	Size 6¾ L-500	Size 7½ L-510	Size 10 L-502
500	$13.50	$17.25	$18.50
1000	24.25	28.80	34.55
2000	45.15	50.15	59.30
5000	98.25	110.85	132.75

HAMMERMILL BOND RAISED-PRINTED

Quantity	Size 6¾ PE-220	Size 7½ PE-192	Size 10 PE-190
500	$16.00	$20.50	$21.25
1000	26.30	28.90	34.75
2000	45.40	53.35	59.60
5000	99.00	124.25	133.45

25% RAG CONTENT BOND FLAT-PRINTED

Quantity	Size 6¾ NB-800	Size 7½ NB-600	Size 10 NB-700
500	$18.90	$24.55	$25.20
1000	33.40	34.95	44.60
2000	57.80	67.75	76.95
5000	126.50	149.95	171.90

25% RAG CONTENT BOND RAISED-PRINTED

Quantity	Size 6¾ PNB-520	Size 7½ PNB-510	Size 10 PNB-500
500	$21.60	$27.25	$27.90
1000	33.40	39.55	44.70
2000	58.15	70.95	77.20
5000	127.15	152.55	172.60

FIGURE 19-3

JOB SKILL 19-6
Complete an Order Form for Office Supplies

Name _____ Date _____ Score _____

Performance Objective

Task: Complete an order form for office supplies, filling in designated spaces and computing total amount ordered.

Conditions: Need:
- Computer with Internet connection
- Online Form 90 (order form) located at www.cengagebrain.com with student resources
- Calculator
- Pen or pencil

Refer to:
- *Workbook* Appendix A (Medical Practice Reference Material)
- *Textbook* Procedure 19-10 for step-by-step directions

Standards: Complete all steps listed in this skill in _____ minutes with a minimum score of _____.
(Time element and accuracy criteria may be given by instructor.)

Time: **Start:** _____ **Completed:** _____ **Total:** _____ minutes

Scoring: One point for each step performed satisfactorily unless otherwise listed or weighted by instructor.

Directions with Performance Evaluation Checklist

Doctors Fran and Gerald Practon have asked you to order some office supplies. Abstract information within the exercise, and then neatly and accurately complete the order form.

1st Attempt	2nd Attempt	3rd Attempt	
_____	_____	_____	Gather materials (equipment and supplies) listed under *Conditions*.
_____	_____	_____	1. Fill in the customer number (667-32-7118-4006).
____/5	____/5	____/5	2. Complete the customer contact information.
____/7	____/7	____/7	3. Order four 1000 single-sheet cartons of CMS-1500 laser-printed insurance claim forms (8½" by 11"), $29.95/carton, Cat. No. RED-25104, page 53.
____/7	____/7	____/7	4. Order four boxes of end-tab file folders with two fasteners (blue, letter size), ¾" expansions, $40.90/box, Cat No. GLW-FF113, page 32.
____/7	____/7	____/7	5. Order six daily group practice wire-bound appointment books with 15-minute appointments, four columns per page, appointments from 8 a.m. to 7:45 p.m. (11" by 7⅞"), $29.15 each (price break: for each five ordered, one is free), Cat. No. GLW-AB402, page 65.
____/7	____/7	____/7	6. Order five packages of large envelopes (9" by 12") with clasp, 28-lb heavyweight Kraft, 25/pkg., $3.75 pkg., Cat No. 42SH-11, page 61.
____/7	____/7	____/7	7. Order two packages of double-prong clasp envelopes (9" by 12"), reinforced eyelet, gummed flaps, $4.25/pkg., Cat. No. 387-ACJ, page 62.
____/7	____/7	____/7	8. Order two dozen packages of post-it flags, Style No. 680-1 (1" by 1.7"), one dozen red, one dozen yellow, $1.49 pkg., Cat. No. 49WEX-52, page 50.
_____	_____	_____	9. Total order and insert figure.

JOB SKILL 19-6 *(continued)*

_____ _____ _____			10. Calculate and insert sales tax at 6%.

_____ _____ _____ 11. Determine the two-day shipping and handling fee, which is 5% of the total order. This is waived for orders over $400, and a flat fee of $15.00 is charged.

_____ _____ _____ 12. Add the sales tax and shipping and handling fee to determine the total amount for the order; insert this figure on the order form.

____/4 ____/4 ____/4 13. You will be paying for the order with the company credit card, which is a Visa card, number 2222-3333-4444-0000, expiration date August 2017. You have signature authority on the card; complete this section.

_____ _____ _____ Complete within specified time.

____/58 ____/58 ____/58 **Total points earned** (To obtain a percentage score, divide the total points earned by the number of points possible.)

Comments:

Evaluator's Signature: _____ **Need to Repeat:** _____

National Curriculum Competency: CAAHEP: Cognitive: II.C.1, 2   ABHES: 7.f

JOB SKILL 19-7
Perform Mathematic Calculations of an Office Manager

Name _____ Date _____ Score _____

Performance Objective

Task: Perform basic mathematic calculations when ordering supplies to determine the cost, taking advantage of special discounts, and applying sales tax.

Conditions: Need:
- Calculator
- Paper
- Pencil

Standards: Complete all steps listed in this skill in _____ minutes with a minimum score of _____.
(Time element and accuracy criteria may be given by instructor.)

Time: Start: _____ Completed: _____ Total: _____ minutes

Scoring: One point for each step performed satisfactorily unless otherwise listed or weighted by instructor.

Directions with Performance Evaluation Checklist

The office manager may be responsible for ordering supplies, and he or she should be able to perform basic mathematics to calculate discounts and sales tax amounts. Wise purchasing and correct math procedures can save the office added expense. Solve the following problems, assuming that you pay all bills within the discount period stated. Discounts are subtracted before sales tax is added.

1st Attempt	2nd Attempt	3rd Attempt	
_____	_____	_____	Gather materials (equipment and supplies) listed under *Conditions*.
___/2	___/2	___/2	1. The laundry bill is $33.80. If paid within 10 days, the company allows a 2.5% discount. Calculate the amount of the bill. $ _____
___/5	___/5	___/5	2. Mr. Carl McFadden had five office visits at $25 each, three injections at $8.50 each, an x-ray at $26.60, and a home visit at $40.00. He has a $4.60 credit on his account. What will be the amount of his next bill? $ _____
___/2	___/2	___/2	3. Mr. Bill Nelson is scheduled to have a corrective surgery, which will be $385. He is asked to make a down payment of $50 before the operation, and then his payments will be divided into six equal installments. What will be the amount of each installment? $ _____
___/10	___/10	___/10	4. The following items are on an invoice that arrived today. You are required to check to see that the bill is correct and that the supplies received are the ones ordered. The physician will receive a 3% discount, and sales tax is 6%. The total shown on the invoice is $26.14. Calculate and verify that the amount is correct. $ _____

4 bottles rubbing alcohol @ $2.25 each

3 thermometers @ $1.95 each

6 boxes cotton @ $.29 each

6 bottles mouthwash @ $.89 each

JOB SKILL 19-7 (*continued*)

11 cartons cotton swabs @ $.39 each

3 hypodermic needles @ $.39 each

List the correct amount for which the check
would be written. $ _____

_____/5 _____/5 _____/5 5. Paper towels are sold at the rate of $6.50 per dozen rolls.
Figure the cost of 10 dozen rolls of towels with a 3.5%
discount and a 6% sales tax. $ _____

_____/6 _____/6 _____/6 6. Dr. Fran Practon needs 500 needles priced
at $2.60 per hundred. If she pays within 10 days,
she receives a 2% discount; sales tax is 5.5%.
What amount would you pay with the discount? $ _____

_____/6 _____/6 _____/6 7. An advertisement states that eight thermometers
cost $12.42 minus a 3% discount. Dr. Practon wants
to order a dozen to take advantage of the savings;
sales tax is 5%. What would the cost be? $ _____

_____/3 _____/3 _____/3 8. Robert Mason's account of $98.50 has been delinquent
for 3 months. According to the office procedures manual,
after 90 days a 2% service charge, compounded monthly,
is added to future bills. What will be the amount owed
after 9 months? $ _____

_____/2 _____/2 _____/2 9. Steri-Strips cost $4.95 per box; there are 100 in a box. $ _____

a. How much would 300 Steri-Strips cost? $ _____

b. How much would 700 Steri-Strips cost? $ _____

_____/12 _____/12 _____/12 10. If the Steri-Strips are purchased in large lots of 1000
or more, the manufacturer allows a discount of 15%.

a. How much would 3000 Steri-Strips cost? $ _____

b. How much would 14,000 Steri-Strips cost? $ _____

c. If an orthopedic surgical group uses 200 Steri-Strips
a month, how much would be saved in a year by
making a single purchase for a year's supply rather
than 12 monthly purchases? $ _____

_____ _____ _____ Complete within specified time.

_____/55 _____/55 _____/55 **Total points earned** (To obtain a percentage score, divide the total points
earned by the number of points possible.)

Comments:

Evaluator's Signature: _____ **Need to Repeat:** _____

National Curriculum Competency: CAAHEP: Cognitive: II.C.1, 2

JOB SKILL 19-8
Prepare Two Order Forms

Name _____ Date _____ Score _____

Performance Objective

Task: Key or type two order forms for medical supplies using the given information, and determine the total amount owed after taking advantage of all discounts.

Conditions: Need:

- Computer with Internet connection
- Online Forms 90 and 91 (order forms) located at www.cengagebrain.com with student resources
- Calculator
- Pen or pencil

Refer to:

- *Workbook* Appendix A (Medical Practice Reference Material)
- *Textbook* Figure 19-8 for a visual example
- *Textbook* Procedure 19-10 for step-by-step directions

Standards: Complete all steps listed in this skill in _____ minutes with a minimum score of _____. (Time element and accuracy criteria may be given by instructor.)

Time: **Start:** _____ **Completed:** _____ **Total:** _____ minutes

Scoring: One point for each step performed satisfactorily unless otherwise listed or weighted by instructor.

Directions with Performance Evaluation Checklist

Use the following information to order office and medical supplies. Determine the total for all merchandise, subtract the physician's discount, and then add the sales tax. The supplies are to be shipped to Practon Medical Group, Inc. Note: *Photocopies would be made before sending off the order; all prices are fictitious.*

1st Attempt	2nd Attempt	3rd Attempt	
_____	_____	_____	Gather materials (equipment and supplies) listed under *Conditions*.
___/10	___/10	___/10	1. Complete the "Bill to" information on both order forms.
___/2	___/2	___/2	2. Fill in the email address for Practon Medical Group, Inc. (PMGI@aol.com), on both forms.
___/2	___/2	___/2	3. Indicate "SAME" in the "Ship to" location on both order forms.
___/4	___/4	___/4	4. Fill in the customer order number (0001002345) and the source code (BTGF) from the catalog.
___/4	___/4	___/4	5. List your name as the person to call for questions and the office telephone number; you are at extension 12.
___/2	___/2	___/2	6. List the practice specialty and number of doctors.
___/2	___/2	___/2	7. Indicate the method of shipping as UPS 2nd Day.

ORDER NO. 1

___/6	___/6	___/6	8. Order four reams of white 8½" by 11" bond paper, 20# weight, catalog number P20, unit price $12.95.
___/5	___/5	___/5	9. Order five boxes security-lined envelopes, 500/box, No. 6¾, catalog number E60, unit price 19.99.

JOB SKILL 19-8 (*continued*)

____/5 ____/5 ____/5   10. Order 1500 large No. 10 envelopes, catalog number E10, unit price $5.50M*.

____/5 ____/5 ____/5   11. Order six boxes red fine-line ballpoint pens, catalog number B23, unit price $3.95.

_____ _____ _____   12. Subtotal the merchandise order and insert figure on line 5 of the order form (e.g., Subtotal 123.45).

_____ _____ _____   13. Calculate 2% discount and insert figure. Write this figure on line 6 of the order form (e.g., Less 2% discount 1.23)

_____ _____ _____   14. Subtract discount from subtotal.

_____ _____ _____   15. Insert total on order form.

_____ _____ _____   16. Calculate 5.5% sales tax and insert figure.

_____ _____ _____   17. Add the sales tax and insert total for order.

ORDER NO. 2

____/4 ____/4 ____/4   18. Order three surgeon's blade handles (Model No. B872C), catalog number BH3, unit price $2.95.

____/4 ____/4 ____/4   19. Order two dozen scalpel blades (No. F112), 12 to a box, catalog number SB2, unit price $1.39.

____/4 ____/4 ____/4   20. Order four Oval Duplex thermometers, rectal, catalog number T66, unit price $2.95.

____/4 ____/4 ____/4   21. Order 3M* tongue blades, catalog number RB2, unit price $2.50M*.

____/8 ____/8 ____/8   22. Order 5000 laser (8.5" by 11"), OCR-scannable red ink insurance claim forms (single sheets) for Dr. Fran Practon. Catalog number CMS29, unit prices: $43.99/1,000; $77.99/2,000; $144.99/5,000; $239.99/10,000; $389.99/20,000.

_____ _____ _____   23. Subtotal the merchandise order and insert this figure on line 6 of the order form (e.g., Subtotal 123.45).

_____ _____ _____   24. Calculate a 3% discount and subtract it from the subtotal. Write this figure on line 7 of the order form (e.g., Less 3% discount 1.23).

_____ _____ _____   25. List the merchandise total.

_____ _____ _____   26. Calculate 4% sales tax and insert figure.

_____ _____ _____   27. Add the sales tax to the total of the order and insert figure.

_____ _____ _____   Complete within specified time.

____/84 ____/84 ____/84   **Total points earned** (To obtain a percentage score, divide the total points earned by the number of points possible.)

Comments:

*M is the Roman numeral that means 1000.

Evaluator's Signature: _____   **Need to Repeat:** _____

National Curriculum Competency: CAAHEP: Cognitive: II.C.1, 2   ABHES: 7.f

JOB SKILL 19-9
Prepare a Travel Expense Report

Name _____ Date _____ Score _____

Performance Objective

Task: Complete a travel expense report for the accountant.

Conditions: Need:

- Computer with Internet connection
- Online Form 92 (Travel Expense Report) located at www.cengagebrain.com with student resources
- Calculator
- Pen or pencil

Refer to:

- *Textbook* Figure 19-14 for a visual example
- *Textbook* Procedure 19-13 for step-by-step directions

Standards: Complete all steps listed in this skill in _____ minutes with a minimum score of _____. (Time element and accuracy criteria may be given by instructor.)

Time: Start: _____ Completed: _____ Total: _____ minutes

Scoring: One point for each step performed satisfactorily unless otherwise listed or weighted by instructor.

Directions with Performance Evaluation Checklist

Dr. Gerald Practon presented a research paper at a medical convention in Boston, Massachusetts. He kept a detailed record of all expenses for the week of May 9 (Sat.) through May 16 (Sat.). Set up a travel expense report, transferring the figures that follow by placing them in the proper columns. Calculate totals.

1st Attempt	2nd Attempt	3rd Attempt	
_____	_____	_____	Gather materials (equipment and supplies) listed under *Conditions*.
____/2	____/2	____/2	1. Enter beginning and ending dates of trip.
____/8	____/8	____/8	2. Record dates for column headings that will be used on the travel report.
_____	_____	_____	3. Record parking fees for Monday: $5.20.
_____	_____	_____	4. Record parkway toll fees for Monday: $4.00.
____/5	____/5	____/5	5. Record tips for the week: $2 on Saturday, $3 on Sunday, $6 on Wednesday, $5.50 on Friday, and $6.25 on Saturday.
____/7	____/7	____/7	6. Record the discounted Hertz car rental, which was $25 per day for seven days.
____/2	____/2	____/2	7. Record gasoline expenses, which were $30.90 on Monday and $44.20 on Saturday.
____/7	____/7	____/7	8. Record the hotel expenses: Conroy Hotel was $150 per night for the first four nights, Commonwealth Hotel was $135 per night for the next two nights, and Shoreham Hotel was $165 per night for the last night.
_____	_____	_____	9. Record one telephone call ($1.91) on Sunday, May 10, which was made to confirm the time for the speaking engagement.

JOB SKILL 19-9 (*continued*)

___/16   ___/16   ___/16   10. Record all meal expenses.

Day	Breakfast	Lunch	Dinner
Sunday	$8.90	$15.40	$36.20
Monday	5.10	—	26.14
Tuesday	3.40	10.90	31.50
Wednesday	—	13.98	48.14
Thursday	9.15	10.00	20.02
Friday	10.82	22.08	36.33

___/7   ___/7   ___/7   11. Calculate and record total for Lodging.

___/5   ___/5   ___/5   12. Calculate and record total for Breakfasts.

___/5   ___/5   ___/5   13. Calculate and record total for Lunches.

___/6   ___/6   ___/6   14. Calculate and record total for Dinners.

___   ___   ___   15. Calculate and record total for Local Fares.

___/7   ___/7   ___/7   16. Calculate and record total for Auto Expenses.

___   ___   ___   17. Calculate and record total for Parking Fees.

___   ___   ___   18. Calculate and record total for Phone and Email.

___   ___   ___   19. Calculate and record total for Entertainment.

___/5   ___/5   ___/5   20. Calculate and record total for Tips.

___   ___   ___   21. Calculate and record total for Toll Charges.

___/2   ___/2   ___/2   22. Calculate and record total for Other/Miscellaneous.

___/3   ___/3   ___/3   23. Calculate and record total for May 9.

___/7   ___/7   ___/7   24. Calculate and record total for May 10.

___/7   ___/7   ___/7   25. Calculate and record total for May 11.

___/5   ___/5   ___/5   26. Calculate and record total for May 12.

___/5   ___/5   ___/5   27. Calculate and record total for May 13.

___/5   ___/5   ___/5   28. Calculate and record total for May 14.

___/6   ___/6   ___/6   29. Calculate and record total for May 15.

___/2   ___/2   ___/2   30. Calculate and record total for May 16.

___/10   ___/10   ___/10   31. Add and record all totals in the right column.

___/8   ___/8   ___/8   32. Add and record all totals listed for each day and verify against the figure obtained in step 31; they should be the same. If not, recalculate and compare again.

___/2   ___/2   ___/2   33. Write a brief description for the purpose of the trip and enter on report.

___   ___   ___   Complete within specified time.

___/154   ___/154   ___/154   **Total points earned** (To obtain a percentage score, divide the total points earned by the number of points possible.)

JOB SKILL 19-9 (*continued*)

Comments:

Financial Management of the Medical Practice

STOP AND THINK CASE SCENARIOS

Refer to the end of Chapter 20 in the *textbook* for the following scenarios:

- Prepare an Analysis to Determine the Effectiveness of Capitated Plans

- Determine Payroll Category and Frequency for Deductions

EXAM-STYLE REVIEW QUESTIONS

Refer to the end of Chapter 20 in the *textbook*.

Abbreviation and Spelling Review

Read the patients' chart notes and write the meanings for the abbreviations following each note. To decode any abbreviations you do not understand or that appear unfamiliar to you, refer to the list of abbreviations in Appendix B of this *Workbook*. Step-by-step directions for this exercise are found in Procedure 1-1 of Chapter 1 in the *textbook*. Medical terms in the chart note are italicized; study them for spelling. Use your medical dictionary to look up their definitions. Your instructor may give a spelling and definition test that includes these words and abbreviations.

Bernice Saxon

April 10, 20XX Pt had closed reduction of *telescoping* nasal *ethmoidal fracture* with sutures and application of an *external nasal* splint. When pt ret'nd from surg, she was given 100 mg of *Demerol* q. 3h. IM. Her vital signs were taken q.i.d. for the first 2 days & then b.i.d. p̄ that. Sleeping medication was given h.s. She will be seen in the office in 4 days for follow-up.

Gerald Practon, MD
Gerald Practon, MD

---

pt	_____	IM	_____
ret'nd	_____	q.i.d.	_____
surg	_____	b.i.d.	_____
mg	_____	p̄	_____
q. 3h.	_____	h.s.	_____

Lucy Corsentino

July 7, 20XX Pt, a 3-year-old, has had temp 100.1° for 2 days. Exam reveals strep throat. DX: Acute *streptococcal pharyngitis*. Plan: *Penicillin* V *potassium* 250 mg/tsp to be taken in a dose of 1 tsp q.i.d. × 10 days, *Tylenol* up to 1 gm q. 4h. for pain & fever. Mother advised not to give ASA.

Fran Practon, MD
Fran Practon, MD

---

pt	_____	1 gm	_____
DX	_____	q. 4h.	_____
mg/tsp	_____	ASA	_____
q.i.d. × 10 days	_____		

Review Questions

Review the objectives, glossary, and chapter information before completing the following review questions.

1. List several ways a computerized financial management system benefits a medical practice.

    a. _____

    b. _____

    c. _____

    d. _____

    e. _____

2. What projection does the office manager look at to determine how much actual cash should be available each month? _____

    _____

3. Income received and expenses paid are presented in a report called a _____

    _____

4. What system contains computerized database files that include demographic and billing information used in the preparation of patient statements, insurance forms, and management reports including the breakdown of the accounts receivable? _____

    _____

5. Explain an insurance aging report and list ways it can be broken down for analysis. _____

   _____

   _____

   _____

   _____

6. What are some of the things that are looked at and learned when an office manager analyzes a medical practice's productivity?

   a. _____

   b. _____

   c. _____

7. To track the accounts payable, expenditures are recorded in a _____.

8. Name some responsibilities of the office manager or medical assistant when he or she is in complete charge of the payroll.

   a. _____

   b. _____

   c. _____

   d. _____

9. What law covers minimum wage and overtime standards? _____

10. The office manager must post notices in the medical office according to the _____.

11. Explain how to obtain a tax identification number for a physician-employer.

    _____

    _____

12. What form is used for employers to verify that all employees hired (citizens and noncitizens) are

    authorized to work? _____

13. Why do you have an employee complete an Employee's Withholding Allowance Certificate, Form W-4?

    _____

14. Under the Federal Insurance Contributions Act (FICA), both the _____ and

    _____ contribute at a rate specified by law.

15. Name three programs financed under Social Security (FICA) from one payroll tax, and list what they provide.

    a. Program 1: _____

       Provides: _____

    b. Program 2: _____

       Provides: _____

    c. Program 3: _____

       Provides: _____

16. List three names used for state disability insurance deductions.

    a. _____

    b. _____

    c. _____

17. List several optional payroll deductions, also called _____.

    a. _____

    b. _____

    c. _____

    d. _____

    e. _____

18. How often must employers report payments by using Form 940?

    _____

19. In what publication does the Department of the Treasury, Internal Revenue Service, publish submission guidelines and requirements for quarterly reports, federal tax deposits, and unemployment tax payments?

    _____

20. The employer's quarterly federal tax return must be filed by an employer on or before _____, _____, _____, and _____ on Form _____.

21. Spell out the following payroll abbreviations.

    FICA _____

    FUTA _____

    UCD _____

22. Agnes Baker terminated her employment with Dr. Jeffries on August 31. What document must be given to her by the employer and what is the time limit?

    _____

    _____

✘ Critical Thinking Exercises

1. Why is it a federal requirement that the Wage and Tax Statement (W-2) tax form be sent by the employer to both the IRS and to each employee? _____

    _____

2. State the deductions from a payroll check required in your state.

    a. _____

    b. _____

    c. _____

    d. _____

    e. _____

3. In the following list, check the correct definitions. Use logic to determine those not mentioned in the *textbook*.

Biyearly _____ a. twice a year   Semiannually _____ a. every six months

_____ b. once a year   _____ b. every two years

_____ c. every two years   _____ c. once a year

Biweekly _____ a. twice a week   Semimonthly _____ a. every half month

_____ b. every two weeks   _____ b. twice a month

_____ c. semiweekly   _____ c. every other month

Quarterly _____ a. twice a year   Weekly _____ a. every day

_____ b. every four weeks   _____ b. once a week

_____ c. four times a year   _____ c. every week

4. Looking ahead to when you are employed as an administrative medical assistant, list what kind of fringe benefits you would prefer and why.

_____

_____

JOB SKILL 20-1
Perform Accounts Payable Functions:
Write Checks and Record Disbursements

Name _____ Date _____ Score _____

Performance Objective

Task: Write checks for disbursement, enter transactions on the check register, and post deposits.

Conditions: Need:

• Computer with Internet connection

• Online Forms 93, 94, and 95 (check register) located at www.cengagebrain.com with student resources

• Online Forms 96 through 99 (four sheets with 12 checks)

• Calculator

• Pencil

Refer to:

• *Textbook* Procedure 20-1 for step-by-step directions

Note: *Job Skills 20-1, 20-2, 20-3, and 20-4 will use the same information and check register.*

Standards: Complete all steps listed in this skill in _____ minutes with a minimum score of _____. (Time element and accuracy criteria may be given by instructor.)

Time: Start: _____ Completed: _____ Total: _____ minutes

Scoring: One point for each step performed satisfactorily unless otherwise listed or weighted by instructor.

Directions with Performance Evaluation Checklist

Read the entire job skill before beginning. You may complete the online forms (93, 94, and 95) electronically or print them and enlarge them onto legal size paper to make it easier to handwrite entries. Another option would be to complete the job skill on the computer using an Excel spreadsheet.

Check Stub: List date and record deposit(s), and then add to the balance forward; list the check amount and a brief description subtracting the amount to determine the checkbook balance; *always carry the balance forward to the next check.*

Check Entries: Write out the amount of the check and enter the numerical figure in the "Check Amount." Record the company name and address to which the check is written; use the date indicated.

Check Register:

PAGE 1: Fill in the company name that the check was written to in the "Paid to" column and indicate the date written in the "Date" column. Write the amount of the check in the "Gross Amount" column and in the "Amount of Check" column. Indicate the check number.

PAGE 2: Bank Account Balance and Bank Deposits: Enter the starting balance of the checking account in the "Bank Balance" column. Enter all money deposited in the "Bank Deposit" column.

PAGES 2 and 3: Study the column headings to familiarize yourself with the various categories. Then, post each check amount on the appropriate line in the correct disbursement column of the check register.

1st Attempt	2nd Attempt	3rd Attempt	
_____	_____	_____	Gather materials (equipment and supplies) listed under *Conditions*.
_____/5	_____/5	_____/5	1. Prepare pages 1, 2, and 3 of the check register (Online Forms 93, 94, and 95) for checks drawn on "The First National Bank" for the month of June 20XX.

JOB SKILL 20-1 (*continued*)

____/2   ____/2   ____/2   2. Record the beginning checkbook balance of $9745.45 on the first check stub (No. 479) and on page 2 of the check register bank deposit slip.

____/2   ____/2   ____/2   3. Record a deposit of $130 on June 1, 20XX, on the first check stub (No. 479) and on the bank deposit slip.

____/8   ____/8   ____/8   4. Make out check No. 479 on June 1, 20XX, for rent to Security Pacific Company, 2091 Mission Street, Woodland Hills, XY 12345, in the amount of $1900.00, and make the appropriate calculations on the check stub.

____/6   ____/6   ____/6   5. Record check No. 479 on the check register.

____/2   ____/2   ____/2   6. Record a deposit of $95 on June 3, 20XX, on check stub No. 480 and on the bank deposit slip.

____/8   ____/8   ____/8   7. Make out check No. 480 on June 3, 20XX, for medical supplies to Central Laboratories, 351 Robin Avenue, Woodland Hills, XY 12345, in the amount of $74.50, and make the appropriate calculations on the check stub.

____/6   ____/6   ____/6   8. Record check No. 480 on the check register.

____/8   ____/8   ____/8   9. Make out check No. 481 on June 3, 20XX, for parking fees to Broadway Garage, 4560 Broad Avenue, Woodland Hills, XY 12345, in the amount of $300.00, and make the appropriate calculations on the check stub.

____/6   ____/6   ____/6   10. Record check No. 481 on the check register.

____/2   ____/2   ____/2   11. Record a deposit of $195 on June 4, 20XX, on check stub No. 482 and on the bank deposit slip.

____/8   ____/8   ____/8   12. Make out check No. 482 on June 4, 20XX, for diesel fuel to Union Oil Company, PO Box 232, Woodland Hills, XY 12345, in the amount of $87.75, and make the appropriate calculations on the check stub.

____/6   ____/6   ____/6   13. Record check No. 482 on the check register.

____/2   ____/2   ____/2   14. Record a deposit of $80 on June 15, 20XX, on check stub No. 483 and on the bank deposit slip.

____/8   ____/8   ____/8   15. Make out check No. 483 on June 15, 20XX, for quarterly city tax to Woodland Hills Tax Commission, 2200 James Street, Woodland Hills, XY 12345, in the amount of $162.00, and make the appropriate calculations on the check stub.

____/6   ____/6   ____/6   16. Record check No. 483 on the check register.

____/8   ____/8   ____/8   17. Make out check No. 484 on June 15, 20XX, for medications to Eli Lilly and Company, Lilly Corporate Center, Indianapolis, IN 46285, in the amount of $226.00, and make the appropriate calculations on the check stub.

____/6   ____/6   ____/6   18. Record check No. 484 on the check register.

____/2   ____/2   ____/2   19. Record a deposit of $160 on June 20, 20XX, on check stub No. 485 and on the bank deposit slip.

____/8   ____/8   ____/8   20. Make out check No. 485 on June 20, 20XX, for utilities to Woodland Hills Gas Company, 50 South M Street, Woodland Hills, XY 12345, in the amount of $87.80, and make the appropriate calculations on the check stub.

____/6   ____/6   ____/6   21. Record check No. 485 on the check register.

____/8   ____/8   ____/8   22. Make out check No. 486 on June 20, 20XX, for drugs and medical supplies to Sargents Pharmacy, 711 Wheeler Road, Woodland Hills, XY 12345, in the amount of $38.75, and make the appropriate calculations on the check stub.

JOB SKILL 20-1 *(continued)*

____/6 ____/6 ____/6   23. Record check No. 486 on the check register.

____/8 ____/8 ____/8   24. Make out check No. 487 on June 20, 20XX, for a donation to United Fund, PO Box 400, New York, NY 10015, in the amount of $200.00, and make the appropriate calculations on the check stub.

____/6 ____/6 ____/6   25. Record check No. 487 on the check register.

____/2 ____/2 ____/2   26. Record a deposit of $105 on June 25, 20XX, on check stub No. 488 and on the bank deposit slip.

____/8 ____/8 ____/8   27. Make out check No. 488 on June 25, 20XX, for utilities to Woodland Hills Telephone Company, 505 Peppermint Street, Woodland Hills, XY 12345, in the amount of $79.60, and make the appropriate calculations on the check stub.

____/6 ____/6 ____/6   28. Record check No. 488 on the check register.

____/8 ____/8 ____/8   29. Make out check No. 489 on June 25, 20XX, for utilities to Woodland Hills Electric Company, 320 Banyon Avenue, Woodland Hills, XY 12345, in the amount of $85.78, and make the appropriate calculations on the check stub.

____/6 ____/6 ____/6   30. Record check No. 489 on the check register.

____/8 ____/8 ____/8   31. Make out check No. 490 on June 25, 20XX, for office linens to Rite-Way Laundry, 2500 Torrance Way, Woodland Hills, XY 12345, in the amount of $45.00, and make the appropriate calculations on the check stub.

____/6 ____/6 ____/6   32. Record check No. 490 on the check register.

_____ _____ _____   Complete within specified time.

__/189 __/189 __/189   **Total points earned** (To obtain a percentage score, divide the total points earned by the number of points possible.)

Comments:

Evaluator's Signature: _____   **Need to Repeat:** _____

National Curriculum Competency: CAAHEP: Cognitive: II.C.1 Psychomotor: VII.P.2

JOB SKILL 20-2
Pay Bills and Record Expenditures

Name _____ Date _____ Score _____

Performance Objective

Task: Write checks for invoices received, complete the check register, and enter the deposit.

Conditions: Need:

- Computer with Internet connection
- Online Forms 93, 94, and 95 (check register used in Job Skill 20-1)
- Online Forms 100 and 101 (four checks) located at www.cengagebrain.com with student resources
- *Workbook* Figure 20-1 (four invoices)
- Calculator
- Pencil

Refer to:

- *Textbook* Procedure 20-1 for step-by-step directions

Standards: Complete all steps listed in this skill **in** _____ minutes with a minimum score of _____.
(Time element and accuracy criteria may be given by instructor.)

Time: **Start:** _____ **Completed:** _____ **Total:** _____ minutes

Scoring: One point for each step performed satisfactorily unless otherwise listed or weighted by instructor.

Directions with Performance Evaluation Checklist

Read the entire job skill before beginning. Use the date June 30, 20XX. If possible, copy the invoices on the following page and cut them apart.

1st Attempt	2nd Attempt	3rd Attempt	
_____	_____	_____	Gather materials (equipment and supplies) listed under *Conditions*.
_____	_____	_____	1. Carry the checkbook balance forward from the previous job skill to check No. 491 ($7223.27).
____/6	____/6	____/6	2. You have deposited money on the following dates for the amounts listed: 6/28 $410.99, 6/29 $70, 6/30 $95. Include these deposits on the first check stub that you will be using (No. 491) and on page 2 of the check register bank deposit slip.
____/3	____/3	____/3	3. Cut the invoices apart in *Workbook* Figure 20-1.
____/56	____/56	____/56	4. Write checks for the invoices shown in Figure 20-1 and record the information on the check register as in Job Skill 20-1.
____/12	____/12	____/12	5. Indicate the following on each invoice: date paid, check number, and check amount.
_____	_____	_____	Complete within specified time.
____/80	____/80	____/80	**Total points earned** (To obtain a percentage score, divide the total points earned by the number of points possible.)

JOB SKILL 20-2 (*continued*)

Central Medical Supply Company
859 East Santa Clara Drive
Woodland Hills, XY 12345-0012

STATEMENT

20XX
6-15   Ophthalmoscope $350.00
                      tax   24.50
        Shipping & handling   10.00
        BALANCE DUE $384.50

Thrifty Drug Store
540 West Main Street
Woodland Hills, XY 12345-6785

STATEMENT

20XX

6-20   1 roll bandages $6.50
       2 boxes tissues   3.00
       1 box cotton swabs   4.50
                    tax   .98
            TOTAL $14.98

Prudential Life Insurance
2603 Underpass Street
Woodland Hills, XY 12345-9822

INVOICE

20XX

6-30   Gerald Practon
       Life Insurance
       6 months premium

PLEASE PAY $1969.42

ABC MOTORS
610 Main Street
Woodland Hills, XY 12345-2389

INVOICE

20XX

6-15   Lube and oil
       1998 Toyota $65.00
       5 qts oil   10.00
       filter   5.00
       TOTAL BALANCE DUE $80.00

FIGURE 20-1

Comments:

Evaluator's Signature: _____   **Need to Repeat:** _____

National Curriculum Competency: CAAHEP: Cognitive: II.C.1 Psychomotor: VII.P.2

JOB SKILL 20-3
Replenish and Balance the Petty Cash Fund

Name _____ Date _____ Score _____

Performance Objective

Task: Record entries on a petty cash envelope, calculate totals, balance the cash drawer, and write a check to replenish the petty cash fund.

Conditions: Need:
- Computer with Internet connection
- Online Forms 93, 94, and 95 (check register used in Job Skills 20-1 and 20-2)
- Online Form 102 (one check No. 495) located at www.cengagebrain.com with student resources
- Online Form 103 (petty cash envelope)
- Calculator
- Pencil

Refer to:

Textbook Procedure 20-1 for step-by-step instructions

Standards: Complete all steps listed in this job skill in _____ minutes with a minimum score of _____. (Time element and accuracy criteria may be given by instructor.)

Time: Start: _____ Completed: _____ Total: _____ minutes

Scoring: One point for each step performed satisfactorily unless otherwise listed or weighted by instructor.

Directions with Performance Evaluation Checklist

1st Attempt	2nd Attempt	3rd Attempt	
_____	_____	_____	Gather materials (equipment and supplies) listed under *Conditions*.
___/2	___/2	___/2	1. Indicate in the middle of the petty cash receipt envelope (Form 103) the office fund beginning petty cash amount of $100 for June 1, 20XX; this envelope will be used for the entire month of June.
___/30	___/30	___/30	2. Enter the following expenses that occurred during the month of June on the top portion of the petty cash receipt envelope listing the date paid, voucher number, to whom it was paid, a brief description of the item, under which account heading it would be listed (i.e., office supplies, postage, medical supplies, and miscellaneous), and the amount.

Date	Voucher	Vendor	Item	Amount
6/3/XX	103	Crown Stationers	stationery supplies	$2.70
6/7/XX	104	U.S. Postal Service	postage due	.95
6/15/XX	105	Thrifty Drug Store	medical supplies	7.32
6/20/XX	106	TG & Y Store	miscellaneous (office plant)	3.40
6/22/XX	107	U.S. Postal Service	postage	45.00
6/27/XX	108	Thrifty Drug Store	medical supplies	2.62

| ___/6 | ___/6 | ___/6 | 3. Total the amount of all items and record on the last line of the top portion of the envelope. |

JOB SKILL 20-3 (*continued*)

_____/4 _____/4 _____/4   4. List the following headings in the first line of the "Distribution of Petty Cash": Office Supplies, Postage, Medical Supplies, Miscellaneous.

_____/6 _____/6 _____/6   5. Itemize each of the expenditures under the correct heading.

_____/4 _____/4 _____/4   6. Total each column under "Distribution of Petty Cash" and list the total on the last line.

_____/4 _____/4 _____/4   7. Add all totals listed and record in the right column on the last line under "Totals." This number should be the same as the total in step 3.

_____ _____ _____   8. List the dollar amount of all vouchers paid under "Receipts Paid."

_____ _____ _____   9. Count the cash in the cash drawer and list under "Cash on Hand."

_____/2 _____/2 _____/2   10. Add the receipts paid and the cash on hand; it should equal the beginning amount listed in the "Office Fund Amount."

_____ _____ _____   11. List this amount in "Total Receipts and Cash."

_____/2 _____/2 _____/2   12. Subtract the "Total Receipts and Cash" from the "Office Fund Amount" and list the amount of money that is over or short.

_____/6 _____/6 _____/6   13. Write check No. 495, made out to "Petty Cash," for the amount necessary to replenish the petty cash.

_____ _____ _____   14. Bring down the checkbook balance forward from the previous check (No. 494).

_____ _____ _____   15. List and subtract the amount of the check written to Petty Cash and record the balance.

_____/5 _____/5 _____/5   16. Record the check information and list the amount of the check on page 1 of the Check Register.

_____ _____ _____   17. Indicate at the top of the "Petty Cash Receipt Envelope" the check number used to replenish the petty cash fund.

_____/11 _____/11 _____/11   18. List petty cash amounts on pages 1 and 2 of the check register. Note: *Add together items in the same category; office supplies and postage will be combined and listed under "Office Supplies."*

_____ _____ _____   Complete within specified time.

_____/90 _____/90 _____/90   **Total points earned** (To obtain a percentage score, divide the total points earned by the number of points possible.)

Comments:

Evaluator's Signature: _____   **Need to Repeat:** _____

National Curriculum Competency: CAAHEP: Cognitive: II.C.1 Psychomotor: VII.P.2

JOB SKILL 20-4
Balance a Check Register

Name _____ Date _____ Score _____

Performance Objective

Task: Total all columns (pages 1, 2, and 3) and balance the check register.

Conditions: Need:

- Online Forms 93, 94, and 95 (check register with figures entered that were used in Job Skills 20-1, 20-2, and 20-3)
- Calculator
- Pencil

Refer to:

- *Textbook* Procedure 20-1 for step-by-step directions

Standards: Complete all steps listed in this job skill in _____ minutes with a minimum score of _____.
(Time element and accuracy criteria may be given by instructor.)

Time: **Start:** _____ **Completed:** _____ **Total:** _____ minutes

Scoring: One point for each step performed satisfactorily unless otherwise listed or weighted by instructor.

Directions with Performance Evaluation Checklist

1st Attempt	2nd Attempt	3rd Attempt	
_____	_____	_____	Gather materials (equipment and supplies) listed under *Conditions*.
___/20	___/20	___/20	1. Page 1: Total both columns of the check register and record at the bottom of the form; they should equal.
___/8	___/8	___/8	2. Page 2: Total the bank deposit and all columns of the check register and record at the bottom of the form.
___/6	___/6	___/6	3. Page 3: Total all columns of the check register and record at the bottom of the form.
___/14	___/14	___/14	4. Balance the check register: Add all disbursement column totals on pages 2 and 3; they should equal the total listed on page 1 (c).
_____	_____	_____	Complete within specified time.
___/50	___/50	___/50	**Total points earned** (To obtain a percentage score, divide the total points earned by the number of points possible.)

Comments:

Evaluator's Signature: _____ **Need to Repeat:** _____

National Curriculum Competency: CAAHEP: Cognitive: II.C.1 Psychomotor: VII.P.2

JOB SKILL 20-5
Reconcile a Bank Statement

Name _____ Date _____ Score _____

Performance Objective

Task: Reconcile a bank statement.

Conditions: Need:

- Computer with Internet connection
- Online Form 104 (one bank account reconciliation form) located at www.cengagebrain.com with student resources
- Checkbook stubs completed in Job Skills 20-1, 20-2, and 20-3
- *Workbook* Figure 20-2 (bank statement)
- Calculator
- Pen or pencil

Refer to:

- *Textbook* Procedure 14-3 in Chapter 14 to review the steps for reconciling a bank statement

Standards: Complete all steps listed in this skill in _____ minutes with a minimum score of _____.
(Time element and accuracy criteria may be given by instructor.)

Time: **Start:** _____ **Completed:** _____ **Total:** _____ minutes

Scoring: One point for each step performed satisfactorily unless otherwise listed or weighted by instructor.

Directions with Performance Evaluation Checklist

You have received the bank statement from The First National Bank for June 20XX. Use the checks written in the previous job skills for the month of June 20XX (No. 479 through 495) and the bank statement shown in *Workbook* Figure 20-2 to reconcile the bank statement.

1st Attempt	2nd Attempt	3rd Attempt	
_____	_____	_____	Gather materials (equipment and supplies) listed under *Conditions*.
___/9	___/9	___/9	1. Mark off all checks made out during the month of June that have been returned by the bank and appear on the bank statement.
___/16	___/16	___/16	2. List all checks that have not been returned on the reconciliation form under "Outstanding Checks or Other Withdrawals."
___/8	___/8	___/8	3. Add all outstanding checks and record the total on the reconciliation form.
___/6	___/6	___/6	4. Check off all deposits that have been made during the month of June that appear on the bank statement.
___/6	___/6	___/6	5. List all deposits that do not appear on the statement on the reconciliation form under "Deposits Not Credited."
___/3	___/3	___/3	6. Add all deposits not credited to the account and record the total on the reconciliation form.
___/4	___/4	___/4	7. Balance the checking account using the steps indicated on the reconciliation form under "Balance Your Account."
___/2	___/2	___/2	8. Compare this figure with the ending figure in the checkbook (see check No. 495); they should match. If it does not balance, recalculate figures in the checkbook and on the bank reconciliation form.

JOB SKILL 20-5 (*continued*)

_____ _____ _____ Complete within specified time.

___/56 ___/56 ___/56 **Total points earned** (To obtain a percentage score, divide the total points earned by the number of points possible.)

Account Statement ⬡ THE FIRST NATIONAL BANK

CHECKING ACCOUNT # 00012345   WOODLAND HILLS 140

                                                                    0020
                                                                    100

PRACTON MEDICAL GROUP, INC   140
4567 BROAD AVENUE
WOODLAND HILLS XY   12345

CHECKING ACCOUNT SUMMARY AS OF 06-27-20XX   3

BEGINNING BALANCE	TOTAL DEPOSITS	TOTAL WITHDRAWALS	SERVICE CHARGES	ENDING BALANCE
9,745 45	765 00	3076 80	00	7,433 65

– – – – – – – – – – – – – – –CHECKING ACCOUNT TRANSACTIONS– – – – – – – – – – – – – – –

DEPOSITS	DATE	AMOUNT
BRANCH DEPOSIT	06-01	130.00
BRANCH DEPOSIT	06-03	95.00
BRANCH DEPOSIT	06-04	195.00
BRANCH DEPOSIT	06-15	80.00
BRANCH DEPOSIT	06-20	160.00
BRANCH DEPOSIT	06-25	105.00

– – – –CHECKS– – – –			– – – –CHECKS– – – –			– – – –BALANCES– – – –	
ITEM	DATE	AMOUNT	ITEM	DATE	AMOUNT	DATE	BALANCES
479	06-01	1,900.00	484	06-15	226.00	06-01	7,975.45
480	06-03	74.50	485	06-20	87.80	06-03	7,695.95
481	06-03	300.00	486	06-20	38.75	06-04	7,803.20
482	06-04	87.75	487	06-20	200.00	06-15	7,495.20
483	06-15	162.00				06-20	7,328.65
						06-25	7,433.65

FIGURE 20-2

Comments:

Evaluator's Signature: _____   **Need to Repeat:** _____

National Curriculum Competency: CAAHEP: Cognitive: II.C.1

JOB SKILL 20-6
Prepare Payroll

Name _____ Date _____ Score _____

Performance Objective

Task: Prepare payroll for seven employees; calculate gross pay and all deductions to determine net pay.

Conditions: Need:
- *Workbook* Figure 20-3 through Figure 20-11 (income tax tables)
- Calculator
- Pen or pencil

Refer to:
- *Textbook* Procedure 20-2 for step-by-step directions
- *Textbook* Figure 20-13 and Figure 20-14 for examples of a completed employee earning record and monthly payroll register

Standards: Complete all steps listed in this skill in _____ minutes with a minimum score of _____. (Time element and accuracy criteria may be given by instructor.)

Time: **Start:** _____ **Completed:** _____ **Total:** _____ minutes

Scoring: One point for each step performed satisfactorily unless otherwise listed or weighted by instructor.

Directions with Performance Evaluation Checklist

It is May 28, 20XX, and you will be preparing the payroll for seven employees. Note: *Hourly pay and salaries are used as examples only and do not indicate current pay rates for medical assistants.* Following are payroll guidelines and instructions:

Frequency of pay:
1. Hourly employees are paid once each month, on the first. To determine the gross pay, multiply the amount paid per hour by the number of hours worked (e.g., $12 per hour × 160 hours = $1920).
2. Salaried employees are paid semimonthly. To determine the gross pay, divide the salary per month by two (e.g., $2000 per month divided by 2 = $1000).

Employee status:
3. Divorced persons are considered "single" on federal tax tables and "head of household" on state tax tables that appear in this exercise.
4. Single persons with a dependent parent are considered "unmarried head of household" with the state.

Payroll deductions:
5. A few employees have elected to pay 2% of their gross pay into the Practon Medical Group, Inc., insurance plan.
6. If you reside in California, Hawaii, New Jersey, New York, Puerto Rico, or Rhode Island, assume state disability insurance is 1% of gross pay; in all other states, disregard this deduction.
7. Calculate FICA deductions at 6.2% of gross earnings.
8. Calculate Medicare deductions at 1.45% of gross earnings.
9. To calculate deductions, multiply the gross salary by the percent of deductions (e.g., $1920 [gross salary] × .062 [FICA deduction] = $119.04).

Instructions:
10. Read the following scenarios and refer to these directions while using the worksheet provided.
11. Deixtermine whether the employee is on salary or paid hourly and number of hours worked; then calculate the gross pay.
12. Next, indicate whether the person is single (S), married (M), or divorced (D); the number of exemptions claimed; and frequency of pay (e.g., semimonthly, monthly).

JOB SKILL 20-6 (*continued*)

13. Refer to the tax tables that follow this exercise to determine federal and state deductions. If the amount of income is shown on two lines (e.g., at least $540 but less than $560 and at least $560 but less than $580), use the higher deduction.

14. Round off numbers to the highest digit.

1st Attempt	2nd Attempt	3rd Attempt	
_____	_____	_____	Gather materials (equipment and supplies) listed under *Conditions*.
___/13	___/13	___/13	1. Prepare payroll for Hillary Sheehan who is the physician's bookkeeper. She is married and claims herself as an exemption. She earns $13 an hour and worked 168 hours this month with no overtime.

Status	Exemptions	Salary/Hrs Worked	Frequency of Pay
S M D	0 1 2 3	_____	Monthly/Semimonthly

| Gross Pay | FICA | Fed. Inc. Tax | State Inc. Tax | SDI | Medicare | Other | Total Deduc. | Net Pay |

___/13	___/13	___/13	2. Prepare payroll for Roger Young, who works part-time as a custodian on weekends. He is single and claims himself and a dependent mother. He is paid $7.50 per hour. He worked 18 hours this month.

Status	Exemptions	Salary/Hrs Worked	Frequency of Pay
S M D	0 1 2 3	_____	Monthly/Semimonthly

| Gross Pay | FICA | Fed. Inc. Tax | State Inc. Tax | SDI | Medicare | Other | Total Deduc. | Net Pay |

___/13	___/13	___/13	3. Prepare payroll for Kelley Jones, who is the office receptionist. She is single and claims herself only. She is paid $1650 per month, and she elected not to enroll in the hospital insurance plan.

Status	Exemptions	Salary/Hrs Worked	Frequency of Pay
S M D	0 1 2 3	_____	Monthly/Semimonthly

| Gross Pay | FICA | Fed. Inc. Tax | State Inc. Tax | SDI | Medicare | Other | Total Deduc. | Net Pay |

___/13	___/13	___/13	4. Prepare payroll for Maryjane Moran, who works part-time doing insurance. She is paid hourly and earns $12.50 per hour. She is married and claims no dependents because her husband claims her. She worked 80 hours this month.

Status	Exemptions	Salary/Hrs Worked	Frequency of Pay
S M D	0 1 2 3	_____	Monthly/Semimonthly

| Gross Pay | FICA | Fed. Inc. Tax | State Inc. Tax | SDI | Medicare | Other | Total Deduc. | Net Pay |

JOB SKILL 20-6 *(continued)*

___/13 ___/13 ___/13 5. Prepare payroll for Carla O'Hare, who is the administrative medical assistant. She is divorced and has three children. She claims herself and her children. She is paid $1675 a month, and she is a member of the hospital insurance plan.

Status	Exemptions	Salary/Hrs Worked	Frequency of Pay
S M D	0 1 2 3	_____	Monthly/Semimonthly

Gross Pay	FICA	Fed. Inc. Tax	State Inc. Tax	SDI	Medicare	Other	Total Deduc.	Net Pay

___/13 ___/13 ___/13 6. Prepare payroll for Amy Seaforth, who is a part-time laboratory technician. She is married; her husband does not claim her, and she does not wish to claim herself either. She joined the hospital insurance plan. She is paid a salary of $145 per week plus car expense figured at $0.34 per mile. She drove 36 miles this pay period. Amy is a new employee hired on May 1, 20XX. You will be completing an employee earning record card for her in a future job skill. Her address is 29926 West Ridgeway Avenue, Woodland Hills, XY 12345; telephone 555-692-4408; Social Security number XXX-XX-1945; birth date 08-04-50.

Status	Exemptions	Salary/Hrs Worked	Frequency of Pay
S M D	0 1 2 3	_____	Monthly/Semimonthly

Gross Pay	FICA	Fed. Inc. Tax	State Inc. Tax	SDI	Medicare	Other	Total Deduc.	Net Pay

___/13 ___/13 ___/13 7. Prepare payroll for Lisa Adams, who is the clinical medical assistant. She is married and has one child, whom she claims along with herself as deductions. She is paid $1750 per month, and she joined the hospital insurance plan.

Status	Exemptions	Salary/Hrs Worked	Frequency of Pay
S M D	0 1 2 3	_____	Monthly/Semimonthly

Gross Pay	FICA	Fed. Inc. Tax	State Inc. Tax	SDI	Medicare	Other	Total Deduc.	Net Pay

_____ _____ _____ Complete within specified time.

___/93 ___/93 ___/93 **Total points earned** (To obtain a percentage score, divide the total points earned by the number of points possible.)

Comments:

Evaluator's Signature: _____ **Need to Repeat:** _____

National Curriculum Competency: CAAHEP: Cognitive: II.C.1

JOB SKILL 20-6 (*continued*)

SINGLE Persons—SEMI-MONTHLY Payroll Period											FEDERAL
And the wages are–		**And the number of withholding allowances claimed is—**									
At least	But less than	0	1	2	3	4	5	6	7	8	9	10
		The amount of income tax to be withheld is —										
$ 800	$ 820	$ 91	$ 68	$ 44	$ 26	$ 11	$ 0	$ 0	$ 0	$ 0	$ 0	$ 0
820	840	94	71	47	28	13	0	0	0	0	0	0
840	860	97	74	50	30	15	0	0	0	0	0	0
860	880	100	77	53	32	17	1	0	0	0	0	0
880	900	103	80	56	34	19	3	0	0	0	0	0
900	920	106	83	59	36	21	5	0	0	0	0	0
920	940	109	86	62	39	23	7	0	0	0	0	0
940	960	112	89	65	42	25	9	0	0	0	0	0
960	980	115	92	68	45	27	11	0	0	0	0	0
980	1,000	118	95	71	48	29	12	0	0	0	0	0
1,000	1,020	121	98	74	51	31	15	0	0	0	0	0
1,020	1,040	124	101	77	54	33	17	2	0	0	0	0
1,040	1,060	127	104	80	57	35	19	4	0	0	0	0
1,060	1,080	130	107	83	60	37	21	6	0	0	0	0
1,080	1,100	133	110	86	63	40	23	8	0	0	0	0
1,100	1,120	136	113	89	66	43	25	10	0	0	0	0
1,120	1,140	139	116	92	69	46	27	12	0	0	0	0
1,140	1,160	142	119	95	72	49	29	14	0	0	0	0
1,160	1,180	145	122	98	75	52	31	16	0	0	0	0
1,180	1,200	148	125	101	78	55	33	18	2	0	0	0
1,200	1,220	151	128	104	81	58	35	20	4	0	0	0
1,220	1,240	154	131	107	84	61	38	22	6	0	0	0
1,240	1,260	157	134	110	87	64	41	24	8	0	0	0
1,260	1,280	160	137	113	90	67	44	26	10	0	0	0
1,280	1,300	163	140	116	93	70	47	28	12	0	0	0
1,300	1,320	166	143	119	96	73	50	30	14	0	0	0
1,320	1,340	169	146	122	99	76	53	32	16	1	0	0
1,340	1,360	172	149	125	102	79	56	34	18	3	0	0
1,360	1,380	175	152	128	105	82	59	36	20	5	0	0
1,380	1,400	178	155	131	108	85	62	39	22	7	0	0
1,400	1,420	181	158	134	111	88	65	42	24	9	0	0
1,420	1,440	184	161	137	114	91	68	45	26	11	0	0
1,440	1,460	184	164	140	117	94	71	48	28	13	0	0
1,460	1,480	190	167	143	120	97	74	51	30	15	0	0
1,480	1,500	193	170	146	123	100	77	54	32	17	2	0
1,500	1,520	196	173	149	126	103	80	57	34	19	4	0
1,520	1,540	199	176	152	129	106	83	60	37	21	6	0
1,540	1,560	204	179	155	132	109	86	63	40	23	8	0
1,560	1,580	209	182	158	135	112	89	66	43	25	10	0
1,580	1,600	214	185	161	138	115	92	69	46	27	12	0
1,600	1,620	219	188	164	141	118	95	72	49	29	14	0
1,620	1,640	224	191	167	144	121	98	75	52	31	16	0
1,640	1,660	229	194	170	147	124	101	78	55	33	18	2
1,660	1,680	234	197	173	150	127	104	81	58	35	20	4
1,680	1,700	239	201	176	153	130	107	84	61	38	22	6
1,700	1,720	244	206	179	156	133	110	87	64	41	24	8
1,720	1,740	249	211	182	159	136	113	90	67	44	26	10
1,740	1,760	254	216	185	162	139	116	93	70	47	28	12
1,760	1,780	259	221	188	165	142	119	96	73	50	30	14
1,780	1,800	264	226	191	168	145	122	99	76	53	32	16
1,800	1,820	269	231	194	171	148	125	102	79	56	34	18
1,820	1,840	274	236	197	174	151	128	105	82	59	36	20
1,840	1,860	279	241	202	177	154	131	108	85	62	39	22
1,860	1,880	284	246	207	180	157	134	111	88	65	42	24
1,880	1,900	289	251	212	183	160	137	114	91	68	45	26
1,900	1,920	294	256	217	186	163	140	117	94	71	48	28
1,920	1,940	299	261	222	189	166	143	120	97	74	51	30
1,940	1,960	304	266	227	192	169	146	123	100	77	54	32
1,960	1,980	309	271	232	195	172	149	126	103	80	57	34
1,980	2,000	314	276	237	199	175	152	129	106	83	60	36
2,000	2,020	319	281	242	204	178	155	132	109	86	63	39
2,020	2,040	324	286	247	209	181	158	135	112	89	66	42
2,040	2,060	329	291	252	214	184	161	138	115	92	69	45
2,060	2,080	334	296	257	219	187	164	141	118	95	72	48
2,080	2,100	339	301	262	224	190	167	144	121	98	75	51
2,100	2,120	344	306	267	229	198	170	147	124	101	78	54
2,120	2,140	349	311	272	234	196	173	150	127	104	81	57

FIGURE 20-3

JOB SKILL 20-6 (*continued*)

And the wages are—		SINGLE Persons—MONTHLY Payroll Period										FEDERAL
		And the number of withholding allowances claimed is—										
At least	But less than	0	1	2	3	4	5	6	7	8	9	10
		The amount of income tax to be withheld is —										
$ 0	$ 220	$ 0	$ 0	$ 0	$ 0	$ 0	$ 0	$ 0	$0	$0	$0	$0
220	230	5	0	0	0	0	0	0	0	0	0	0
230	240	6	0	0	0	0	0	0	0	0	0	0
240	250	7	0	0	0	0	0	0	0	0	0	0
250	260	8	0	0	0	0	0	0	0	0	0	0
260	270	9	0	0	0	0	0	0	0	0	0	0
270	280	10	0	0	0	0	0	0	0	0	0	0
280	290	11	0	0	0	0	0	0	0	0	0	0
290	300	12	0	0	0	0	0	0	0	0	0	0
300	320	14	0	0	0	0	0	0	0	0	0	0
320	340	16	0	0	0	0	0	0	0	0	0	0
340	360	18	0	0	0	0	0	0	0	0	0	0
360	380	20	0	0	0	0	0	0	0	0	0	0
380	400	22	0	0	0	0	0	0	0	0	0	0
400	420	24	0	0	0	0	0	0	0	0	0	0
420	440	26	0	0	0	0	0	0	0	0	0	0
440	460	28	0	0	0	0	0	0	0	0	0	0
460	480	30	0	0	0	0	0	0	0	0	0	0
480	500	32	1	0	0	0	0	0	0	0	0	0
500	520	34	3	0	0	0	0	0	0	0	0	0
520	540	36	5	0	0	0	0	0	0	0	0	0
540	560	38	7	0	0	0	0	0	0	0	0	0
560	580	40	9	0	0·	0	0	0	0	0	0	0
580	600	42	11	0	0	0	0	0	0	0	0	0
600	640	45	14	0	0	0	0	0	0	0	0	0
640	680	49	18	0	0	0	0	0	0	0	0	0
680	720	53	22	0	0	0	0	0	0	0	0	0
720	760	57	26	0	0	0	0	0	0	0	0	0
760	800	61	30	0	0	0	0	0	0	0	0	0
800	840	65	34	3	0	0	0	0	0	0	0	0
840	880	69	38	7	0	0	0	0	0	0	0	0
880	920	73	42	11	0	0	0	0	0	0	0	0
920	960	79	46	15	0	0	0	0	0	0	0	0
960	1,000	85	50	19	0	0	0	0	0	0	0	0
1,000	1,040	91	54	23	0	0	0	0	0	0	0	0
1,040	1,080	97	58	27	0	0	0	0	0	0	0	0
1,080	1,120	103	62	31	0	0	0	0	0	0	0	0
1,120	1,160	109	66	35	4	0	0	0	0	0	0	0
1,160	1,200	115	70	39	8	0	0	0	0	0	0	0
1,200	1,240	121	75	43	12	0	0	0	0	0	0	0
1,240	1,280	127	81	47	16	0	0	0	0	0	0	0
1,280	1,320	133	87	51	20	0	0	0	0	0	0	0
1,320	1,360	139	93	55	24	0	0	0	0	0	0	0
1,360	1,400	145	99	59	28	0	0	0	0	0	0	0
1,400	1,440	151	105	63	32	1	0	0	0	0	0	0
1,440	1,480	157	111	67	36	5	0	0	0	0	0	0
1,480	1,520	163	117	71	40	9	0	0	0	0	0	0
1,520	1,560	169	123	77	44	13	0	0	0	0	0	0
1,560	1,600	175	129	83	48	17	0	0	0	0	0	0
1,600	1,640	181	135	89	52	21	0	0	0	0	0	0
1,640	1,680	187	141	95	56	25	0	0	0	0	0	0
1,680	1,720	193	147	101	60	29	0	0	0	0	0	0
1,720	1,760	199	153	107	64	33	2	0	0	0	0	0
1,760	1,800	205	159	113	68	37	6	0	0	0	0	0
1,800	1,840	211	165	119	73	41	10	0	0	0	0	0
1,840	1,880	217	171	125	79	45	14	0	0	0	0	0
1,880	1,920	223	177	131	85	49	18	0	0	0	0	0
1,920	1,960	229	183	137	91	53	22	0	0	0	0	0
1,960	2,000	235	189	143	97	57	26	0	0	0	0	0
2,000	2,040	241	195	149	103	61	30	0	0	0	0	0
2,040	2,080	247	201	155	109	65	34	4	0	0	0	0
2,080	2,120	253	207	161	115	69	38	8	0	0	0	0
2,120	2,160	259	213	167	121	74	42	12	0	0	0	0
2,160	2,200	265	219	173	127	80	46	16	0	0	0	0
2,200	2,240	271	225	179	133	86	50	20	0	0	0	0
2,240	2,280	277	231	185	139	92	54	24	0	0	0	0
2,280	2,320	283	237	191	145	98	58	28	0	0	0	0
2,320	2,360	289	243	197	151	104	62	32	1	0	0	0
2,360	2,400	295	249	203	157	110	66	36	5	0	0	0

FIGURE 20-4

JOB SKILL 20-6 (*continued*)

		MARRIED Persons—MONTHLY Payroll Period										FEDERAL
And the wages are–		And the number of withholding allowances claimed is—										
At least	But less than	0	1	2	3	4	5	6	7	8	9	10
		The amount of income tax to be withheld is —										
$ 0	$ 680	$ 0	$ 0	$ 0	$ 0	$ 0	$ 0	$ 0	$ 0	$ 0	$ 0	$ 0
680	720	4	0	0	0	0	0	0	0	0	0	0
720	760	8	0	0	0	0	0	0	0	0	0	0
760	800	12	0	0	0	0	0	0	0	0	0	0
800	840	16	0	0	0	0	0	0	0	0	0	0
840	880	20	0	0	0	0	0	0	0	0	0	0
880	920	24	0	0	0	0	0	0	0	0	0	0
920	960	28	0	0	0	0	0	0	0	0	0	0
960	1,000	32	1	0	0	0	0	0	0	0	0	0
1,000	1,040	36	5	0	0	0	0	0	0	0	0	0
1,040	1,080	40	9	0	0	0	0	0	0	0	0	0
1,080	1,120	44	13	0	0	0	0	0	0	0	0	0
1,120	1,160	48	17	0	0	0	0	0	0	0	0	0
1,160	1,200	52	21	0	0	0	0	0	0	0	0	0
1,200	1,240	56	25	0	0	0	0	0	0	0	0	0
1,240	1,280	60	29	0	0	0	0	0	0	0	0	0
1,280	1,320	64	33	3	0	0	0	0	0	0	0	0
1,320	1360	68	37	7	0	0	0	0	0	0	0	0
1360	1,400	72	41	11	0	0	0	0	0	0	0	0
1,400	1,440	76	45	15	0	0	0	0	0	0	0	0
1,440	1,480	80	49	19	0	0	0	0	0	0	0	0
1,480	1,520	84	53	23	0	0	0	0	0	0	0	0
1,520	1,560	88	57	27	0	0	0	0	0	0	0	0
1,560	1,600	92	61	31	0	0	0	0	0	0	0	0
1,600	1,640	96	65	35	4	0	0	0	0	0	0	0
1,640	1,680	100	69	39	8	0	0	0	0	0	0	0
1,680	1,720	104	73	43	12	0	0	0	0	0	0	0
1,720	1,760	108	77	47	16	0	0	0	0	0	0	0
1,760	1,800	112	81	51	20	0	0	0	0	0	0	0
1,800	1,840	116	85	55	24	0	0	0	0	0	0	0
1,840	1,880	120	89	59	28	0	0	0	0	0	0	0
1,880	1,920	124	93	63	32	1	0	0	0	0	0	0
1,920	1,960	128	97	67	36	5	0	0	0	0	0	0
1,960	2,000	132	101	71	40	9	0	0	0	0	0	0
2,000	2,040	136	105	75	44	13	0	0	0	0	0	0
2,040	2,080	140	109	79	48	17	0	0	0	0	0	0
2,080	2,120	145	113	83	52	21	0	0	0	0	0	0
2,120	2,160	151	117	87	56	25	0	0	0	0	0	0
2,160	2,200	157	121	91	60	29	0	0	0	0	0	0
2,200	2,240	163	125	95	64	33	2	0	0	0	0	0
2,240	2,280	169	129	99	68	37	6	0	0	0	0	0
2,280	2,320	175	133	103	72	41	10	0	0	0	0	0
2,320	2,360	181	137	107	76	45	14	0	0	0	0	0
2,360	2,400	187	141	111	80	49	18	0	0	0	0	0
2,400	2,440	193	147	115	84	53	22	0	0	0	0	0
2,440	2,480	199	153	119	88	57	26	0	0	0	0	0
2,480	2,520	205	159	123	92	61	30	0	0	0	0	0
2,520	2,560	211	165	127	96	65	34	3	0	0	0	0
2,560	2,600	217	171	131	100	69	38	7	0	0	0	0
2,600	2,640	223	177	135	104	73	42	11	0	0	0	0
2,640	2,680	229	183	139	108	77	46	15	0	0	0	0
2,680	2,720	235	189	143	112	81	50	19	0	0	0	0
2,720	2,760	241	195	149	116	85	54	23	0	0	0	0
2,760	2,800	247	201	155	120	89	58	27	0	0	0	0
2,800	2,840	253	207	161	124	93	62	31	0	0	0	0
2,840	2,880	259	213	167	128	97	66	35	4	0	0	0
2,880	2,920	265	219	173	132	101	70	39	8	0	0	0
2,920	2,960	271	225	179	136	105	74	43	12	0	0	0
2,960	3,000	277	231	185	140	109	78	47	16	0	0	0
3,000	3,040	283	237	191	145	113	82	51	20	0	0	0
3,040	3,080	289	243	197	151	117	86	55	24	0	0	0
3,080	3,120	295	249	203	157	121	90	59	28	0	0	0
3,120	3,160	301	255	209	163	125	94	63	32	2	0	0
3,160	3,200	307	261	215	169	129	98	67	36	6	0	0
3,200	3,240	313	267	221	175	133	102	71	40	10	0	0
3,240	3,280	319	273	227	181	137	106	75	44	14	0	0
3,280	3,320	325	279	233	187	141	110	79	48	18	0	0
3,320	3,360	331	285	239	193	146	114	83	52	22	0	0
3,360	3,400	337	291	245	199	152	118	87	56	26	0	0

FIGURE 20-5

JOB SKILL 20-6 (*continued*)

		And the number of withholding allowances claimed is—										
MARRIED Persons—**SEMI-MONTHLY** Payroll Period											**FEDERAL**	
And the wages are–		0	1	2	3	4	5	6	7	8	9	10
At least	But less than	The amount of income tax to be withheld is —										
$ 0	$ 330	$ 0	$ 0	$0	$ 0	$ 0	$ 0	$ 0	$0	$ 0	$0	$0
330	340	1	0	0	0	0	0	0	0	0	0	0
340	350	2	0	0	0	0	0	0	0	0	0	0
350	360	3	0	0	0	0	0	0	0	0	0	0
360	370	4	0	0	0	0	0	0	0	0	0	0
370	380	5	0	0	0	0	0	0	0	0	0	0
380	390	6	0	0	0	0	0	0	0	0	0	0
390	400	7	0	0	0	0	0	0	0	0	0	0
400	410	8	0	0	0	0	0	0	0	0	0	0
410	420	9	0	0	0	0	0	0	0	0	0	0
420	430	10	0	0	0	0	0	0	0	0	0	0
430	440	11	0	0	0	0	0	0	0	0	0	0
440	450	12	0	0	0	0	0	0	0	0	0	0
450	460	13	0	0	0	0	0	0	0	0	0	0
460	470	14	0	0	0	0	0	0	0	0	0	0
470	480	15	0	0	0	0	0	0	0	0	0	0
480	490	16	0	0	0	0	0	0	0	0	0	0
490	500	17	1	0	0	0	0	0	0	0	0	0
500	520	18	3	0	0	0	0	0	0	0	0	0
520	540	20	5	0	0	0	0	0	0	0	0	0
540	560	22	7	0	0	0	0	0	0	0	0	0
560	580	24	9	0	0	0	0	0	0	0	0	0
580	600	26	11	0	0	0	0	0	0	0	0	0
600	620	28	13	0	0	0	0	0	0	0	0	0
620	640	30	15	0	0	0	0	0	0	0	0	0
640	660	32	17	1	0	0	0	0	0	0	0	0
660	680	34	19	3	0	0	0	0	0	0	0	0
680	700	36	21	5	0	0	0	0	0	0	0	0
700	720	38	23	7	0	0	0	0	0	0	0	0
720	740	40	25	9	0	0	0	0	0	0	0	0
740	760	42	27	11	0	0	0	0	0	0	0	0
760	780	44	29	13	0	0	0	0	0	0	0	0
780	800	46	31	15	0	0	0	0	0	0	0	0
800	820	48	33	17	2	0	0	0	0	0	0	0
820	840	50	35	19	4	0	0	0	0	0	0	0
840	860	52	37	21	6	0	0	0	0	0	0	0
860	880	54	39	23	8	0	0	0	0	0	0	0
880	900	56	41	25	10	0	0	0	0	0	0	0
900	920	58	43	27	12	0	0	0	0	0	0	0
920	940	60	45	29	14	0	0	0	0	0	0	0
940	960	62	47	31	16	0	0	0	0	0	0	0
960	980	64	49	33	18	2	0	0	0	0	0	0
980	1,000	66	51	35	20	4	0	0	0	0	0	0
1,000	1,020	68	53	37	22	6	0	0	0	0	0	0
1,020	1,040	70	55	39	24	8	0	0	0	0	0	0
1,040	1,060	73	57	41	26	10	0	0	0	0	0	0
1,060	1,080	76	59	43	28	12	0	0	0	0	0	0
1,080	1,100	79	61	45	30	14	0	0	0	0	0	0
1,100	1,120	82	63	47	32	16	1	0	0	0	0	0
1,120	1,140	85	65	49	34	18	3	0	0	0	0	0
1,140	1,160	88	67	51	36	20	5	0	0	0	0	0
1,160	1,180	91	69	53	38	22	7	0	0	0	0	0
1,180	1,200	94	71	55	40	24	9	0	0	0	0	0
1,200	1,220	97	74	57	42	26	11	0	0	0	0	0
1,220	1,240	100	77	59	44	28	13	0	0	0	0	0
1,240	1,260	103	80	61	46	30	15	0	0	0	0	0
1,260	1,280	106	83	63	48	32	17	2	0	0	0	0
1,280	1,300	109	86	65	50	34	19	4	0	0	0	0
1,300	1,320	112	89	67	52	36	21	6	0	0	0	0
1,320	1,340	115	92	69	54	38	23	8	0	0	0	0
1,340	1,360	118	95	71	56	40	25	10	0	0	0	0
1,360	1,380	121	98	74	58	42	27	12	0	0	0	0
1,380	1,400	124	101	77	60	44	29	14	0	0	0	0
1,400	1,420	127	104	80	62	46	31	16	0	0	0	0
1,420	1,440	130	107	83	64	48	33	18	2	0	0	0
1,440	1,460	133	110	86	66	50	35	20	4	0	0	0
1,460	1,480	136	113	89	68	52	37	22	6	0	0	0
1,480	1,500	139	116	92	70	54	39	24	8	0	0	0

FIGURE 20-6

JOB SKILL 20-6 (*continued*)

SINGLE persons, dual income MARRIED
or MARRIED with multiple employers—SEMIMONTHLY payroll period

		And the number of withholding allowances claimed is...										**STATE**

If wages are...

At least	But less than	0	1	2	3	4	5	6	7	8	9	10 Or more
		...The amount of income tax to be withheld shall be ...										
$1	$300											
300	320	1.74										
320	340	1.94										
340	360	2.14										
360	380	2.34										
380	400	2.54										
400	420	2.86										
420	440	3.26										
440	460	3.66	0.03									
460	480	4.06	0.43									
480	500	4.46	0.83									
500	540	5.06	1.43									
540	580	5.86	2.23									
580	620	6.66	3.03									
620	660	7.46	3.83	0.20								
660	700	8.26	4.63	1.00								
700	740	9.06	5.43	1.80								
740	780	9.87	6.24	2.61								
780	820	11.47	7.84	4.21	0.58							
820	860	13.07	9.44	5.81	2.18							
860	900	14.67	11.04	7.41	3.78	0.15						
900	940	16.27	12.64	9.01	5.38	1.75						
940	980	17.87	14.24	10.61	6.98	3.35						
980	1020	19.47	15.84	12.21	8.58	4.95	1.32					
1020	1060	21.07	17.44	13.81	10.18	6.55	2.92					
1060	1100	22.67	19.04	15.41	11.78	8.15	4.52	0.89				
1100	1140	24.27	20.64	17.01	13.38	9.75	6.12	2.49				
1140	1180	26.66	23.03	19.40	15.77	12.14	8.51	4.88	1.25			
1180	1220	29.06	25.43	21.80	18.17	14.54	10.91	7.28	3.65	0.02		
1220	1260	31.46	27.83	24.20	20.57	16.94	13.31	9.68	6.05	2.42		
1260	1300	33.86	30.23	26.60	22.97	19.34	15.71	12.08	8.45	4.82	1.19	
1300	1340	36.26	32.63	29.00	25.37	21.74	18.11	14.48	10.85	7.22	3.59	
1340	1380	38.66	35.03	31.40	27.77	24.14	20.51	16.88	13.25	9.62	5.99	2.36
1380	1420	41.06	37.43	33.80	30.17	26.54	22.91	19.28	15.65	12.02	8.39	4.76
1420	1460	43.46	39.83	36.20	32.57	28.94	25.31	21.68	18.05	14.42	10.79	7.16
1460	1500	45.86	42.23	38.60	34.97	31.34	27.71	24.08	20.45	16.82	13.19	9.56
1500	1540	48.60	44.97	41.34	37.71	34.08	30.45	26.82	23.19	19.56	15.93	12.30
1540	1580	51.80	48.17	44.54	40.91	37.28	33.65	30.02	26.39	22.76	19.13	15.50
1580	1620	55.00	51.37	47.74	44.11	40.48	36.85	33.22	29.59	25.96	22.33	18.70
1620	1660	58.20	54.57	50.94	47.31	43.68	40.05	36.42	32.79	29.16	25.53	21.90
1660	1700	61.40	57.77	54.14	50.51	46.88	43.25	39.62	35.99	32.36	28.73	25.10
1700	1750	65.00	61.37	57.74	54.11	50.48	46.85	43.22	39.59	35.96	32.33	28.70
1750	1800	69.00	65.37	61.74	58.11	54.48	50.85	47.22	43.59	39.96	36.33	32.70
1800	1850	73.00	69.37	65.74	62.11	58.48	54.85	51.22	47.59	43.96	40.33	36.70
1850	1900	77.15	73.52	69.89	66.26	62.63	59.00	55.37	51.74	48.11	44.48	40.85
1900	1950	81.80	78.17	74.54	70.91	67.28	63.65	60.02	56.39	52.76	49.13	45.50
1950	2000	86.45	82.82	79.19	75.56	71.93	68.30	64.67	61.04	57.41	53.78	50.15
2000	2100	93.43	89.80	86.17	82.54	78.91	75.28	71.65	68.02	64.39	60.76	57.13
2100	2200	102.73	99.10	95.47	91.84	88.21	84.58	80.95	77.32	73.69	70.06	66.43
2200	2300	112.03	108.40	104.77	101.14	97.51	93.88	90.25	86.62	82.99	79.36	75.73
2300	2400	121.33	117.70	114.07	110.44	106.81	103.18	99.55	95.92	92.29	88.66	85.03
2400 and over		(Table Amount PLUS 9.3 Percent of the Amount Over 2350)										

FIGURE 20-7

JOB SKILL 20-6 (*continued*)

MARRIED persons—SEMIMONTHLY payroll period												
If wages are...		And the number of withholding allowances claimed is...										**STATE**
At least	But less than	0	1	2	3	4	5	6	7	8	9	10 Or more
		...The amount of income tax to be withheld shall be...										
$1	$300											
300	320	1.74										
320	340	1.94										
340	360	2.14										
360	380	2.34										
380	400	2.54										
400	420	2.74										
420	440	2.94										
440	460	3.14										
460	480	3.34										
480	500	3.54										
500	520	3.74	0.11									
520	540	3.94	0.31									
540	560	4.14	0.51									
560	580	4.34	0.71									
580	600	4.54	0.91									
600	620	4.74	1.11									
620	640	4.94	1.31									
640	660	5.14	1.51									
660	680	5.43	1.80									
680	700	5.83	2.20									
700	720	6.23	2.60									
720	740	6.63	3.00									
740	760	7.03	3.40									
760	780	7.43	3.80									
780	800	7.83	4.20									
800	820	8.23	4.60									
820	840	8.63	5.00									
840	860	9.03	5.40									
860	880	9.43	5.80									
880	900	9.83	6.20									
900	920	10.23	6.60	0.26								
920	940	10.63	7.00	0.66								
940	960	11.03	7.40	1.06								
960	980	11.43	7.80	1.46								
980	1000	11.83	8.20	1.86								
1000	1040	12.43	8.80	2.46								
1040	1080	13.23	9.60	3.26								
1080	1120	14.03	10.40	4.06	0.43							
1120	1160	14.83	11.20	4.86	1.23							
1160	1200	15.63	12.00	5.66	2.03							
1200	1240	16.43	12.80	6.46	2.83							
1240	1280	17.23	13.60	7.26	3.63							
1280	1320	18.03	14.40	8.06	4.43	0.80						
1320	1360	18.83	15.20	8.86	5.23	1.60						
1360	1400	19.63	16.00	9.66	6.03	2.40						
1400	1440	21.16	17.53	10.46	6.83	3.20						
1440	1480	22.76	19.13	11.26	7.63	4.00	0.37					
1480	1520	24.36	20.73	12.06	8.43	4.80	1.17					
1520	1560	25.96	22.33	13.27	9.64	6.01	2.38					
1560	1600	27.56	23.93	14.87	11.24	7.61	3.98	0.35				

FIGURE 20-8

JOB SKILL 20-6 *(continued)*

UNMARRIED head of household—SEMIMONTHLY payroll period

If wages are...   And the number of withholding allowances claimed is...   **STATE**

At least	But less than	0	1	2	3	4	5	6	7	8	9	10 Or more
		...The amount of income tax to be withheld is...										
$1	$600											
600	620	3.39										
620	640	3.59										
640	660	3.79	0.16									
660	680	3.99	0.36									
680	700	4.19	0.56									
700	720	4.39	0.76									
720	740	4.59	0.96									
740	760	4.79	1.16									
760	780	4.99	1.36									
780	800	5.19	1.56									
800	820	5.51	1.88									
820	840	5.91	2.28									
840	860	6.31	2.68									
860	880	6.71	3.08									
880	900	7.11	3.48									
900	920	7.51	3.88	0.25								
920	940	7.91	4.28	0.65								
940	960	8.31	4.68	1.05								
960	980	8.71	5.08	1.45								
980	1000	9.11	5.48	1.85								
1000	1025	9.56	5.93	2.30								
1025	1050	10.06	6.43	2.80								
1050	1075	10.56	6.93	3.30								
1075	1100	11.06	7.43	3.80	0.17							
1100	1125	11.56	7.93	4.30	0.67							
1125	1150	12.06	8.43	4.80	1.17							
1150	1175	12.56	8.93	5.30	1.67							
1175	1200	13.06	9.43	5.80	2.17							
1200	1225	13.56	9.93	6.30	2.67							
1225	1250	14.06	10.43	6.80	3.17							
1250	1275	14.56	10.93	7.30	3.67	0.04						
1275	1300	15.06	11.43	7.80	4.17	0.54						
1300	1325	15.56	11.93	8.30	4.67	1.04						
1325	1350	16.06	12.43	8.80	5.17	1.54						
1350	1375	16.56	12.93	9.30	5.67	2.04						
1375	1400	17.06	13.43	9.80	6.17	2.54						
1400	1450	17.81	14.18	10.55	6.92	3.29						
1450	1500	18.81	15.18	11.55	7.92	4.29	0.66					
1500	1550	19.92	16.29	12.66	9.03	5.40	1.77					
1550	1600	21.92	18.29	14.66	11.03	7.40	3.77	0.14				
1600	1650	23.92	20.29	16.66	13.03	9.40	5.77	2.14				
1650	1700	25.92	22.29	18.66	15.03	11.40	7.77	4.14	0.51			
1700	1750	27.92	24.29	20.66	17.03	13.40	9.77	6.14	2.51			
1750	1800	29.92	26.29	22.66	19.03	15.40	11.77	8.14	4.51	0.88		
1800	1850	31.92	28.29	24.66	21.03	17.40	13.77	10.14	6.51	2.88		
1850	1900	33.92	30.29	26.66	23.03	19.40	15.77	12.14	8.51	4.88	1.25	
1900	2000	38.32	34.69	31.06	27.43	23.80	20.17	16.54	12.91	9.28	5.65	2.02
2000	2100	44.32	40.69	37.06	33.43	29.80	26.17	22.54	18.91	15.28	11.65	8.02
2100	2200	50.32	46.69	43.06	39.43	35.80	32.17	28.54	24.91	21.28	17.65	14.02
2200	2300	56.32	52.69	49.06	45.43	41.80	38.17	34.54	30.91	27.28	23.65	20.02
2300 and over		(Table Amount PLUS 9.3 Percent of the Amount Over 2250)										

FIGURE 20-9

JOB SKILL 20-6 *(continued)*

MARRIED persons—MONTLY payroll period

If wages are...   And the number of withholding allowances claimed is...   **STATE**

...The amount of income tax to be withheld shall be...

At least	But less than	0	1	2	3	4	5	6	7	8	9	10 Or more
$1	$600											
600	640	3.49										
640	680	3.89										
680	720	4.29										
720	760	4.69										
760	800	5.09										
800	840	5.49										
840	880	5.89										
880	920	6.29										
920	960	6.69										
960	1000	7.09										
1000	1040	7.49	0.23									
1040	1080	7.89	0.63									
1080	1120	8.29	1.03									
1120	1160	8.69	1.43									
1160	1200	9.09	1.83									
1200	1240	9.49	2.23									
1240	1280	9.89	2.63									
1280	1320	10.29	3.03									
1320	1360	10.86	3.60									
1360	1400	11.66	4.40									
1400	1440	12.46	5.20									
1440	1480	13.26	6.00									
1480	1520	14.06	6.80									
1520	1560	14.86	7.60									
1560	1600	15.66	8.40									
1600	1640	16.46	9.20									
1640	1680	17.26	10.00									
1680	1720	18.06	10.80									
1720	1760	18.86	11.60									
1760	1800	19.66	12.40									
1800	1840	20.46	13.20	0.51								
1840	1880	21.26	14.00	1.31								
1880	1920	22.06	14.80	2.11								
1920	1960	22.86	15.60	2.91								
1960	2000	23.66	16.40	3.71								
2000	2040	24.46	17.20	4.51								
2040	2080	25.26	18.00	5.31								
2080	2140	26.26	19.00	6.31								
2140	2200	27.46	20.20	7.51	0.25							
2200	2260	28.66	21.40	8.71	1.45							
2260	2320	29.86	22.60	9.91	2.65							
2320	2380	31.06	23.80	11.11	3.85							
2380	2440	32.26	25.00	12.31	5.05							
2440	2500	33.46	26.20	13.51	6.25							
2500	2560	34.66	27.40	14.71	7.45	0.19						
2560	2620	35.86	28.60	15.91	8.65	1.39						
2620	2680	37.06	29.80	17.11	9.85	2.59						
2680	2740	38.26	31.00	18.31	11.05	3.79						
2740	2800	39.51	32.25	19.51	12.25	4.99						
2800	2860	41.91	34.65	20.71	13.45	6.19						

FIGURE 20-10

JOB SKILL 20-6 (*continued*)

UNMARRIED head of household—MONTHLY payroll period

If wages are...   And the number of withholding allowances claimed is...   **STATE**

At least	But less than	0	1	2	3	4	5	6	7	8	9	10 Or more
					... The amount of income tax to be withheld shall be...							
$1	1400											
1400	1420	8.68	1.42									
1420	1440	8.88	1.62									
1440	1460	9.08	1.82									
1460	1480	9.28	2.02									
1480	1500	9.48	2.22									
1500	1520	9.68	2.42									
1520	1540	9.88	2.62									
1540	1560	10.08	2.82									
1560	1580	10.28	3.02									
1580	1600	10.48	3.22									
1600	1620	10.81	3.55									
1620	1640	11.21	3.95									
1640	1660	11.61	4.35									
1660	1680	12.01	4.75									
1680	1720	12.61	5.35									
1720	1760	13.41	6.15									
1760	1800	14.21	6.95									
1800	1840	15.01	7.75	0.49								
1840	1880	15.81	8.55	1.29								
1880	1920	16.61	9.35	2.09								
1920	1960	17.41	10.15	2.89								
1960	2000	18.21	10.95	3.69								
2000	2040	19.01	11.75	4.49								
2040	2080	19.81	12.55	5.29								
2080	2120	20.61	13.35	6.09								
2120	2160	21.41	14.15	6.89								
2160	2200	22.21	14.95	7.69	0.43							
2200	2250	23.11	15.85	8.59	1.33							
2250	2300	24.11	16.85	9.59	2.33							
2300	2350	25.11	17.85	10.59	3.33							
2350	2400	26.11	18.85	11.59	4.33							
2400	2450	27.11	19.85	12.59	5.33							
2450	2500	28.11	20.85	13.59	6.33							
2500	2550	29.11	21.85	14.59	7.33	0.07						
2550	2600	30.11	22.85	15.59	8.33	1.07						
2600	2650	31.11	23.85	16.59	9.33	2.07						
2650	2700	32.11	24.85	17.59	10.33	3.07						
2700	2800	33.61	26.35	19.09	11.83	4.57						
2800	2900	35.61	28.35	21.09	13.83	6.57						
2900	3000	37.61	30.35	23.09	15.83	8.57	1.31					
3000	3100	39.85	32.59	25.33	18.07	10.81	3.55					
3100	3200	43.85	36.59	29.33	22.07	14.81	7.55	0.29				
3200	3300	47.85	40.59	33.33	26.07	18.81	11.55	4.29				
3300	3400	51.85	44.59	37.33	30.07	22.81	15.55	8.29	1.03			
3400	3500	55.85	48.59	41.33	34.07	26.81	19.55	12.29	5.03			
3500	3600	59.85	52.59	45.33	38.07	30.81	23.55	16.29	9.03	1.77		
3600	3800	65.85	58.59	51.33	44.07	36.81	29.55	22.29	15.03	7.77	0.51	
3800	4000	76.64	69.38	62.12	54.86	47.60	40.34	33.08	25.82	18.56	11.30	4.04
4000	4200	88.64	81.38	74.12	66.86	59.60	52.34	45.08	37.82	30.56	23.30	16.04
4200	4400	100.64	93.38	86.12	78.86	71.60	64.34	57.08	49.82	42.56	35.30	28.04
4400 and over		(Table Amount PLUS 9.3 Percent of the Amount Over 4300)										

FIGURE 20-11

JOB SKILL 20-7
Complete a Payroll Register

Name _____ Date _____ Score _____

Performance Objective

Task: Insert employee payroll data to complete a payroll register.

Conditions: Need:

- Computer with Internet connection
- Online Form 105 (one payroll register) located at www.cengagebrain.com with student resources
- Payroll information obtained for seven employees from Job Skill 20-6
- Pen or pencil

Refer to:

- *Textbook* Procedure 20-2 for step-by-step directions
- *Textbook* Figure 20-14 for a visual example

Standards: Complete all steps listed in this skill in _____ minutes with a minimum score of _____. (Time element and accuracy criteria may be given by instructor.)

Time: **Start:** _____ **Completed:** _____ **Total:** _____ minutes

Scoring: One point for each step performed satisfactorily unless otherwise listed or weighted by instructor.

Directions with Performance Evaluation Checklist

Refer to the employees in Job Skill 20-6. Alphabetize their names (last name first), and record the information in the payroll register.

1st Attempt	2nd Attempt	3rd Attempt	
_____	_____	_____	Gather materials (equipment and supplies) listed under *Conditions*.
___/14	___/14	___/14	1. Complete payroll register information for employee Lisa Adams.
___/13	___/13	___/13	2. Complete payroll register information for employee Kelley Jones.
___/13	___/13	___/13	3. Complete payroll register information for employee Maryjane Moran.
___/13	___/13	___/13	4. Complete payroll register information for employee Carla O'Hare.
___/14	___/14	___/14	5. Complete payroll register information for employee Amy Seaforth.
___/13	___/13	___/13	6. Complete payroll register information for employee Hillary Sheehan.
___/11	___/11	___/11	7. Complete payroll register information for employee Roger Young.
_____	_____	_____	Complete within specified time.
___/93	___/93	___/93	**Total points earned** (To obtain a percentage score, divide the total points earned by the number of points possible.)

Comments:

Evaluator's Signature: _____ **Need to Repeat:** _____

National Curriculum Competency:

JOB SKILL 20-8
Complete an Employee Earning Record

Name _____ Date _____ Score _____

Performance Objective

Task: Complete an employee earning record for Amy Seaforth.

Conditions: Need:

- Computer with Internet connection
- Online Form 106 (one employee earning record) located at www.cengagebrain.com with student resources
- Information from Job Skill 20-6
- Pen or pencil

Standards: Complete all steps listed in this skill in _____ minutes with a minimum score of _____. (Time element and accuracy criteria may be given by instructor.)

Time: Start: _____ Completed: _____ Total: _____ minutes

Scoring: One point for each step performed satisfactorily unless otherwise listed or weighted by instructor.

Directions with Performance Evaluation Checklist

Refer to Amy Seaforth's employment information in Job Skill 20-6 and complete an employee earning record; she is a new employee.

1st Attempt	2nd Attempt	3rd Attempt	
_____	_____	_____	Gather materials (equipment and supplies) listed under *Conditions*.
____/5	____/5	____/5	1. Fill in the employee's name, address, telephone number, and Social Security number.
____/8	____/8	____/8	2. Fill in the employee's date of hire, birth date, position, number of exemptions, and rate of pay indicating (with a circle) whether she is part-time or full-time; single or married; and paid hourly, weekly, or monthly.
____/12	____/12	____/12	3. Complete all line items in the earning record that are applicable to Amy Seaforth for May 28, 20XX.
_____	_____	_____	Complete within specified time.
____/27	____/27	____/27	**Total points earned** (To obtain a percentage score, divide the total points earned by the number of points possible.)

Comments:

Evaluator's Signature: _____ **Need to Repeat:** _____

National Curriculum Competency:

JOB SKILL 20-9
Complete an Employee's Withholding Allowance Certificate

Name _____ Date _____ Score _____

Performance Objective

Task: Complete an employee's withholding allowance certificate.

Conditions: Need:

- Computer with Internet connection
- Online Form 107 (Employee's Withholding Allowance Certificate) located at www.cengagebrain.com with student resources
- Pen or pencil

Refer to:

- *Workbook* Appendix A (physician information)
- *Textbook* Figure 20-8 for an illustration of a completed W-4 form

Standards: Complete all steps listed in this skill in _____ minutes with a minimum score of _____. (Time element and accuracy criteria may be given by instructor.)

Time: Start: _____ Completed: _____ Total: _____ minutes

Scoring: One point for each step performed satisfactorily unless otherwise listed or weighted by instructor.

Directions with Performance Evaluation Checklist

Complete an Employee's Withholding Allowance Certificate for yourself as if you were being hired by Drs. Gerald and Fran Practon.

1st Attempt	2nd Attempt	3rd Attempt	
_____	_____	_____	Gather materials (equipment and supplies) listed under *Conditions*.
____/5	____/5	____/5	1. Read through Items A through G, and mark which allowances you would like to claim.
_____	_____	_____	2. Total all deductions and enter in Line H.
____/4	____/4	____/4	3. Fill in your last name, first name, and address.
_____	_____	_____	4. Fill in your Social Security number. You may use a mock SSN or the last four digits for confidentiality.
_____	_____	_____	5. Indicate whether you are single, married, or married and withholding at a higher single rate.
_____	_____	_____	6. Verify your last name with that appearing on your Social Security card and indicate if it is different.
_____	_____	_____	7. Indicate the number of allowances in Item 5.
_____	_____	_____	8. Read Items 6 and 7 and mark if applicable.
____/2	____/2	____/2	9. Sign and date the form.
____/3	____/3	____/3	10. Complete the employer's name and address in Item 8.
_____	_____	_____	11. Fill in the Employer Identification Number (EIN) for Practon Medical Group, Inc., in Item 10.

JOB SKILL 20-9 *(continued)*

_____ _____ _____   Complete within specified time.

____/23 ____/23 ____/23   **Total points earned** (To obtain a percentage score, divide the total points earned by the number of points possible.)

Comments:

Evaluator's Signature: _____ **Need to Repeat:** _____

National Curriculum Competency:

JOB SKILL 20-10
Complete an Employee Benefit Form

Name _____ Date _____ Score _____

Performance Objective

Task: Extract information from the case scenario, calculate employee benefits, and complete an employee benefit form.

Conditions: Need:
- Computer with Internet connection
- Online Form 108 (employee benefit form) located at www.cengagebrain.com with student resources
- Calculator
- Pen or pencil

Refer to:
- *Textbook* Figure 20-10 for an illustration of a completed benefit form

Standards: Complete all steps listed in this skill in _____ minutes with a minimum score of _____.
(Time element and accuracy criteria may be given by instructor.)

Time: **Start:** _____ **Completed:** _____ **Total:** _____ minutes

Scoring: One point for each step performed satisfactorily unless otherwise listed or weighted by instructor.

Directions with Performance Evaluation Checklist

Extract information for the following case scenario and complete an employee benefit form.

Scenario: You have just been hired by Drs. Gerald and Fran Practon as a full-time administrative medical assistant, and they have agreed to pay you $1760 per month, which amounts to approximately $10 per hour. You receive six paid holidays per year and one week (5 days) paid vacation after the first year. You have 10 sick days per year and $150 yearly uniform allowance. There are no retirement benefits; there may be an incentive bonus if the practice does well. The practice pays for your medical insurance, which costs $60 per month, and you elect to get life insurance at your own expense, at $12 per month for $100,000 coverage. You also elect to get accident insurance at an additional $4.60 per month for $200,000 coverage. Drs. Practon pay $15.35 per month for your workers' compensation insurance and an additional $17.60 per month for your disability insurance. They pay for your dues to the American Association of Medical Assistants, which are $90 per year.

1st Attempt	2nd Attempt	3rd Attempt	
_____	_____	_____	Gather materials (equipment and supplies) listed under *Conditions*.
_____	_____	_____	1. Calculate the employer/employee benefits for medical insurance.
_____	_____	_____	2. Calculate the employer/employee benefits for life insurance.
_____	_____	_____	3. Calculate the employer/employee benefits for accident insurance.
_____	_____	_____	4. Calculate the employer/employee benefits for disability insurance.
_____	_____	_____	5. Calculate the employer/employee benefits for workers' compensation.
_____	_____	_____	6. Calculate the employer/employee benefits for holidays.
_____	_____	_____	7. Calculate the employer/employee benefits for vacation.
_____	_____	_____	8. Calculate the employer/employee benefits for sick leave.

JOB SKILL 20-10 (*continued*)

_____	_____	_____	9. Complete the employer/employee benefits for personal leave.
_____	_____	_____	10. Complete the employer/employee benefits for education.
_____	_____	_____	11. Complete the employer/employee benefits for incentive bonus.
_____	_____	_____	12. Complete the employer/employee benefits for retirement.
_____	_____	_____	13. Complete the employer/employee benefits for uniforms.
_____	_____	_____	14. Complete other employer/employee benefits.
_____	_____	_____	15. Total all employer-paid benefits.
_____	_____	_____	16. Total all employee-paid benefits.
_____	_____	_____	17. Fill in the wage of the employee.
_____	_____	_____	18. Calculate the gross wage for the year.
___/6	___/6	___/6	19. Calculate the amount for the total employee package paid by the employer.
___/5	___/5	___/5	Complete within specified time.
___/30	___/30	___/30	**Total points earned** (To obtain a percentage score, divide the total points earned by the number of points possible.)

Comments:

Evaluator's Signature: _____   **Need to Repeat:** _____

National Curriculum Competency: CAAHEP: Cognitive: II.C.1   ABHES: 7.a

Practon Medical Group, Inc.

- **Introduction**
- **Medical Practice Reference Material**
- **Office Policies**
- **Payment Policies and Health Insurance Protocol**
- **Fee Schedule**
- *CPT* **Modifiers**
- *HCPCS Level II* **Codes**

INTRODUCTION

To gain practical experience and put theory to work, assume that you have been hired to work as an administrative medical assistant for a husband-and-wife team; Dr. Fran T. Practon is a family practitioner (FP) and Dr. Gerald M. Practon is a general practitioner (GP). Their practice is called Practon Medical Group, Inc., and they are on the staff of College Hospital. You will be presented with realistic scenarios and will perform tasks in the *Workbook* Job Skills as if you were employed in their office. Use this reference material for data required in the assignments.

MEDICAL PRACTICE REFERENCE MATERIAL

Practon Medical Group, Inc.
4567 Broad Avenue
Woodland Hills, XY 12345-4700
Telephone Number: (555) 486-9002
Fax Number: (555) 488-7815
Email: PMGI@aol.com
Group National Provider Identification Number (NPI): 36640210XX
Group Tax Employer Identification Number (EIN): 20-8765432
Medicare Durable Medical Equipment (DME) Supplier Number: 33420985XX

Fran T. Practon, MD
State License Number: C 1503X
National Provider Identification Number (NPI): 65499947XX
Federal Tax Employer Identification Number (EIN): 73-40313XX

Gerald M. Practon, MD
State License Number: C 1402X
National Provider Identification Number (NPI): 46278897XX
Federal Tax Employer Identification Number (EIN): 78-51342XX

College Hospital
4500 Broad Avenue
Woodland Hills, XY 12345-4700
Telephone Number: (555) 487-6789
Fax Number: (555) 487-6790
Hospital National Provider Identification Number (NPI): 54378601XX

OFFICE POLICIES

The office policies set by Drs. Fran and Gerald Practon appear on the next several pages. Refer to them for daily routines, office hours, appointment scheduling, telephone procedures, and filling practices as you complete the *Workbook* Job Skills. Account information is also included to help determine fees and office policies regarding charges.

Daily Routine

Both physicians prefer that the medical assistant call the answering service for messages right after the office is opened and office machines are turned on. Incoming mail should be opened and sorted when it arrives. Correspondence is to be mailed the same day it is dictated. Chart notes are to be transcribed electronically or placed in each patient's medical record as soon as possible after the dictation is received, typically within 72 hours.

Office Hours

Office hours are 9:00 a.m. to 5:00 p.m. Monday through Friday. The lunch hour is from 12:00 noon to 1:00 p.m. Both physicians leave the office at 3:00 p.m. on Wednesdays and reserve one morning each week for surgery and additional hospital responsibilities. Gerald reserves Tuesday mornings and Fran reserves Thursday mornings. Each physician covers the office while the other is at the hospital. No elective appointments are scheduled between 11:30 a.m. and noon or between 4:30 p.m. and 5:00 p.m. to allow time for callbacks, work-ins, emergencies, and dictation. An asterisk (*) distinguishes Fran's patients from Gerald's when physician verification is necessary. *Record office hours' information on a 3" by 5" card for easy reference.*

Appointments

Both physicians work by appointment. New patients receiving a complete physical examination or consultation are scheduled for one hour. Routine follow-up appointments for established patients are scheduled for half an hour. Brief office visits for services such as suture removals, cast checks, dressing changes, injections, and blood pressure checks are scheduled for 15-minute appointments. Appointments should be scheduled at the earliest time available and consecutively when possible. Check with the physician regarding time frames for office procedures and hospital surgeries. House calls are discouraged but, if necessary, are made after 5:00 p.m.

Patients should be specific in outlining the nature of their medical problem so appropriate time is allowed. If multiple problems exist and are made known by the patient, additional time will be allotted. There is no charge if appointments are cancelled 24 hours in advance; uncancelled appointments are billed at one-half the usual fee. *Record appointment information on the back of the office hours 3" by 5" card for easy reference.* Refer to Table B-2 and B-3 in Appendix B of the *Workbook* for appointment terms and their abbreviations.

Telephone Procedures

The medical assistant answers most inquiries so the physicians need not leave patients during examinations to answer the telephone. When a medical emergency arises or a telephone call is received from another physician, it may be necessary to knock on the door of the treatment room and advise the physician of the urgency of the telephone call or ask the physician if he or she wishes to take the call. When the assistant is unable to give a complete answer to a question asked via telephone, the physician is consulted and typically reviews the medical record and either calls back the same day or has a member of the staff make the callback. Routine calls that the physicians personally return are made after 11:30 a.m., during the lunch hour, or after 4:30 p.m. Generally, there is no charge for telephone calls.

Filing Procedures

The "Patient Information" (registration) form is stapled to the left inside area of the file folder. Folders are filed alphabetically according to rules established by the Association of Records Managers and Administrators (ARMA), and material is filled chronologically within each section—on the right side of the file folder. In lieu of file folder dividers, sections may be indicated with a colored sheet of paper, titled according to the section. Sections include the following (starting from the front of the chart):

- Progress notes
- Consultations
- Operative reports
- Laboratory test reports
- Radiology reports

History and physical reports for new patients or yearly examinations and progress notes for established patients are filed under "Progress Notes". Correspondence and telephone communication in reference to patients are also filed under the patient's name, in chronological order under "Progress notes."

The history and physical report as well as the discharge summary are filed along with the operative report for the patient's hospital encounter.

Ledger cards are kept alphabetically in a special file container; however, in our mock situation, place them in front of the patient's file folder behind the "Patient Information" form.

PAYMENT POLICIES AND HEALTH INSURANCE PROTOCOL

After a patient is seen, the fee is determined by referring to the *CPT** code listing and the correct column in the fee schedule. The fee is posted to the patient's account (ledger card) and entered on the daily journal (daysheet). All monies received by mail are posted in the same manner on the day they arrive. The first statement is given to the patient at the time of service or sent shortly thereafter. Successive statements are sent every 30 days according to a schedule set by the first date of service.

Uninsured patients are expected to pay at the time of service. The office accepts cash, checks, and debit/credit cards. Professional discounts are not typically allowed; however, uninsured or cash patients who pay the entire bill in cash at the time of service are allowed a 20% discount. If either physician treats an uninsured physician, a professional discount or no charge is considered. Financial hardship cases are reviewed case by case.

Patients who have health insurance coverage are expected to pay copayments prior to services being rendered. Insured patients are responsible for the total amount of the bill at the time services are rendered and will receive regular statements after the date of service; however, their insurance company is billed by Practon Medical Group, Inc., and patients can wait until the insurance company pays their portion before paying the coinsurance amount. If the insurance payment is delayed, the patient is responsible for paying the bill and contacting the insurance company to help resolve the problem.

When coding insurance claims, use codes from the Standard Code Set, which has been developed by the Centers for Medicare and Medicaid Services (CMS). Codes in this standard that apply to billing outpatient medical claims include the following:

- *International Classification of Diseases, 10th Revision, Clinical Modification (ICD-10-CM)*—diagnostic codes
- *Current Procedural Terminology (CPT)**—also referred to as *HCPCS Level I* codes for procedures and services
- *Healthcare Common Procedure Coding System (HCPCS)—HCPCS Level II* codes

When coding diagnoses using *ICD-10-CM*, refer to the following example, which illustrates how to locate a code by the main term found in the diagnostic statement.

Note: To identify the main term, ask "What is wrong with the patient?" The additional term may state where the problem is (anatomic site), identify the *time frame* in which the patient is experiencing the problem (e.g., acute, subacute, or chronic), or further define the *type* of problem (e.g., *alcoholic* liver disease).

*2017 Current Procedural Terminology only © 2016 American Medical Association. All rights reserved.

Example of Main Terms			
Diagnostic Statement	**Main Term**	***ICD-10-CM* Codes**	**Additional Term**
muscle atrophy	atrophy	M62.50	muscle—where
chronic bronchitis	bronchitis	J42	chronic—time frame
allergic conjunctivitis (chronic)	conjunctivitis	H10.45	allergic—type
recurrent depression	depression	F33.9	recurrent—time frame
nasal (bone) fracture	fracture	S02.2xxA	nasal—where

For information regarding filing health insurance claim forms, refer to Chapter 18 and the CMS-1500 Field-by-Field Instructions in Appendix A of the *textbook*. Both physicians bill using their group tax EIN (see Field 25) and their group NPI number (see Field 33), *not independently*.

FEE SCHEDULE

Following is Figure A-1, the fee schedule for Practon Medical Group, Inc. Fees are listed numerically according to *CPT** code number as found in the codebook. Section titles of the codebook and subsection titles of the Surgery section are included for easy reference. All fees listed are examples only. Fees can vary according to the region of the United States (West, Midwest, South, and East), the type of community (urban, suburban, or rural), the type of practice (solo, group, and so forth), and the specialty of the practitioner, as well as the practice overhead, expense, and a number of other factors.

The seven columns in the fee schedule are as follows:

- **Column 1 (*CPT* Code Number)** lists selected code numbers from 2017 *CPT*.*
- **Column 2 (*CPT* Code Description)** contains abbreviated descriptions of procedures and services.

2017 Current Procedural Terminology only © 2016 American Medical Association. All rights reserved.

- **Column 3 (Mock Fee)** shows the physician's standard fees. These are used to bill private patients as well as those on Medicaid, TRICARE, and workers' compensation.
- **Column 4 (Medicare—Participating)** lists the allowed amounts Medicare approves for a physician with a contract. Medicare pays 80% of this fee, the patient pays 20%, and the difference between the allowed amount and the charged amount is written off the books as a courtesy adjustment.
- **Column 5 (Medicare—Nonparticipating)** shows the allowed amounts Medicare approves for non-contracted physicians. Medicare pays 80% of this fee, and 20% is collected from the patient (see comments under Limiting Charge).
- **Column 6 (Limiting Charge)** lists the highest amounts that a nonparticipating physician is allowed to bill for the service rendered. In addition to the 20% collected from the nonparticipating physician's allowed amount, the noncontracted physician can also collect the difference between the nonparticipating fee (charged amount) and the limiting charge from the patient.
- **Column 7 (Follow-Up Days)** lists the number of global follow-up days included in a surgical package.

Drs. Gerald and Fran Practon are both contracted with Medicare and use the participating fee unless otherwise stated.

FIGURE A-1 Fee schedule for Practon Medical Group, Inc., for reference when completing *Workbook* Job Skills.

FRAN T. PRACTON, M.D.	GERALD M. PRACTON, M.D.
Family Practice	General Practice

Practon Medical Group, Inc.
4567 Broad Avenue
Woodland Hills, XY 12345-4700

FEE SCHEDULE

		Medicare		
CPT Code No. and Description	Mock Fees	Participating	Nonparticipating	Limiting Charge
EVALUATION AND MANAGEMENT*				
OFFICE **New Patient**				
99201 Level I	33.25	30.43	28.91	33.25
99202 Level II	51.91	47.52	45.14	51.91
99203 Level III	70.92	64.92	61.67	70.92
99204 Level IV	106.11	97.13	92.27	106.11
99205 Level V	132.28	121.08	115.03	132.38
Established Patient				
99211 Level I	16.07	14.70	13.97	16.07
99212 Level II	28.55	26.14	24.83	28.55
99213 Level III	40.20	36.80	34.96	40.20
99214 Level IV	61.51	56.31	53.49	61.51
99215 Level V	96.97	88.76	84.32	96.97
HOSPITAL Observation Services (new or established patient)				
99217 Discharge, other than initial date of observation status	66.88	61.22	58.16	66.88
99218 Initial observation care (D/C hx/exam SF/LC DM)	74.22	67.91	64.54	74.22
99219 Initial observation care (C hx/exam MC DM)	117.75	107.78	102.39	117.75
99220 Initial observation care (C hx/exam HC DM)	147.48	134.99	128.24	147.48
Initial Hospital Care (new or established patient)				
99221 30 min	73.00	66.82	63.48	73.00
99222 50 min	120.80	110.57	105.04	120.80
99223 70 min	152.98	140.03	133.03	152.98
Subsequent Hospital Care				
99231 15 min	37.74	34.55	32.82	37.74
99232 25 min	55.56	50.85	48.31	55.56
99233 35 min	76.97	70.45	66.93	76.97

(continues)

*See Tables 16-2 and 16-3 in Chapter 16 of the *textbook* for more description of E/M codes. Descriptions here include levels of E/M codes (e.g., Level I, Level II, etc.), which correspond with the last digit of the code, and abbreviations for the level of history, examination, and medical decision-making (e.g., problem focused [PF], expanded problem focused [EPF], and/or straightforward [SF]).

2017 Current Procedural Terminology only © 2016 American Medical Association. All rights reserved.

FIGURE A-1 Fee schedule (*continued*)

			Medicare		
CPT Code No. and Description		Mock Fees	Participating	Nonparticipating	Limiting Charge
Subsequent Hospital Care (*continued*)					
99238	Discharge (30 min or less)	65.26	59.74	56.75	65.26
99239	more than 30 min				
CONSULTATIONS office (new or established patient)					
99241	Level I	51.93	47.54	45.16	51.93
99242	Level II	80.24	73.44	69.77	80.24
99243	Level III	103.51	94.75	90.01	103.51
99244	Level IV	145.05	132.77	126.13	145.05
99245	Level V	195.48	178.93	169.98	195.48
Inpatient (new/established patient)					
99251	Level I	53.29	48.78	46.34	53.29
99252	Level II	80.56	73.74	70.05	80.56
99253	Level III	106.10	97.12	92.26	106.10
99254	Level IV	145.26	132.96	126.31	145.26
99255	Level V	196.55	179.91	170.91	196.55
EMERGENCY DEPARTMENT (new/established patient)					
99281	PF hx/exam SF DM	24.32	22.26	21.15	24.32
99282	EPF hx/exam LC DM	37.02	33.88	32.19	37.02
99283	EPF hx/exam MC DM	66.23	60.62	57.59	66.23
99284	D hx/exam MC DM	100.71	92.18	87.57	100.71
99285	C hx/exam HC DM	158.86	145.41	138.14	158.86
CRITICAL CARE SERVICES					
99291	First 30–74 min	208.91	191.22	181.66	208.91
+99292*	Each addl 30 min	102.02	92.46	87.84	102.02
NURSING FACILITY (initial new/established patient)					
99304	D/C hx/exam SF/LC DM	64.11	58.68	55.75	64.11
99305	C hx/exam MC DM	90.55	82.88	78.74	90.55
99306	C hx/exam HC DM	136.76	125.18	118.92	136.76
Subsequent (new/est pt)					
99307	PF hx/exam SF DM	37.95	34.74	33.00	37.95
99308	EPF hx/exam LC DM	55.11	50.44	47.92	55.11
99309	D hx/exam MC DM	69.61	63.72	60.53	69.61
99310	C hx/exam HC DM	83.12	77.11	74.88	83.12
DOMICILIARY, REST HOME, CUSTODIAL CARE New patient					
99324	PF hx/exam SF DM	46.10	42.20	40.09	46.10
99325	EPF hx/exam LC DM	65.02	59.52	56.54	65.02
99326	D hx/exam MC DM	86.18	78.88	74.94	86.18
99327	C hx/exam MC DM	105.77	113.54	109.40	105.77
99328	C hx/exam HC DM	123.98	131.06	127.62	123.98
Established patient					
99334	PF hx/exam SF DM	37.31	34.15	32.44	37.31
99335	EPF hx/exam LC DM	49.22	45.05	42.80	49.22

(*continues*)

*The symbol + indicates an add-on code in *CPT* 2017.

FIGURE A-1 Fee schedule (*continued*)

CPT Code No. and Description		Mock Fees	Medicare* Participating	Medicare* Nonparticipating	Medicare* Limiting Charge
99336	D hx/exam MC DM	60.61	55.47	52.70	60.61
99337	C hx/exam MC/HC DM	72.03	77.65	74.12	72.03
HOME SERVICES New patient					
99341	PF hx/exam SF DM	70.32	64.37	61.15	70.32
99342	EPF hx/exam LC DM	91.85	84.07	79.87	91.85
99343	D hx/exam MC DM	120.24	110.06	104.56	120.24
99344	C hx/exam MC DM	131.04	122.16	116.98	131.04
99345	C hx/exam HC DM	148.67	132.59	124.88	148.67
Established patient					
99347	PF hx/exam SF DM	54.83	50.19	47.68	54.83
99348	EPF hx/exam LC DM	70.06	64.13	60.92	70.06
99349	D hx/exam MC DM	88.33	80.85	76.81	88.33
99350	C hx/exam M//HC DM	101.36	94.54	88.21	101.36
PROLONGED SERVICES WITH CONTACT Outpatient					
+99354	E/M or Psychotherapy; first hour	96.67	88.76	84.32	96.97
+99355	Each addl 30 min	96.97	88.76	84.32	96.97
Inpatient					
+99356	First hour	96.42	88.25	83.84	96.42
+99357	Each addl 30 min	96.42	88.25	83.84	96.42
PROLONGED SERVICES WITHOUT DIRECT CONTACT					
99358	First hour	90.00			
+99359	Each addl 30 min	90.00			
STANDBY SERVICES					
99360	Each 30 min	95.00			
CASE MANAGEMENT SERVICES					
Team Conferences					
99366	Face-to-face; health care prof 30 min	102.00			
99367	Non-face-to-face; health care prof 30 min; physician	93.00			
99368	nonphysician prof	85.00			
CARE PLAN OVERSIGHT SERVICES					
99374	Home health pt 15–29 min	93.40	85.49	81.22	93.40
99375	greater than 30 min	118.00			
PREVENTIVE MEDICINE New Patient					
99381	Infant under age 1 year	50.00			
99382	1–4 years	50.00			
99383	5–11 years	45.00			
99384	12–17 years	45.00			

(continues)

*Some services and procedures may not be considered a benefit under the Medicare program; however, it is important to include these codes when billing because Medicare policies may change. For this reason, some of the services shown in this mock fee schedule do not have any amounts listed under the three Medicare columns.

2017 Current Procedural Terminology only © 2016 American Medical Association. All rights reserved.

FIGURE A-1 Fee schedule (*continued*)

CPT Code No. and Description		Mock Fees	Medicare*		
			Participating	Nonparticipating	Limiting Charge
PREVENTIVE MEDICINE New Patient (*continued*)					
99385	18–39 years	50.00			
99386	40–64 years	50.00			
99387	65 years and over	55.00			
Established Patient					
99391	Infant under age 1 year	35.00			
99392	1–4 years	35.00			
99393	5–11 years	30.00			
99394	12–17 years	30.00			
99395	18–39 years	35.00			
99396	40–64 years	35.00			
99397	65 years and over	40.00			
COUNSELING (new/established patient)					
Individual—Preventive Medicine					
99401	15 min	35.00			
99402	30 min	50.00			
99403	45 min	65.00			
99404	60 min	80.00			
Group—Preventive Medicine					
99411	30 min	30.00			
99412	60 min	50.00			
Other Preventive Medicine Services					
99429	Unlisted preventive med serv	variable			
NON-FACE-TO-FACE-PHYSICIAN SERVICES					
Telephone Services					
99441	Simple/brief (5–10 min)	30.00			
99442	Intermediate (11–20 min)	40.00			
99443	Complex (21–30 min)	60.00			
NEWBORN CARE (evaluation)					
99460	Initial hosp or birthing center care	102.15	93.50	88.83	102.15
99461	other than hosp or birth room (per day)	110.16	100.83	95.79	110.16
99462	Subsequent hospital care	54.02	49.44	46.97	54.02
99463	Initial hospital or birthing center care, per day; discharge same day	240.55	220.18	209.17	240.55
99464	Newborn stabilization	248.97	239.22	231.23	248.97
99465	Newborn resuscitation	255.98	234.30	222.59	255.98

(continues)

*Some services and procedures may not be considered a benefit under the Medicare program; however, it is important to include these codes when billing because Medicare policies may change. For this reason, some of the services shown in this mock fee schedule do not have any amounts listed under the three Medicare columns.

2017 Current Procedural Terminology only © 2016 American Medical Association. All rights reserved.

FIGURE A-1 Fee schedule (*continued*)

CPT Code No. and Description		Mock Fees	Medicare*		
			Participating	Nonparticipating	Limiting Charge
NEONATAL AND PEDIATRIC INTENSIVE CARE					
99468	Initial (28 days or younger)	933.89	887.20	1,020.28	933.89
99469	Subsequent (28 days or younger)	410.80	390.26	448.80	410.80
99471	Initial (29 days–24 mo)	784.38	745.16	856.93	784.38
99472	Subsequent (29 days–24 mo)	399.77	379.78	436.75	399.77
99475	Initial (2–5 yrs)	565.70	537.42	618.03	565.70
99476	Subsequent (2–5 yrs)	343.00	325.85	374.73	343.00

ANESTHESIOLOGY

Anesthesiology fees are presented here for *CPT* codes. However, each case would require unit values indicating time, for example, every 15 minutes would be worth $55. Some anesthetists may list a surgical code with a modifier indicating "anesthesiologist" for carriers that do not acknowledge anesthesia codes.

QUALIFYING CIRCUMSTANCES

+99100	Anes for pt under 1 yr/ over 70	55.00
+99116	Anes complicated by use of total hypothermia	275.00
+99135	Anes complicated by use of hypotension	275.00
+99140	Anes complicated by emer cond	110.00

PHYSICAL STATUS MODIFIER CODES

P-1	Normal healthy patient	variable
P-2	Patient with mild systemic disease	variable
P-3	Patient with severe systemic disease	55.00
P-4	Patient with severe systemic disease (constant threat to life)	110.00
P-5	Moribund pt not expected to survive without the operation	165.00
P-6	Declared brain-dead, pt organs being removed for donor	variable

HEAD

00160	Anes for proc nose & accessory sinuses: NOS	275.00
00172	Anes repair cleft palate	165.00

(continues)

*Some services and procedures may not be considered a benefit under the Medicare program; however, it is important to include these codes when billing because Medicare policies may change. For this reason, some of the services shown in this mock fee schedule do not have any amounts listed under the three Medicare columns.

2017 Current Procedural Terminology only © 2016 American Medical Association. All rights reserved.

FIGURE A-1 Fee schedule (*continued*)

CPT Code No. and Description		Mock Fees	Medicare*		
			Participating	Nonparticipating	Limiting Charge
THORAX					
00400	Anes for proc integumentary system extremities, ant trunk, and perineum	165.00			
00402	Breast reconstruction	275.00			
00546	Anes pulmonary resection with thoracoplasty	275.00			
SPINE AND SPINAL CORD					
00600	Anes cervical spine and cord	550.00			
LOWER ABDOMEN					
00800	Anes for proc lower ant abdominal wall	165.00			
00840	Anes intraperitoneal proc lower abdomen: NOS	330.00			
00842	Amniocentesis	220.00			
PERINEUM					
00914	Anes TURP	275.00			
00942	Anes colpotomy, vaginectomy, colporrhaphy, open urethral proc	220.00			
UPPER LEG					
01210	Anes open proc, hip	330.00			
01214	total hip replacement	440.00			
UPPER ARM AND ELBOW					
01740	Anes open/arthroscopic proc upper arm/elbow; NOS	220.00			
01758	Anes open/arthoscopic proc on elbow; exc cyst/tumor humerus	275.00			
RADIOLOGIC PROCEDURES					
01922	Anes noninvasive imaging/radiation therapy	385.00			

(*continues*)

*Some services and procedures may not be considered a benefit under the Medicare program; however, it is important to include these codes when billing because Medicare policies may change. For this reason, some of the services shown in this mock fee schedule do not have any amounts listed under the three Medicare columns.

2017 Current Procedural Terminology only © 2016 American Medical Association. All rights reserved.

FIGURE A-1 Fee schedule (*continued*)

CPT Code No. and Description	Mock Fees	Medicare		Limiting Charge	Follow-Up Days*
		Participating	Nonparticipating		
INTEGUMENTARY SYSTEM					
10060 I & D furuncle, cyst, paronychia; single	75.92	69.49	66.02	75.92	10
11100 Biopsy of skin, SC tissue &/or mucous membrane; 1 lesion	65.43	59.89	56.90	65.43	0
11200 Removal skin tags; up to 15	55.68	50.97	48.42	55.68	10
11401 Exc benign lesion, 0.6–1.0 cm; trunk, arms, legs	95.62	87.53	83.15	96.62	10
11402 1.1–2.0 cm	121.52	111.23	105.67	121.52	10
11403 2.1–3.0 cm	151.82	138.97	132.02	151.82	10
11420 Exc benign lesion, 0.5 cm or less; scalp, neck, hands, feet, genitalia	75.44	69.05	65.60	75.44	10
11422 1.1–2.0 cm	131.35	120.23	114.22	131.35	10
11441 Exc benign lesion face, ears, eyelids, nose, lips, or mucous membrane; 0.6–1.0 cm dia or less	119.08	109.00	103.55	119.08	10
11602 Exc malignant lesion, trunk, arms, or legs; 1.1–2.0 cm dia	195.06	178.55	169.62	195.06	10
11720 Debridement of nails; 1–5	32.58	29.82	28.33	32.58	0
11721 6 or more	32.58	29.82	28.33	32.58	0
11730 Avulsion nail plate, partial or complete, simple; single	76.91	70.40	66.88	76.91	0

(*continues*)

Global Period

Various services are associated with an operative procedure when they are considered integral parts of that procedure. The global period refers to the time frame during which all services integral to the surgical procedure are covered by a single payment.

0   Services provided the day of the procedure are included in the fee schedule amount.

10   Services provided the day of and during the 10-day period following the surgical procedure are included in the fee schedule amount.

90   Services provided the day before, the day of, and during the 90-day period following the surgical procedure are included in the fee schedule amount.

INC   Services are included in the global period of another related service.

N/A   Not applicable

*Timeframes for the surgical follow-up days may vary according to insurance carrier and are listed as examples only.

2017 Current Procedural Terminology only © 2016 American Medical Association. All rights reserved.

FIGURE A-1 Fee schedule (*continued*)

CPT Code No. and Description	Mock Fees	Medicare			
		Participating	Nonparticipating	Limiting Charge	Follow-Up Days*
INTEGUMENTARY SYSTEM (continued)					
11750 Exc nail or nail matrix, partial or complete; permanent	193.45	177.07	168.22	193.45	10
12001 Simple repair (scalp, neck, axillae, ext genitalia, trunk, or extremities incl hands & feet); 2.5 cm or less	91.17	83.45	79.82	91.17	10
12011 Simple repair (face, ears, eyelids, nose, lips, or mucous membranes); 2.5 cm or less	101.44	92.85	88.21	101.44	10
12013 2.6–5.0 cm	123.98	113.48	107.81	123.98	10
12032 Repair, scalp axillae, trunk (intermediate) 2.6–7.5 cm	169.73	155.36	147.59	169.73	10
12034 7.6–12.5 cm	214.20	196.06	186.26	214.20	10
12051 Repair, intermediate, layer closure of wounds (face, ears, eyelids, nose, lips, or mucous membranes); 2.5 cm or less	167.60	153.41	145.74	167.60	10
17000 Destruction benign or premalignant lesion, first	37.38	34.58	32.85	37.38	10
+ 17003 2–14 lesions, each	19.41	17.77	16.88	19.41	NA
17110 Destruction benign lesions, other than skin tags (laser, electro-, cryo-, chemosurgery, curettement); up to 14 lesions	77.05	70.53	67.00	77.05	10
17111 15 or more lesions	88.92	81.39	77.32	88.92	10
19020 Mastotomy, drainage /exploration; deep	237.36	217.26	206.40	237.36	90
19100 Biopsy, breast, needle core	96.17	88.03	83.63	96.17	0
19101 open, incisional	281.51	257.67	244.79	281.51	10
MUSCULOSKELETAL SYSTEM					
20610 Arthrocentesis, aspiration, or injection; major joint (shoulder, hip, knee) or bursa	52.33	47.89	45.50	52.33	0

(continues)

*Timeframes for the surgical follow-up days may vary according to insurance carrier and are listed as examples only.

2017 Current Procedural Terminology only © 2016 American Medical Association. All rights reserved.

FIGURE A-1 Fee schedule (*continued*)

CPT Code No. and Description		Mock Fees	Medicare Participating	Nonparticipating	Limiting Charge	Follow-Up Days*
21330	Nasal fracture, open treatment complicated	599.46	548.71	521.27	599.46	90
24066	Biopsy, soft tissue, upper arm, elbow; superficial deep	383.34	350.88	333.34	383.34	90
27455	Osteotomy, proximal tibia	1248.03	1142.36	1085.24	1248.03	90
27500	Treatment closed femoral shaft fracture without manipulation	554.90	507.92	482.52	554.90	90
27530	Treatment closed tibial fracture, proximal, without manipulation	344.24	315.90	299.34	344.24	90
27750	Treatment closed tibial shaft fracture without manipulation	400.94	366.99	348.64	400.94	90
27752	with manipulation	531.63	486.62	462.29	531.63	90
29345	Appl long leg cast (thigh to toes)	123.23	112.80	107.16	123.23	0
29355	walker or ambulatory type	133.75	122.42	116.30	133.75	0
29425	Appl short leg walking cast	102.10	93.45	88.78	102.10	0
RESPIRATORY SYSTEM						
30110	Excision, nasal polyp; simple	145.21	132.92	126.27	145.21	10
30520	Septoplasty	660.88	604.93	574.68	660.88	90
30903	Control nasal hemorrhage; anterior; complex	118.17	108.17	102.76	118.17	0
30905	Control nasal hemorrhage, posterior with posterior nasal packs; initial	190.57	174.43	165.71	190.57	0
30906	subsequent	173.01	158.36	150.44	173.01	0
31625	Bronchoscopy with biopsy; single/ multiple	312.87	286.38	272.06	312.87	0
32310	Pleurectomy, parietal	1234.79	1130.24	1073.73	1234.79	90
32440	Pneumonectomy, total	1972.10	1805.13	1714.87	1972.10	90

(continues)

*Timeframes for the surgical follow-up days may vary according to insurance carrier and are listed as examples only.

2017 Current Procedural Terminology only © 2016 American Medical Association. All rights reserved.

FIGURE A-1 Fee schedule (*continued*)

CPT Code No. and Description		Mock Fees	Medicare			
			Participating	Nonparticipating	Limiting Charge	Follow-Up Days*
CARDIOVASCULAR SYSTEM						
33020	Pericardiotomy	1289.25	1180.09	1121.09	1289.25	90
33206	Insertion of pacemaker; atrial	728.42	666.75	633.41	728.42	90
33208	AV	751.57	687.89	653.50	751.57	90
35301	Thromboend-arterectomy, inc patch graft; carotid, vertebral, subclavian by neck incision	1585.02	1450.82	1378.28	1585.02	90
36005	Intravenous injection for contrast venography; extremity	59.18	54.17	51.46	59.18	0
36245	Catheter placement (selective) arterial system, ea first order	68.54	62.74	59.60	68.54	NA
36415	Routine venipuncture for collection of specimen(s)	10.00	—	—	—	XXX
38101	Splenectomy, partial	994.44	910.24	864.73	994.44	90
38510	Biopsy, open excision, deep cervical lymph node(s)	327.42	299.69	284.71	327.42	10
MEDIASTINUM/DIAPHRAGM/DIGESTIVE SYSTEM						
42820	T & A under age 12 years	341.63	312.71	297.07	341.63	90
42821	over age 12 years	410.73	375.96	357.16	410.73	90
43213	Esophagoscopy with dilation	201.86	184.77	175.53	201.86	0
43235	Esophagogastro-duodenoscopy; diag inc collection of specimen by brushing or washing (sep proc)	238.92	218.69	207.76	238.92	0
43239	with biopsy, single or multiple	254.52	232.97	221.32	254.52	0
43334	Repair hiatal hernia1	436.50	1314.87	1249.13	1436.50	90
43820	Gastrojejunostomy	971.86	889.58	845.10	971.86	90
44150	Colectomy, total, abdominal	1757.81	1608.98	1528.53	1757.81	90
44320	Colostomy or skin cecostomy	966.25	884.44	840.22	966.25	90

(continues)

*Timeframes for the surgical follow-up days may vary according to insurance carrier and are listed as examples only.

2017 Current Procedural Terminology only © 2016 American Medical Association. All rights reserved.

FIGURE A-1 Fee schedule (*continued*)

CPT Code No. and Description		Mock Fees	Medicare			
			Participating	Nonparticipating	Limiting Charge	Follow-Up Days*
44950	Appendectomy	568.36	520.24	494.23	568.36	90
45308	Proctosigmoidoscopy with removal of single tumor/polyp	135.34	123.88	117.69	135.34	0
45315	multiple tumors /polyps	185.12	169.44	160.97	185.12	0
45330	Sigmoidoscopy, diagnostic, with /without collection of specimen (by brushing or washing)	95.92	87.80	83.41	95.92	0
45380	Colonoscopy with biopsy; single /multiple	382.35	349.98	332.48	382.35	0
46255	Hemorrhoidectomy int & ext, single	503.57	460.94	437.89	503.57	90
46258	with fistulectomy	636.02	582.17	553.06	636.02	90
46600	Anoscopy; diagnostic	32.86	30.07	28.57	32.86	0
46614	with control of bleeding	182.10	166.68	158.35	182.10	0
46700	Anoplasty for stricture, adult	657.39	601.73	571.64	657.39	90
47600	Cholecystectomy	937.74	858.35	815.43	937.74	90
49505	Inguinal hernia repair, age 5 or over	551.07	504.41	479.19	551.07	90
49520	Repair, inguinal hernia, any age; recurrent	671.89	615.00	584.25	671.89	90
URINARY SYSTEM						
50080	Nephrostolithotomy, percutaneous	1323.93	1211.83	1151.24	1323.93	90
50780	Ureteroneocystostomy	1561.23	1429.84	1357.59	1561.23	90
51900	Closure of vesicovaginal fistula, abdominal approach	1196.32	1095.48	1040.71	1196.82	90
52000	Cystourethroscopy	167.05	152.90	145.26	167.05	0
52601	Transurethral electrosurgical resection of prostate	888.87	813.61	772.93	888.87	90
53040	Drainage of deep periurethral abscess	520.11	476.07	452.27	520.11	90

(continues)

*Timeframes for the surgical follow-up days may vary according to insurance carrier and are listed as examples only.

2017 Current Procedural Terminology only © 2016 American Medical Association. All rights reserved.

FIGURE A-1 Fee schedule (*continued*)

CPT Code No. and Description		Mock Fees	Medicare			
			Participating	Nonparticipating	Limiting Charge	Follow-Up Days*
URINARY SYSTEM (*continued*)						
53230	Excision, female diverticulum (urethral)	859.69	786.91	747.56	859.69	90
53240	Marsupialization of urethral diverticulum, M or F	520.11	476.07	452.27	520.11	90
53620	Dilation, urethra, male; initial	100.73	92.20	87.59	100.73	0
53660	Dilation, urethra, female; initial	48.32	44.23	42.02	48.32	0
MALE/FEMALE GENITAL SYSTEM						
54150	Circumcision—clamp type	111.78	102.32	97.20	111.78	10
54520	Orchiectomy, simple	523.92	479.56	455.58	523.92	90
55700	Biopsy of prostate, needle or punch; single/multiple	156.22	142.99	135.84	156.22	0
55801	Prostatectomy, perineal subtotal	1466.56	1342.39	1275.27	1466.56	90
57265	Colporrhaphy AP with enterocele repair	902.24	825.85	784.56	902.24	90
57452	Colposcopy, cervix	84.18	77.05	73.20	84.18	0
57511	Cryocauterization of cervix	195.83	179.25	170.29	195.83	10
57520	Conization of cervix, with/without D & C, cold knife/laser	387.08	354.30	336.59	387.08	90
58100	Endometrial biopsy	71.88	65.79	62.50	71.88	0
58120	D & C diagnostic and/or therapeutic (nonOB)	272.83	249.73	237.24	272.83	10
58150	TAH w/without salpingo-oophorectomy	1167.72	1068.85	1015.41	1167.72	90
58200	TAH, including partial vaginectomy, w/lymph node sampling	1707.24	1562.69	1484.56	1707.24	90
58210	Radical TAH w/ttl pelvic lymphadenectomy & lymph node sampling	2160.78	1977.83	1878.94	2160.78	90
58300	Insertion of intrauterine device	100.00	—	—	—	NA

(*continues*)

*Timeframes for the surgical follow-up days may vary according to insurance carrier and are listed as examples only.

2017 Current Procedural Terminology only © 2016 American Medical Association. All rights reserved.

FIGURE A-1 Fee schedule (*continued*)

CPT Code No. and Description		Mock Fees	Medicare			
			Participating	Nonparticipating	Limiting Charge	Follow-Up Days*
58340	Hysterosalpingography with inj proc	73.06	66.87	63.53	73.06	0
58720	Salpingo-oophorectomy, complete/partial, uni-/bilateral	732.40	670.39	636.87	732.40	90
MATERNITY CARE AND DELIVERY						
59120	Surgical treatment of ectopic pregnancy; salpingectomy and/or oophorectomy	789.26	722.43	686.31	789.26	90
59121	without salpingectomy and /or oophorectomy	638.84	584.75	555.51	638.84	90
59130	abdominal pregnancy	699.12	639.93	607.93	699.12	90
59135	interstitial, uterine pregnancy rq ttl hysterectomy	1154.16	1056.44	1003.62	1154.16	90
59136	partial uterine resection, interstitial uterine pregnancy	772.69	707.26	671.90	772.69	90
59140	cervical, with evacuation	489.68	448.22	425.81	489.68	90
59160	Curettage; postpartum	293.46	268.61	255.18	293.46	10
59400	OB care—routine with vag dlvy, inc antepartum /postpartum care	1864.30	1706.45	1621.13	1864.30	NA
59510	C-section, inc antepartum and postpartum care	2102.33	1924.33	1828.11	2102.33	NA
59515	C-section, inc postpartum care	1469.80	1345.36	1278.09	1469.80	NA
59812	Surgical treatment of incompl abortion, any trimester	357.39	327.13	310.77	357.39	90
NERVOUS SYSTEM						
61314	Craniotomy; extradural or subdural	2548.09	2332.35	2215.73	2548.09	90
62270	Spinal puncture, lumbar; diagnostic	77.52	70.96	67.41	77.52	0

(continues)

*Timeframes for the surgical follow-up days may vary according to insurance carrier and are listed as examples only.

2017 Current Procedural Terminology only © 2016 American Medical Association. All rights reserved.

FIGURE A-1 Fee schedule (*continued*)

CPT Code No. and Description		Mock Fees	Medicare			
			Participating	Nonparticipating	Limiting Charge	Follow-Up Days*
EYE AND OCULAR ADNEXA						
65091	Excision of eye, without implant	708.22	648.25	615.84	708.22	90
65205	Removal of foreign body, ext eye	56.02	51.27	48.71	56.02	0
65222	corneal, with slit lamp	73.81	67.56	64.18	73.81	0
69420	Myringotomy	97.76	89.48	85.01	97.76	10
RADIOLOGY, NUCLEAR MEDICINE, AND DIAGNOSTIC ULTRASOUND						
70120	X-ray mastoids, 1–2 views p/side	38.96	35.66	33.88	38.96	
70130	3 plus views p/side	56.07	51.33	48.76	56.07	
71010	X-ray chest, 1 view	31.95	29.24	27.78	31.95	
71020	2 views	40.97	37.50	35.63	40.97	
71030	compl, 4 views	54.02	49.44	46.97	54.02	
72100	X-ray spine, lumbosacral, 2–3 views	43.23	39.57	37.59	43.23	
72114	complete, incl bending views, minimum 6	74.97	68.62	65.19	74.97	
73100	X-ray wrist, 2 views	31.61	28.94	27.49	31.61	
73501	X-ray hip, 1 view	31.56	28.88	27.44	31.56	
73502	X-ray pelvis & hips, infant or child, 2 views	37.94	34.73	32.99	37.94	
73590	X-ray tibia & fibula, 2 views	33.35	30.53	29.00	33.35	
73620	Radiologic exam, foot; 2 views	31.61	28.94	27.49	31.61	
73650	X-ray calcaneus, min 2 views	30.71	28.11	26.70	30.71	
74241	Radiologic exam, upper GI tract, with/ without delayed images, with KUB	108.93	99.71	94.72	108.93	
74245	with small bowel; multiple images	161.70	148.01	140.61	161.70	
74270	Barium enema; w/wo KUB	118.47	108.44	103.02	118.47	
74290	Oral cholecystography	52.59	48.14	45.73	52.59	

(*continues*)

*Timeframes for the surgical follow-up days may vary according to insurance carrier and are listed as examples only.

2017 Current Procedural Terminology only © 2016 American Medical Association. All rights reserved.

FIGURE A-1 Fee schedule (*continued*)

CPT Code No. and Description		Mock Fees	Medicare* Participating	Medicare* Nonparticipating	Medicare* Limiting Charge
74400	Urography (pyelography), intravenous, with or without KUB	104.78	95.90	91.11	104.78
74410	Urography, infusion	116.76	106.87	101.53	116.76
74420	Urography, retrograde; w/wo KUB	138.89	127.13	120.77	138.89
76805	Ultrasound, pregnant uterus, real time; after first trimester; sngl or 1st gestation	154.18	141.13	134.07	154.18
+ 76810	each additional gestation	306.54	280.59	266.56	306.54
76946	Ultrasonic guidance for amniocentesis; supervision & interpretation	91.22	83.49	79.32	91.22
77065	Mammography, diagnostic, unilateral	62.57	57.27	54.51	62.57
77066	bilateral	82.83	75.82	72.03	82.83
77300	Radiation dosimetry	97.58	89.32	84.85	97.58
77315	Brachytherapy isodose plan, complex	213.59	195.51	185.73	213.59
78104	Bone marrow imaging, whole body	230.56	211.04	200.49	230.56
78215	Liver and spleen imaging	160.44	146.85	139.51	160.44
78800	Tumor localization, limited area	191.53	175.32	166.55	191.53

PATHOLOGY AND LABORATORY**

Laboratory tests done as groups or combination "profiles" performed on multichannel equipment should be billed using the appropriate code number (80047 through 80076). Following is a list of the panels.

80047	Basic metabolic panel (Calcium, ionized)	75.00
80048	Basic metabolic panel (Calcium, total)	75.00
80050	General health panel	50.00
80051	Electrolyte panel	50.00

(continues)

*Some services and procedures may not be considered a benefit under the Medicare program; however, it is important to include these codes when billing because Medicare policies may change. For this reason, some of the services shown in this mock fee schedule do not have any amounts listed under the three Medicare columns.

**Mock fees for laboratory tests presented in this schedule may not be representative of fees in your region due to the variety of insurance contracts and discount policies. Providers must have the CLIA Level of licensure to bill for tests, and test results must be documented.

2017 Current Procedural Terminology only © 2016 American Medical Association. All rights reserved.

FIGURE A-1 Fee schedule (*continued*)

CPT Code No. and Description		Mock Fees	Medicare*		
			Participating	Nonparticipating	Limiting Charge
PATHOLOGY AND LABORATORY (*continued*)					
80053	Comprehensive metabolic panel	200.00			
80055	Obstetric panel	75.00			
80061	Lipid panel	50.00			
80069	Renal function panel	150.00			
80074	Acute hepatitis panel	50.00			
80076	Hepatic function panel	75.00			
81000	Urinalysis (dip stick), non-automated, with microscopy	8.00	7.44	5.98	8.84
81001	automated, with microscopy	8.00	7.44	5.98	8.84
81002	non-automated, without microscopy	8.00	7.44	5.98	8.84
81015	Urinalysis, microscopy only	8.00	7.44	5.98	8.84
81025	Urine pregnancy test; color	10.00			
82565	Creatinine; blood	10.00	9.80	8.88	12.03
82951	Glucose tol test, 3 spec	40.00	41.00	36.80	45.16
+ 82952	each add spec beyond 3	30.00	28.60	25.97	32.16
83020	Hemoglobin, electrophoresis	25.00	20.00	19.94	23.93
83700	Lipoprotein, blood; electrophoretic separation	25.00	20.00	19.94	23.93
84478	Triglycerides, blood	20.00	19.20	15.99	21.87
84480	Triiodothyronine (T-3)	20.00	19.20	15.99	21.87
84520	Urea nitrogen; quantitative	25.00	20.99	19.94	23.93
84550	Uric acid; blood	20.00	19.20	15.99	21.87
84702	Gonadotropin, chorionic; quantitative	20.00	19.20	15.99	21.87
84703	qualitative	20.00	19.20	15.99	21.87

(*continues*)

*Some services and procedures may not be considered a benefit under the Medicare program; however, it is important to include these codes when billing because Medicare policies may change. For this reason, some of the services shown in this mock fee schedule do not have any amounts listed under the three Medicare columns.

2017 Current Procedural Terminology only © 2016 American Medical Association. All rights reserved.

FIGURE A-1 Fee schedule (*continued*)

CPT Code No. and Description		Mock Fees	Medicare		
			Participating	Nonparticipating	Limiting Charge
85018	Blood count, hemoglobin	20.00	19.20	15.99	21.87
85025	Complete blood count (CBC, Hgb, RBC, WBC, and platelet count), automated, differential WBC count	25.00	20.00	19.94	23.93
85032	manual count (each)	25.00	20.00	19.94	23.93
85097	Bone marrow, smear interpretation	73.52	67.29	63.93	73.52
85345	Coagulation time; Lee & White	20.00	19.20	15.99	21.87
86038	Antinuclear antibodies (ANA)	25.00	20.00	19.94	23.93
87081	Culture, screening; pathogenic organisms	25.00	20.00	19.94	23.93
87181	Susceptibility studies, antibiotic; per agent	20.00	19.20	15.99	21.87
87184	disk method, per plate (12 disks or less)	20.00	19.20	15.99	21.87
87210	Smear, primary source; wet mount with simple stain, for infectious agents	35.00	48.35	45.93	55.12
88150	Papanicolaou cytopath, manual screen (vag or cerv); phys supervision	35.00	48.35	45.93	55.12
88302	Surgical pathology (level II), gross & micro exam (skin, fingers, nerve, testis)	24.14	22.09	20.99	24.14
88305	Surgical pathology (level IV); bone marrow, interpret	77.69	71.12	67.56	77.69

(continues)

FIGURE A-1 Fee schedule (*continued*)

CPT Code No. and Description		Mock Fees	Medicare*		
			Participating	Nonparticipating	Limiting Charge
MEDICINE SECTION					
Immunization Administration and Products for Vaccines/Toxoids					
90471	Immunization admin. (inj.); one (single or combination)	2.50			
90473	Immunization admin. intranasal /oral; one (single or combination)	2.50			
90702	Diphtheria & tetanus (younger than 7years)	34.00			
90713	Poliovirus vaccine, SubQ or IM	28.00			
90714	Diphtheria & Tetanus (7 years or older)	34.00			
Psychiatry					
90832	Ind psychotherapy 30 min (pt)	73.70	67.46	64.09	73.30
+90833	with E/M service	82.88	75.86	72.07	82.88
90834	Ind psychotherapy 45 min (pt)	110.23	100.89	95.98	110.23
90853	Group therapy (other than multiple family group)	29.22	26.75	25.41	29.22
Hemodialysis					
90935	Hemodialysis with single eval	117.23	107.31	101.94	117.23
90937	Hemodialysis with repeat eval	206.24	188.78	179.34	206.24
Gastroenterology					
91010	Esophageal motility with interpretation & report	69.82	63.91	60.71	69.82
91030	Esophagus, acid perfusion test	87.41	80.01	16.01	87.41
Ophthalmologic Services					
92004	Comprehensive eye exam; NP	90.86	83.17	79.01	90.86

(continues)

*Some services and procedures may not be considered a benefit under the Medicare program; however, it is important to include these codes when billing because Medicare policies may change. For this reason, some of the services shown in this mock fee schedule do not have any amounts listed under the three Medicare columns.

2017 Current Procedural Terminology only © 2016 American Medical Association. All rights reserved.

FIGURE A-1 Fee schedule (*continued*)

| CPT Code No. and Description | Mock Fees | Medicare | | Limiting Charge |
		Participating	Nonparticipating	
92100 Tonometry (serial)	47.31	43.31	41.14	47.31
92230 Fluorescein angioscopy	55.49	50.79	48.25	55.49
92275 Electroretinography	81.17	74.29	70.58	81.17
92531 Spontaneous nystagmus	26.00			
Audiologic Function Tests				
92557 Comprehensive audiometry	54.33	49.73	47.24	54.33
92596 Ear protector measurements	26.81	24.54	23.31	26.81
Cardiography				
93000 Electrocardiogram (ECG)	34.26	31.36	29.79	34.26
93015 Treadmill ECG, with supervision, interpretation, and report	140.71	128.80	122.36	140.71
93040 Rhythm ECG; 1–3 leads	18.47	16.90	16.06	18.47
Pulmonary				
94010 Spirometry	38.57	35.31	33.54	38.57
94060 Spirometry before and after bronchodilator	71.67	65.60	62.32	71.67
94150 Vital capacity, total	13.82	12.65	12.02	13.82
Allergy and Clinical Immunology				
95024 Intradermal tests, including interpretation and report	6.58	6.02	5.72	6.58
95044 Patch tests (specify number)	8.83	8.08	7.68	8.83
95115 Treatment for allergy, single inj	17.20	15.75	14.96	17.20
95117 two or more inj	22.17	20.29	19.28	22.17
95165 Prof service for super of preparation and antigens for allergen immunotherapy, single or multiple antigens (specify no of doses)	3.63	3.33	3.16	3.63
Neurology and Neuromuscular Procedures				
95812 Electroencephalogram, 41–60 min	129.32	118.37	112.45	129.32

(*continues*)

FIGURE A-1 Fee schedule (*continued*)

CPT Code No. and Description		Mock Fees	Medicare*		
			Participating	Nonparticipating	Limiting Charge
Neurology and Neuromuscular Procedures (*continued*)					
95819	inc recording, awake and asleep	126.81	116.07	110.27	126.81
95860	Electromyography, needle, 1 extremity	88.83	81.31	77.24	88.83
95864	4 extremities	239.99	219.67	208.69	239.99
96102	Psychological testing (per hour)	80.95	74.10	70.39	80.95
Therapeutic Prophylactic and Diagnostic Injections					
96372	Therapeutic, prophylactic, or diagnostic inj; IM or SC	4.77	4.37	4.15	4.77
96374	IV push	21.33	19.53	18.55	21.33
Physical Medicine					
97024	Application of modality (supervised), 1 or more areas; diathermy	14.27	13.06	12.41	14.27
97036	Application of modality (constant attendance); Hubbard tank, each 15 min	24.77	22.67	21.54	24.77
97110	Physical therapy, one or more areas; 15 min	23.89	21.86	20.77	23.89
97140	Manual therapy, one or more areas; 15 min	16.93	15.49	14.72	16.93
Special Services and Reports					
99000	Handling of specimen (transfer from office to lab)	5.00			
99050	Services requested after office hours in addition to basic service	25.00			
99056	Services normally provided in office requested by pt in location other than office	20.00			
99058	Office services provided on an emergency basis, disrupting schedule	65.00			

(continues)

*Some services and procedures may not be considered a benefit under the Medicare program; however, it is important to include these codes when billing because Medicare policies may change. For this reason, some of the services shown in this mock fee schedule do not have any amounts listed under the three Medicare columns.

2017 Current Procedural Terminology only © 2016 American Medical Association. All rights reserved.

FIGURE A-1 Fee schedule (*continued*)

CPT Code No. and Description		Mock Fees	Medicare*		
			Participating	Nonparticipating	Limiting Charge
99070	Supplies and materials over and above those usually required (itemize drugs/materials)	25.00			
99080	Special reports: Insurance forms	10.00			
	Review of data to clarify pt's status	20.00			
	WC reports	50.00			
	WC extensive review report	250.00			

*Some services and procedures may not be considered a benefit under the Medicare program; however, it is important to include these codes when billing because Medicare policies may change. For this reason, some of the services shown in this mock fee schedule do not have any amounts listed under the three Medicare columns.

2017 Current Procedural Terminology only © 2016 American Medical Association. All rights reserved.

CPT MODIFIERS*

–22	Increased procedural services (attach report to claim)
–23	Unusual anesthesia (pt requires general anesthetic instead of none or local anesthesia)
–24	Unrelated evaluation and management service by the same physician during a postoperative period
–25	Significant, separate identifiable evaluation and management service by the same physician on the day of a procedure
–26	Professional component (physician interpretation only, not technical component)
–32	Mandated services (e.g., consult requested by a third-party payor)
–33	Preventive services
–47	Anesthesia by surgeon
–50	Bilateral procedure
–51	Multiple procedures performed on the same day or at the same session
–52	Reduced services
–53	Discontinued procedure
–54	Surgical care only
–55	Postoperative management only
–56	Preoperative management only
–57	Decision for surgery (use with E/M service performed just prior to major surgery)
–58	Staged or related procedure or service by the same physician during the postoperative period
–59	Distinct procedural service
–62	Two surgeons (usually with different skills)
–63	Procedure performed on infants less than 4 kg
–66	Surgical team
–76	Repeat procedure by the same physician or other qualified health care professional
–77	Repeat procedure by another physician or other qualified health care professional
–78	Unplanned return to the operating room for a related procedure during the postoperative period
–79	Unrelated procedure or service by the same physician or other qualified health care professional during the postoperative period
–80	Assistant surgeon
–81	Minimum assistant surgeon
–82	Assistant surgeon (when qualified resident surgeon not available)
–90	Reference (outside) laboratory procedures performed by a lab other than the treating physician
–91	Repeat clinical diagnostic laboratory test
–92	Alternative laboratory platform testing
–95	Synchronous telemedicine service rendered via a real-time interactive audio and video telecommunications system
–99	Multiple modifiers (use of two or more modifiers for a service)

HCPCS Level II CODES**

These codes have been selected from many *HCPCS* codes as examples. The fees stated are only examples.

		FEES
A0422	Ambulance service, oxygen supplies, life sustaining situation	$600.00
A4206	Syringe with needle; 1 cc	10.00
A5051	Ostomy pouch; one piece with barrier attached	15.00
A6410	Eye pad, sterile	15.00
A9150	Nonprescription drugs	10.00
B4034	Enteral feeding supply kit; syringe fed, per day	25.00
E0100	Cane; any material, adjustable or fixed	60.00
E0114	Crutches; underarm, other than wood	100.00
G0008	Administration, influenza virus vaccine	10.00
H0001	Alcohol and/or drug assessment	75.00
J0120	Injection, tetracycline, up to 250 mg	25.00
J0171	Injection, adrenalin, 0.1 mg	25.00
J0558	Injection, penicillin G, 100,000 units	25.00
J1460	Injection, gamma globulin, intramuscular, 1 cc	20.00
L0180	Cervical, multiple post collar	50.00
L3209	Surgical boot, child	50.00
M0075	Cellular therapy	70.00
P3001	Papanicolaou smear screening (up to 3), interpretation by physician	25.00

*For a full description of *CPT* modifiers with examples, see *textbook* Table 16-5.

**2016 HCPCS *Level II* codes used.

2017 Current Procedural Terminology only © 2016 American Medical Association. All rights reserved.

Abbreviation Tables

TABLE B-1
Common Address Abbreviations

Address	Abbreviation	Address	Abbreviation	Address	Abbreviation	Address	Abbreviation
Alley	ALY	East	E	Park	PK	Street	ST
Annex	ANX	Estates	ESTS	Parkway	PKWY	Suite	STE
Apartment	APT	Expressway	EXPY	Place	PL	Summit	SMT
Arcade	ARC	Extension	EXT	Plaza	PLZ	Terrace	TER
Association	ASSN	Freeway	FWY	Point	PT	Track	TRAK
Avenue	AVE	Grove	GRV	Port	PRT	Trail	TRL
Bayou	BYU	Harbor	HBR	Prairie	PR	Tunnel	TUNL
Beach	BCH	Heights	HTS	President	PRES	Turnpike	TPKE
Bend	BND	Hill	HL	Ranch	RNCH	Union	UN
Bluff	BLF	Hospital	HOSP	Rapids	RPDS	Valley	VLY
Bottom	BTM	Institute	INST	Ridge	RDG	Viaduct	VIA
Boulevard	BLVD	Isle	ISLE	River	RIV	Vice	
Branch	BR	Island	IS	Road	RD	President	VP
Bridge	BRG	Junction	JCT	Room	RM	View	VW
Brook	BRK	Lake	LK	Route	RT	Village	VLG
Burg	BG	Lakes	LKS	Row	ROW	Ville	VL
Bypass	BYP	Lane	LN	Run	RUN	Vista	VIS
Camp	CP	Mall	MALL	Rural	R	Walk	WALK
Canyon	CYN	Manager	MGR	Secretary	SECY	Way	WAY
Cape	CPE	Manor	MNR	Shoal	SHL	Wells	WLS
Causeway	CSWY	Mount	MT	Shore	SH	West	W
Center	CTR	Mountain	MTN	South	S		
Circle	CIR	North	N	Southeast	SE		
Cliffs	CLFS	Northeast	NE	Southwest	SW		
Club	CLB	Northwest	NW	Spring	SPG		
Court	CT	Orchard	ORCH	Square	SQ		
Drive	DR	Palms	PLMS	Station	STA		

TABLE B-2
Appointment and Patient Care Abbreviations

Abbreviation	Definition	Abbreviation	Definition
a	allergy; abortion	CI	color index
AB	antibiotic	c m	centimeter
abd, abdom	abdominal, abdomen	CNS	central nervous system
abt	about	CO, C/O	complains of
Acc, acc	accommodation	CO_2, CO2	carbon dioxide
acid	accident	comp	comprehensive
adm	admit; admission; admitted	compl	complete
adv	advice	con, CON,	
aet.	At the age of	Cons, Consult	consultation
$AgNO_3$	silver nitrate	Cont.	continue
AIDS	acquired immune deficiency syndrome	COPD	chronic obstructive pulmonary
alb	albumin		disease
ALL	allergy	CPE, CPX	complete physical examination
a.m., AM	before noon	C section, C/S	cesarean section
AMA	American Medical Association	CT	computerized tomography
an ck	annual check	CV	cardiovascular
an PX	annual physical examination	CVA	costovertebral angle; cardiovascular
ant	anterior		accident; cerebrovascular accident
ante	before	CXR	chest x-ray
A & P	auscultation and percussion	Cysto, cysto	cystoscopy
AP	anterior posterior; anteroposterior;	D & C	dilatation and curettage
	antepartum care	dc	discontinue
AP & L	anteroposterior and lateral	DC	discharge, dressing change
approx.	approximate	del	delivery
apt	apartment	Dg, dg, Dx, dx	diagnosis
ASA	acetylsalicylic acid (Aspirin)	diag.	diagnosis, diagnostic
asap, ASAP	as soon as possible	diam.	diameter
ASCVD	arteriosclerotic cardiovascular	diff.	differential
	disease	dilat	dilate
ASHD	arteriosclerotic heart disease	disch.	discharged
asst	assistant	DNA	does not apply
auto	automobile	DNKA	did not keep appointment
ba	barium	DNS	did not show
BI	biopsy	DOB	date of birth
BM	bowel movement	dr, drsg	dressing
BMR	basal metabolic rate	DSHA	does she have appointment
BP, B/P	blood pressure	DTaP*	diphtheria, tetanus, and pertussis
BP ck, BP ✓	blood pressure check		(vaccine)
breast ck	breast check	Dx, Dg, dx	diagnosis
Brev	Brevital (drug)	E	emergency
BS	blood sugar	ECG	electrocardiogram; electrocardiograph
BUN	blood urea nitrogen	ED	emergency department
Bx, BX	biopsy	EDC	estimated date of confinement;
C	cervical; centigrade; Celsius		due date for baby
C & S	culture and sensitivity	EEG	electroencephalogram;
Ca, CA	cancer, carcinoma		electroencephalograph
canc, cncl	cancel, canceled	EENT	eye, ear, nose, and throat
cast ck	cast check	EKG	electrocardiogram;
Cauc	Caucasian		electrocardiograph
CBC	complete blood count	EMG	electromyogram, electromyelogram
CC	chief complaint	epith.	epithelial
CDC	calculated date of confinement	ER	emergency room
chem.	chemistry	ESR	erythrocyte sedimentation rate
CHF	congestive heart failure	est.	established; estimated
chr	chronic	etiol.	etiology
ck, ✓	check	EU	etiology unknown

*Abbreviation approved by the Joint Commission as the preferred abbreviation.

TABLE B-2
Appointment and Patient Care Abbreviations (*continued*)

Abbreviation	Definition	Abbreviation	Definition
Ex, exam.	examination	int, INT	internal
exc.	excision	intermed	intermediate
ext	external	interpret	interpretation
F	Fahrenheit; French (catheter)	IPPB	intermittent positive pressure breathing
FH	family history	IQ	intelligence quotient
FHS	fetal heart sounds	IUD	intrauterine device
flu syn	influenza syndrome	IV, I.V.	intravenous
fluor	fluoroscopy	IVP	intravenous pyelogram
ft	foot; feet	JVD	jugulovenous distention
FU, F/U	follow-up (visit)	K35	Kollmann (dilator)
FUO	fever of unknown/undetermined origin	KUB	kidneys, ureters, bladder
FX, Fx	fracture	L	left; laboratory; living children; liter
G	gravida (number of pregnancies)	lab, LAB	laboratory
G, gm	gram	lac	laceration
GA	gastric analysis	L&A, l/a	light and accommodation
GB	gallbladder	L&W	living and well
GC	gonorrhea	lat, LAT	lateral
GGE	generalized glandular enlargement	LBP	low back pain
GI	gastrointestinal	lb(s)	pound(s)
GTT	glucose tolerance test	LLL	left lower lobe
GU	genitourinary	LLQ	left lower quadrant
Gyn, GYN	gynecology	LMP	last menstrual period
H	hospital call	lt., LT	left
HA	headache	ltd.	limited
HBP	high blood pressure	LUQ	left upper quadrant
HC	house call; hospital call; hospital consultation	M	medication; married
HCD	house call, day	MA	mental age
HCl	hydrochloric acid	med., MED	medicine
HCN	house call, night	mg	milligram(s)
hct	hematocrit	MH	marital history
HCVD	hypertensive cardiovascular disease	ml	milliliter(s)
HEENT	head, eyes, ears, nose, and throat	mm	millimeter(s)
hgb, Hb	hemoglobin	MM	mucous membrane
hist	history	MMR	measles, mumps, rubella (vaccine)
H₂O, H2O	water	mo	month(s)
hosp	hospital	MRI	magnetic resonance imaging
H&P	history and physical	N	negative
HPI	history of present illness	NA, N/A	not applicable
hr, hrs	hour, hours	NaCl	sodium chloride
HS	hospital surgery	NAD	no appreciable disease
Ht, ht	height	neg.	negative
HV	hospital visit	New OB	new obstetric patient
HX	history	NFA	no future appointment
HX PX	history and physical examination	NP, N/P, (N)	new patient
I	injection	NPN	nonprotein nitrogen
I&D	incision and drainage	N/S, NS	no-show
IC	initial consultation	NTRA	no telephone requests for antibiotics
i.e.	that is	N&V	nausea and vomiting
IM	intramuscular	NYD	not yet diagnosed
imp., IMP	impression	O₂, O2	oxygen
inc	include	OB	obstetrical patient, obstetrics; prenatal care
inf, INF	infection, infected		
inflam., INFL	inflammation	OC	office call
init	initial	occ	occasional
inj., INJ	injection	ofc	office

(continues)

TABLE B-2
Appointment and Patient Care Abbreviations (*continued*)

Abbreviation	Definition	Abbreviation	Definition
OH	occupational history	reg.	regular
OP, op.	operation, operative, outpatient	ret, retn	return
OPD	outpatient department	rev	Review
OR	operating room	Rh-	Rhesus negative (blood)
orig.	original	RHD	rheumatic heart disease
OT	occupational therapy	RLQ	right lower quadrant
OTC	over the counter	RO, R/O	rule out
OV	office visit	ROS	Review of systems
P	pulse; preterm parity or deliveries before term	rt., R	Right
PA	posterior anterior, posteroanterior	RT	respiratory therapy
P&A	percussion and auscultation	RTC	return to clinic
PAP, Pap	Papanicolaou (test/smear)	RTO	return to office
Para I	woman having borne one child (Para II, two children, and so on)	RUQ	right upper quadrant
		RV	return visit
PBI	protein-bound iodine	Rx, RX, ℞	prescription; any medication or treatment ordered
PC	present complaint; pregnancy confirmation		
PD	permanent disability	S	surgery
PE	physical examination	SD	state disability
perf.	Performed	SE	special examination
PERRLA, PERLA	pupils equal, round, react to light and to accommodation	sed rate	sedimentation rate
		sep.	separated
PFT	pulmonary function test	SH	social history
pH	hydrogen ion concentration	SIG, sigmoido	sigmoidoscopy
PH	past history	SLR	straight leg raising
Ph ex	physical examination	slt	slight
phys.	Physical	Smr, sm.	smear
PI	present illness	S, M, W, D	single, married, widowed, divorced
PID	pelvic inflammatory disease	SOB	shortness of breath
p.m., PM	after noon	sp gr	specific gravity
PMH	past medical history	SubQ*	subcutaneous
PND	postnasal drip	SR	suture removal; sedimentation rate
PO	postoperative check, phone order	STAT, stat.	immediately
P Op, Post-op	postoperative check	STD	sexually transmitted disease
pos.	positive	strab	strabismus
post.	posterior	surg.	surgery
postop	postoperative	Sx.	symptoms
PP	postpartum care	T	temperature; term parity or deliveries at term
Pre-op, preop	preoperative (office visit)		
prep	prepare, prepared	T&A	tonsillectomy and adenoidectomy
PRN, p.r.n.	As necessary	Tb, tbc, TB	tuberculosis
procto	proctoscopic (rectal) examination	TD	temporary disability
prog	prognosis	temp.	temperature
P&S	permanent and stationary	TIA	transient ischemic attack
PSP	phenolsulfonphthalein	TMs	tympanic membranes
Pt, pt	patient	TPR	temperature, pulse, respiration
PT	physical therapy	Tr.	treatment
PTR	patient to return	TTD	total temporary disability
PX	physical examination	TURB	transurethral resection of bladder
R	right; residence call; report	TURP	transurethral resection of prostate
RBC, rbc	red blood cell	TX, Tx	treatment
Re:, re:	regarding	U	unit
rec	recommend	Ua, U/A	urinalysis
re ch	recheck	UCHD	usual childhood diseases
re-exam, reex	reexamination	UCR	usual, customary, and reasonable
REF, ref	referral	UGI	upper gastrointestinal

(continues)

TABLE B-2
Appointment and Patient Care Abbreviations (*continued*)

Abbreviation	Definition	Abbreviation	Definition
UPJ	ureteropelvic junction or joint	WF	white female
UR, ur	urine	WI, W/I	walk-in, work-in
URI	upper respiratory infection	wk	week; work
UTI	urinary tract infection	wks	weeks
vac	vaccine	WM, W/M	white male
VD	venereal disease	WNL	within normal limits
VDRL	Venereal Disease Research Laboratory (test for syphilis)	WR	Wassermann reaction (syphilis test)
W	work; white	WT, Wt, wt	weight
WBC, wbc	white blood cell or count; well baby care	x, X	x-ray(s); multiplied by
		XR	x-ray(s)
		yr	year
Symbols			
*	birth	$-\ \bar{o}$	negative
$\bar{c}$, /c, w/	with	$\pm$	negative or positive; indefinite
$\bar{P}$	after	Ⓛ	left
$\bar{s}$, /s, w/o	without	ⓜ	murmur
$\bar{c}c$, $-\bar{c}/c$	with correction (eyeglasses)	Ⓡ	right
		♂	male
$\bar{s}c$, $\bar{s}/c$	without correction (eyeglasses)	♀	female
+	positive	μ	micron

*Abbreviation approved by the Joint Commission as the preferred abbreviation.

TABLE B-3
Appointment Terms and Their Abbreviations

Medical Term	Abbreviation	Medical Term	Abbreviation
abdominal	abd, abdom	immediately	stat
accident	accid	infection	inf
annual check	an ck	influenza syndrome	flu syn
annual physical examination	an PX/PE	injection	inj, INJ
antepartum care	AP	intrauterine device	IUD
blood pressure check	BP	laboratory follow-up	Lab FU, Lab F/U
breast check	breast ck	laceration	lac
cancel, canceled	canc	low back pain	LBP
cast check	cast ck	measles, mumps, rubella vac.	MMR
check	ck	new patient	(N), N/P, NP
chest x-ray	CXR, PA chest, AP chest	new obstetric patient	New OB
complete blood count	CBC	no future appointment	NFA
complete physical examination	CPX, CPE	no-show	N/S, NS
consultation	consult, cons, con	obstetric patient	OB
cystoscopy	cysto	office visit	OV
diagnosis	Dx, dx, dg, diag.	Papanicolaou smear	Pap
did not keep appointment	DNKA	physical examination	PE, PX, Ph ex, phys
did not show	DNS	postoperative check	PO, Post-op
dressing	dr, drsg	postpartum care	PP
dressing change	DC	pregnancy confirmation	PC
electrocardiogram	EKG, ECG	prenatal care	OB
electromyogram,		preoperative office visit	Pre-op, preop
electromyelogram	EMG	proctoscopic examination	procto
emergency	E	referral	REF, ref
emergency room	ER	return to clinic	RTC
follow-up visit	FU	return to office	RTO
fracture	FX, Fx	return visit	RV, ret, retn
glucose tolerance test	GTT	sigmoidoscopy	SIG, sigmoido
gynecological check	Gyn ck, GYN	suture removal	SR
headache	HA	walk-in, work-in	WI, W/I
house call	HC	weight	WT

TABLE B-4
Bookkeeping Abbreviations and Definitions

Abbreviation	Definition	Abbreviation	Definition	Abbreviation	Definition
AC or acct	account	EC, ER	error corrected	pt	patient
A/C	account current	Ex MO	express money order	PVT CK	private check
adj	adjustment			recd, recv'd	received
A/P	accounts payable	FLW/UP	follow-up	ref	refund
A/R	accounts receivable	fwd	forward	req	request
B/B	bank balance	IB	itemized bill	ROA	received on account
Bal fwd, B/F	balance forward	i/f	in full	snt	sent
BD	bad debt	ins, INS	insurance	T	telephoned
BSY	busy	inv	invoice	TB	trial balance
c/a, CS	cash on account	J/A	joint account	UCR	usual, customary, and reasonable
cc	credit card	LTTR	letter		
ck	check	MO	money order	w/o	write off
COINS	coinsurance	mo	month	$	money/cash
Cr	credit	msg	message	—	charge already made
CXL	cancel	NC, N/C	no charge	0	no balance due (zero balance)
DB	debit	NF	no funds		
DED	deductible	NSF	not sufficient funds	✓	posted
def	charge deferred	PD	paid	<$56.78>	credit symbols
disc, discnt	discount	pmt	payment		

TABLE B-5
Collection Abbreviations

Abbreviation	Collection Term	Abbreviation	Collection Term	Abbreviation	Collection Term
B	bankrupt	LMVM	left message voice mail	POW	payment on way
BLG	belligerent			PP	promise to pay
EO	end of month	N1, N2	note one, note two (sent)	S	she or wife
EOW	end of week			SEP	separated
FN	final notice	NA	no answer	SK	skip or skipped
H	he or husband	NF/A	no forwarding address	SOS	same old story
HHCO	have husband call office	NI	not in	STO	she telephoned office
		NLE	no longer employed	T	telephoned
HTO	he telephoned office	NR	no record	TB	telephoned business
L1, L2	letter one, letter two (sent)	NSF	not sufficient funds (check)	TR	telephoned residence
				U/Emp	unemployed
LB	line busy	NSN	no such number	UTC	unable to contact
LD	long distance	OOT	out of town	Vfd/E	verified employment
LMCO	left message, call office	OOW	out of work	Vfd/I	verified insurance
		Ph/Dsc	phone disconnected		

TABLE B-6
Abbreviations for Physician Specialist and Health Care Professionals

Physician Specialist	Abbreviation	Health Care Professional	Abbreviation
Doctor of Chiropractic	DC	Certified Coding Specialist; certified by the American Health Information Management Association	CCS
Doctor of Dental Surgery	DDS		
Doctor of Dental Science	DDSc	Certified First Assistant (surgical)	CFA
Doctor of Emergency Medicine	DEM	Certified Laboratory Assistant; certified by the Registry of American Society of Clinical Pathologists	CLA (ASCP)
Doctor of Hygiene	DHy		
Doctor of Medical Dentistry	DMD		
Doctor of Medicine	MD	Certified Medical Transcriptionist	CMT
Doctor of Optometry	OD	Certified Nurse Midwife	CNM
Doctor of Ophthalmology	OphD	Certified Professional Coder; certified by AAPC (formerly the American Academy of Professional Coders)	CPC
Doctor of Optometry	OD		
Doctor of Osteopathy	DO		
Doctor of Pharmacy	Pharm D	Certified Registered Nurse Anesthetist	CRNA
Doctor of Podiatry	DPM	Certified Surgical Technician (2nd surgical asst.)	CST
Doctor of Public Health	DPH	Emergency Medical Technician	EMT
Doctor of Tropical Medicine	DTM	Health Information Management professional	HIM
Doctor of Veterinary Medicine	DVM		
Doctor of Veterinary Surgery	DVS	Inhalation Therapist	IT
Fellow of the American Academy of Pediatrics	FAAP	Laboratory Technician Assistant	LTA
		Licensed Practical Nurse	LPN
Fellow of the American College of Obstetricians and Gynecologists	FACOG	Licensed Vocational Nurse	LVN
		Master of Public Health	MPH
Fellow of the American College of Surgery	FACS	Medical Technologist	MT (ASCP)
Senior Fellow	SF	Physician's Assistant—Certified	PA-C
		Public Health Nurse	PHN
		Registered Dietitian	RD
		Registered Nurse	RN
		Registered Nurse First Assistant (surgical)	RNFA
		Registered Nurse Practitioner	RNP
		Registered Occupational Therapist	ROT
		Registered Physical Therapist	RPT
		Registered Respiratory Therapist	RRT
		Registered Technologist (Radiology)	RT (R)
		Registered Technologist (Therapy)	RT (T)
		Visiting Nurse	VN

TABLE B-7
Common Prescription Abbreviations* and Symbols

Abbreviation	Definition	Abbreviation	Definition
ā	before	o.m.	every morning
āā	of each	o.n.	every night
a.c.	before meals	OTC	over-the-counter (drugs)
ad lib.	as much as needed	oz	ounce
a.m. or AM	morning	p̄	after
ante	before	p.c.	after meals
aq.	aqueous/water	p.o.	by mouth (per os)
b.i.d.	two times a day	p.r.	per rectum
caps	capsule	p.r.n. or PRN	whenever necessary
c̄	with	**q.	every
**c̄c̄	with meals	**q.a.m.	every morning
comp. or comp	compound	**q.h.	every hour
d	day	**q.h.s.	every night
**DC or D/C	discontinue	q.i.d.	four times a day (not at night)
dos.	doses	**q.n.	every night
DS	double strength	**q.p.m.	every night
DSD	double starting dose	**q.2 h.	every two hours
elix.	elixir	**q.3 h.	every three hours
emul.	emulsion	**q.4 h.	every four hours
et	and	rep, REP	let it be repeated; Latin *repeto*
ext.	extract	Rx	take (recipe), prescription
garg.	gargle	s̄	without
gm or g	gram	sat.	saturated
gr	grain	SC, subc, subcut,	
gt.	drop	subq, SQ	subcutaneous
gtt.	drops	Sig.	write on label; give directions on prescription
h.	hour		
**h.s.	before bedtime (hour of sleep)	SL	sublingual
ID	intradermal	sol.	solution
IM	intramuscular	SR	sustained release
**inj.	injection; to be injected	**ss	one-half
IV or I.V.	intravenous	stat or STAT	immediately
kg	kilogram	syr.	syrup
liq	liquid	tab.	tablet
M or m.	mix	t.i.d.	three times a day
mcg	microgram	top	topically
mg or mgm	milligram (used instead of "cc" for cubic centimeter)	Tr. or tinct.	tincture
		tsp	teaspoon
ml	milliliter	vag.	vagina
N.E. or ne	negative	X or x	times (X10d/times ten days)
noct.	night	i, ii, iii, iv; viii, etc.	1, 2, 3, 4; 8, etc.
NPO or n.p.o.	nothing by mouth	5", 10", 15"	5, 10, 15 minutes, etc.
O₂	oxygen	5°, 10°, 15°, or	5 hours, 10 hours,
**o.d.	once a day	5', 10', 15', etc.	15 hours, etc.
o.h.	every hour	ʒ or dr.	dram (drachm)
oint	ointment	℥ or oz.	ounce

*Many of these abbreviations are derived from Latin; they are usually typed in lowercase and with periods. Periods are especially important because without periods an abbreviation would spell a word; for example, b.i.d. without periods is bid.

**Recommendation: Write out this term or use alternate wording, so an abbreviation error does not occur.

TABLE B-8
Two-Letter State Abbreviations for the United States and Territories and Canadian Provinces

United States and Territories					
Alabama	AL	Kansas	KS	No. Mariana Islands	MP
Alaska	AK	Kentucky	KY	Ohio	OH
American Samoa	AS	Louisiana	LA	Oklahoma	OK
Arizona	AZ	Maine	ME	Oregon	OR
Arkansas	AR	Marshall Islands	MH	Palau	PW
California	CA	Maryland	MD	Pennsylvania	PA
Colorado	CO	Massachusetts	MA	Puerto Rico	PR
Connecticut	CT	Michigan	MI	Rhode Island	RI
Delaware	DE	Minnesota	MN	South Carolina	SC
District of Columbia	DC	Mississippi	MS	South Dakota	SD
Federated States of		Missouri	MO	Tennessee	TN
Micronesia	FM	Montana	MT	Texas	TX
Florida	FL	Nebraska	NE	Utah	UT
Georgia	GA	Nevada	NV	Vermont	VT
Guam	GU	New Hampshire	NH	Virginia	VA
Hawaii	HI	New Jersey	NJ	Virgin Islands, U.S.	VI
Idaho	ID	New Mexico	NM	Washington	WA
Illinois	IL	New York	NY	West Virginia	WV
Indiana	IN	North Carolina	NC	Wisconsin	WI
Iowa	IA	North Dakota	ND	Wyoming	WY

Canadian Provinces					
Alberta	AB	Northwest Territories	NT	Quebec	QC
British Columbia	BC	Nova Scotia	NS	Saskatchewan	SK
Manitoba	MB	Nunavut	NU	Yukon Territory	YT
New Brunswick	NB	Ontario	ON		
Newfoundland and Labrador	NL	Prince Edward Island	PE		